THE HUMAN EMBRYO

Edited by **Shigehito Yamada**
and **Tetsuya Takakuwa**

The Human Embryo

Edited by Shigehito Yamada and Tetsuya Takakuwa

Published by InTech

Janeza Trdine 9, 51000 Rijeka, Croatia

Publishing Process Manager Ivana Zec

Technical Editor Teodora Smiljanic

Cover Designer InTech Design Team

Additional hard copies can be obtained from orders@intechopen.com

The Human Embryo, Edited by Shigehito Yamada and Tetsuya Takakuwa

p. cm.

ISBN 978-953-51-0124-6

For EU product safety concerns:
IN TECH d.o.o., Prolaz Marije Krucifikse Kozulić 3, 51000 Rijeka, Croatia,
info@intechopen.com or visit our website at intechopen.com.

Meet the editors

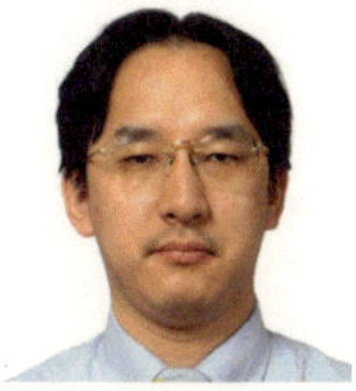

Dr Shigehito Yamada, MD, graduated from the Faculty of Medicine at Kyoto University in 1998. He started his career as a Medical Doctor of Obstetrics and Gynecology and developed an active interest in human embryology, in 1995, when he was a medical student. Dr. Yamada continued his work and received his PhD in 2006 at the Graduate School of Medicine, Kyoto University. His thesis dealt with making tutorial software of clinical embryology. He then took the role of Assistant Professor of Congenital Anomaly Research Center, Kyoto University Graduate School of Medicine, and also became the Research Fellow at the Laboratory of Developmental Biology, NHLBI/NIH, in 2006. He has been the Associate Professor of Congenital Anomaly Research Center, Kyoto University Graduate School of Medicine since 2008.

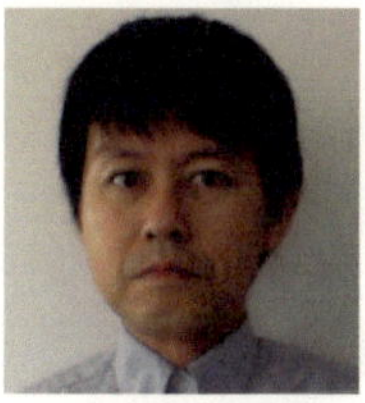

Dr Tetsuya Takakuwa, MD, graduated from University of Tokyo, Faculty of Science in 1986, as well as from Osaka University, Faculty of Medicine in 1990. He worked as an Acute Care Physician at Osaka University Hospital and Critical Care and Emergency center Iwate Medical collage for 8 years. During those years, he got the opportunity to study at Max-Plank Institute for Immuno-biology in Germany. He took the role of the Associate Professor at the Department of Pathology, Osaka University Graduate School of Medicine, in 2002, and received his PhD in 2005. He has been a Professor at Kyoto University Graduate School of Medicine, Department of Human Health Science since 2008.

Contents

Preface

Human embryology is now rapidly moving to a new phase due to recent innovation and advances of life science including ES and iPS technology. This new era also directs a difficult challenge for scientists in terms of technological and ethical issues for future human embryology. However, human embryology is difficult to research due to ethics involved in the collection of human materials. This book traces the early history and provides knowledge on demonstration of principles from ancient to the most recent embryo studies amidst the unresolved scientific and ethical issues.

In the first introductory section, various human embryo collections are summarized with four well-known ones: The Carnegie, the Blechschmidt, the Hinrichsen and the Kyoto collections. Although remarkable progress has been achieved in studying each collection, there are very few reviews available that summarize the past and the present of the collections. Therefore, this book discusses in vivid detail how human embryology has changed since ancient discoveries to most recent research done.

The next section covers "implantation" as a theme. This section reviews the outline of ethical and technical issues related to implantation. In this context, four chapters are included and discussed. The ethical issue and its adaptation depend on the country, region, race and religions. Although this section does not cover all the directions, the chapters are dedicated to all international persons to be free and open discussion for better understanding. We are glad this book will trigger deeper discussions of this issue.

The third section deals with "organogenesis". The techniques and tools for studying morphogenetic changes and fundamental understanding of organogenesis are discussed. In organogenesis, miscarriages often occur and genetic analyses are required for elucidation of the cause and one such paper reviewing cytogenetic aspects of miscarriages is adopted.

In dealing with the special subject of this book, we wish to acknowledge the courtesy of the publishers and everyone involved in Japan and overseas for their valid contribution. We hope this book will help the readers to understand human embryo development better.

Dr. Shigehito Yamada
M.D., Ph.D., Congenital Anomaly Research Center,
Kyoto University, Graduate School of Medicine, Kyoto,
Japan

Co-editor:
Professor Tetsuya Takakuwa,
M.D., Ph.D., Human Health Science,
Kyoto University Graduate School of Medicine, Kyoto,
Japan

Part 1

Introduction

1

Introduction – Developmental Overview of the Human Embryo

Shigehito Yamada[1], and Tetsuya Takakuwa[2]
[1]*Congenital Anomaly Research Center, Kyoto University,*
[2]*Human Health Science, Kyoto University,*
Japan

1. Introduction

In this chapter, we provide a historical background on human embryo collections and describe their significant contribution to the understanding of human ontogenesis. More particularly, an overview of human embryonic development is presented using computer-generated images obtained from embryonic specimens housed at the Kyoto Collection in Japan.

1.1 Human embryology and embryo collections

Historically, several human embryo collections have been created. The Carnegie Collection, the Blechschmidt Collection, the Hinrichsen Collection and the Kyoto Collection are reported as the four famous compendiums of human embryos in the world. The Carnegie Collection is the oldest and was established as early as 1887, while the Blechschmidt collection was created in 1948 by the Göttingen anatomist Erich Blechschmidt, well known for its contribution to the development of novel methods of reconstruction. In 1961, the Kyoto Collection of Human Embryos was instigated, followed by the Hinrichsen Collection in 1969. While the Blechschmidt and the Hinrichsen collections are described in Chapter 2, here, we focus on the Carnegie and the Kyoto Collections.

1.2 The carnegie human embryo collection

The basis of the Carnegie Human Embryo Collection was established by Franklin P. Mall. After earning his medical degree at the University of Michigan in 1883, Mall traveled to Germany to receive a clinical training and there he met Wilhelm His and other eminent biologists. Mall then became aware of the importance of studying human embryology, and initiated a collection of human embryos in 1887. When he returned to the United States and took on a position in the Anatomy department of the Johns Hopkins School of Medicine in Baltimore, Maryland, he already had in his possession several hundreds of specimens. In 1913, as a professor of Anatomy at the Johns Hopkins School of Medicine, Mall applied for a Carnegie grant to support his research on human embryos, was successful in his application and thus, in 1914, became the first director of the Department of Embryology at the Carnegie Institution of Washington, in Baltimore, MD. The collection grew up at a rate of about 400 specimens a year, and the number of samples attained over 8,000 by the early 1940s. The most difficult task, however, was to organize and catalogue the collection. Age or size proved to be a poor way to organize embryos, as embryos could shrink a full 50% in the preserving fluids. Mall devised a better way and based his staging scheme on morphological characteristics instead. To that end, Mall and his colleagues not only prepared and preserved serial sections of the embryos; they also made hundreds of three-dimensional models at different stages of growth. Over 700 wax-based reconstructions were created.

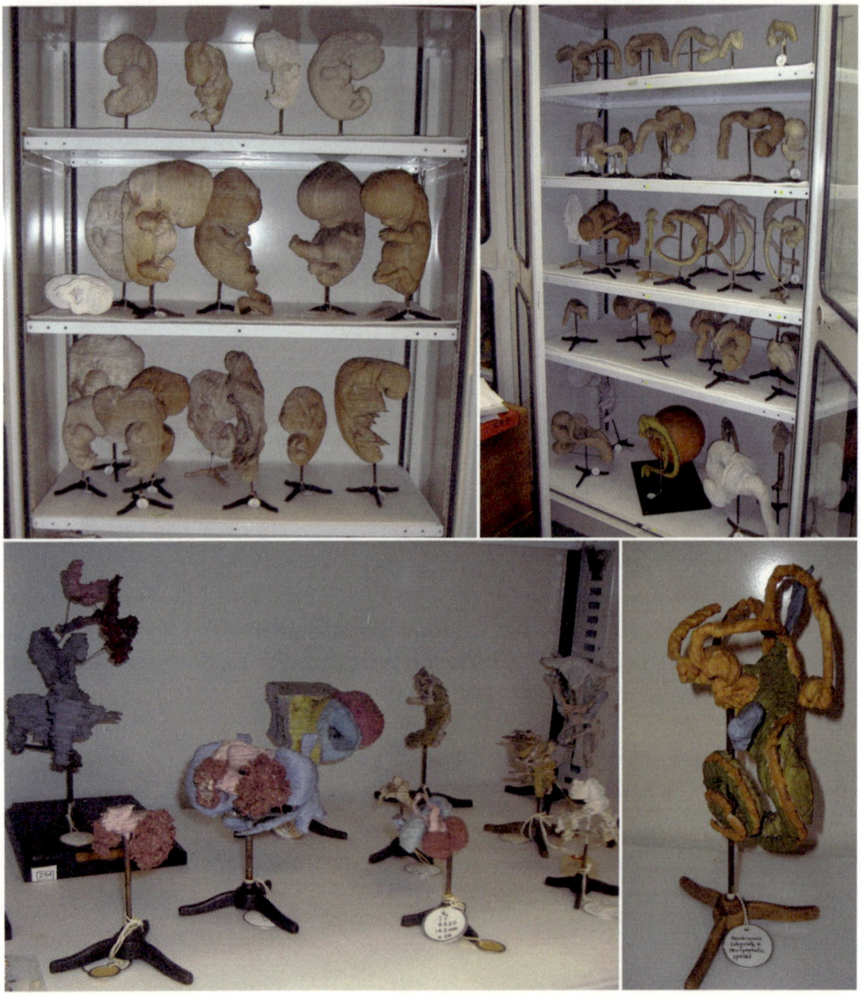

Fig. 1. Wax reconstruction models at the Carnegie Collection, housed at the National Museum of Health and Medicine, Washington, DC. Surface reconstruction of human whole embryos (top left), neural tubes and brains (top right), hearts and great vessels (bottom left), and membranous labyrinth and perilymphatic spaces (bottom right).

Throughout the Mall's era, several members of his department became renowned scientists. George L. Streeter and Franz J. Keibel were both former students of Wilhelm His; Osborne O. Heard worked as an embryo modeler; and James D. Didusch as a scientific illustrator. Mall documented his research in a series of papers compiled in the *Contributions to Embryology of the Carnegie Institution of Washington*, published from 1915 to 1966. Today, these articles are still regarded as textual and visual standards for human embryologists. In 1917, Mall unexpectedly died, and Streeter became the second director of the Department of Embryology. Under his supervision, hundreds of specimens continued to join the collection every year. Notable were the rare, very young normal specimens. At the time, induced abortions were illegal in the United States and miscarriages usually result in abnormal embryos. Streeter was the first to define the 23 Carnegie Stages currently used to classify the developmental stages of the human embryo.

When Streeter retired in 1940, George W. Corner became the third director of the department. Corner was a former Johns Hopkins researcher who discovered the ovarian hormone progesterone. Under his direction, many advances in human reproductive physiology were made. Research in human embryology continued to be actively pursued, but came to an end in 1956 with the succeeding director. In 1973, the Collection was sent to the University of California at Davis Medical School, where the Carnegie Laboratories of Embryology, under the directorship of Ronan O'Rahilly, officially opened in 1976. In 1991, following O'Rahilly's retirement, the collection was donated to the National Museum of Health and Medicine, located at the Walter Reed Army Medical Center in Washington, D.C. The specimens remain available for use by researchers, and are in high demand. Adrianne Noe and colleagues have generated an online database system for easy information access to some 660 embryos from the collection. These embryos were selected to represent the full range of embryonic growth from single cells through to eight weeks of age. The Carnegie Collection forms the centerpiece of the Human Developmental Anatomy Center, and is used by hundreds of researchers every year. Further details of the embryo collection can be found in earlier publications (Brown, 1987, O'Rahilly, 1988) as well as on the web (http://nmhm.washingtondc.museum/ collections/hdac/carnegie_history.htm).

1.3 The Kyoto collection of human embryos

In 1961, Hideo Nishimura, Professor in the Department of Anatomy at Kyoto University School of Medicine, instigated a collection of human conceptuses. Induced abortions were then legal in Japan under the Maternity Protection Law of Japan, therefore, in a great majority of cases; pregnancies were terminated for social reasons during the first trimester. Fifteen years later, the number of specimens reached over 36,000 and the Congenital Anomaly Research Center was created in 1975. Today, the embryo collection comprises over 45,000 specimens, and represents the largest human embryo collection in the world. The specimens were primarily obtained from pregnancies interrupted by dilatation or curettage. Other specimens resulted from spontaneous or threatened abortions. When the aborted materials were brought to our laboratory, the embryos were measured, staged, and examined for gross external abnormalities and signs of intrauterine death under a dissecting microscope. The developmental stage of the embryos (Carnegie stage: CS) was determined according to the criteria proposed by O'Rahilly and Müller (1987). Since the attending obstetricians were not involved in examining the aborted materials, the collection of embryos was not biased by their outcome (e.g., normal or abnormal, live or dead), thus, the embryo collection is considered representative of the total intrauterine population in Japan (Nishimura, 1974, 1975). Using this representative embryo population, it was reported that the incidence of malformations in embryos were more frequent than that in infants (Nishimura et al., 1968), and that embryos with severe malformations were prone to spontaneous abortion at high rates (Shiota, 1991). Of these embryonic malformations, holoprosencephaly (HPE) was observed at a high frequency in the Kyoto Collection. HPE is a group of malformation characterized by specific dysmorphia of the brain and the face. They are caused by an impaired or incomplete midline cleavage of the prosencephalon into cerebral hemispheres. Although HPE is a rather rare anomaly in newborns (1/10,000-20,000), it is encountered much more frequently (1/250 or more) in the unselected early human embryonic population (Matsunaga and Shiota, 1977). This estimation may be lower than the actual prevalence as milder forms of HPE also exist but are more difficult to diagnose (Yamada et al., 2004, Yamada, 2006). Well-preserved samples were stored and some of them were selected to be sectioned serially; a total of 500 normal embryos and 500 abnormal embryos were stored as complete serial sections, including HPE embryos.

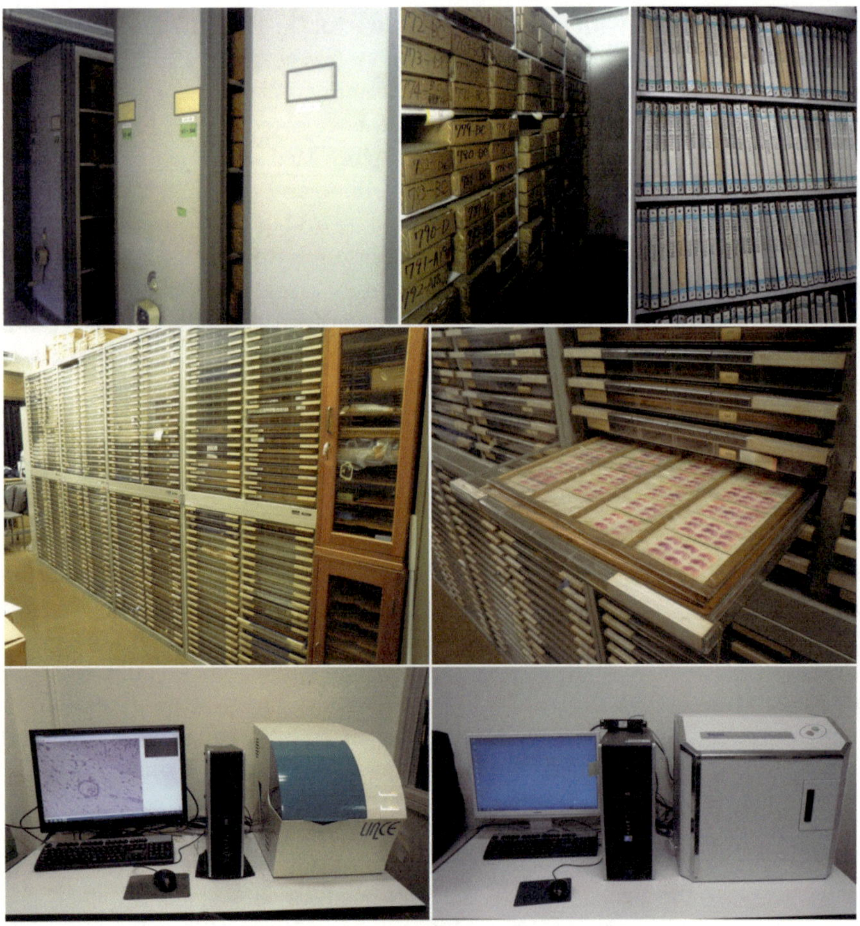

Fig. 2. The Kyoto Collection of Human Embryos. Stock room (top left, top middle), and individual files containing epidemiological data (top right). Histological specimens (middle left, middle right). Digital slide scanners manufactured by Claro Inc. (http://www.claro-inc.com/); LINCE (bottom left) and TOCO (bottom right).

A unique feature of the Kyoto Collection is that maternal epidemiological data and detailed clinical information on the pregnancies were collected in association with every specimen. Based on these epidemiological data, statistical analyses are currently conducted to determine the existence of potential causative links between maternal factors and congenital anomalies (Kameda et al., 2012).

Recently, owing to advances in imaging technologies, embryos can be scanned and 3D digital models can be generated. Using magnetic resonance (MR) microscopes equipped with superconducting magnets ranging from 1.0T to 7.0T, embryos from the Kyoto Collections were imaged (Haishi et al., 2001, Matsuda et al., 2007, Matsuda et al., 2003, Yamada et al., 2010) and morphologically analyzed using 3D reconstruction (Hirose et al., 2011). Episcopic Fluorescence Image Capture (EFIC) and phase-contrast x-ray computed tomography have also been applied to human embryos of the Kyoto Collection (Yamada et al., 2010, Yoneyama et al., 2011). Further details on imaging techniques and reconstruction can be found in Chapter 7. Additionally, a project aiming at digitizing all histological sections comprised in the library is now ongoing. As mentioned earlier, the Kyoto Collection contains a register of 1,000 embryos sectioned serially; half of them are classified as normal and the other half with anomalies. The project is currently focusing on serial sections of normal embryos. Parts of the digitized serial sections are accessible from our website (http://atlas.cac.med.kyoto-u.ac.jp).

2. Human embryonic development

2.1 Developmental overview (Carnegie stages: CS)

Classification into developmental stages is necessary to accurately describe prenatal growth. Embryonic staging of animals was introduced at the end of the 19th century (Hopwood, 2007), and was first applied to human embryology by Mall (1914), as described earlier. At first, human embryos were classified based on their length on the basis of "3-mm stage", but the approach was quickly abandoned due to high inter-individual variations. Subsequently, Streeter (1942, 1945, 1948, 1951) developed a 23-stage developmental scheme of human embryos, commonly known as the Carnegie stages, a staging scheme which remains widely used today. Here below are illustrated all 23 stages using computer graphics either based on photographs acquired in multiple directions, with precise measurements (CS 1-12), or based on data acquired by magnetic resonance microscopy (Yamada et al., 2006, Matsuda et al., 2003).

Relation between the Carnegie stage and estimated age after fertilization (Table 1)

It is accepted that a wide range of normal variations can occur in actual human embryonic age for any given Carnegie stage. The standard criteria proposed by O'Rahilly and Müller (1987) are close to those suggested by Olivier and Pineau (1962). It is also important to point out that Streeter's human series included pathological specimens obtained from spontaneous abortion or ectopic implantation. In the present chapter, the CG models ranging from CS1 to CS11 were based on Carnegie criteria (O'Rahilly and Müller, 1987), while CS13 to CS23 were based on Kyoto Collection samples (Nishimura et al., 1968, Nishimura et al., 1974).

Carnegie stage (CS)	Ovulation age (days)					
	Streeter (1942, 1945, 1948, 1951)	Nishimura (1968, 1974)	Olivier and Pineau (1962)	Iffy et al. (1967)	Jirásek (1971)	O'Rahilly and Müller (1987)
11	24	27	24	-	23-26	23-25
12	26	30	26	-	26-30	25-27
13	28	32	28	28	28-32	28
14	29	34-35	32	32	31-35	32
15	31.5	36	33	34.5	35-38	33
16	33	38	37	37	37-42	37
17	35	40	41	40	42-44	41
18	37	42	44	43	44-48	44
19	39	44	47.5	45	48-51	47-48
20	41	46	50.5	47	51-53	50-51
21	43	48	52	48.5	53-54	52
22	45	50	54	50	54-56	54
23	47	52	56.5	52	56-60	56-57

Table 1. Estimated ovulation age (days) based on developmental stages (CS) of human embryos, according to various authors. Modified from Nishimura (1983).

Carnegie stage 1: Fertilized ovum
1 day after fertilization, 0.1 mm in diameter

The oocyte is 120-150 μm in diameter and is surrounded by the zona pellucida. The second maturation division of the oocyte completes as the sperm penetrates the egg (fertilization). The sperm head and the nucleus of the oocyte then swell to form the male and female pronuclei, respectively. Once they unite, the resultant diploid cell is called the zygote. The first mitotic division soon begins.

Carnegie stage 2: Cleavage
1.5-3 days after fertilization, 0.1-0.2 mm in diameter

The conceptus is composed of two to 16 cells but has no blastocystic cavity yet and the zona pellucida can still be easily recognized. The size of the embryo is 0.1-0.2 mm in diameter. The cell division at this stage is called cleavage since furrows (clefts) appear as the cytoplasm divides. The daughter cells are called blastomeres. An embryo with 16-32 cells is called a morula.

Carnegie stage 3: Free blastocyst
4 days after fertilization, 0.1-0.2 mm in diameter

The conceptus is a free (unattached) blastocyst. The blastocyst is a hollow mass of cells characterized by the blastocystic cavity. The blastocystic cavity begins by the coalescence of intercellular spaces when the embryo has acquired about 32 cells. The blastomeres segregate into an internally situated inner cell mass and an outer trophoblast. The trophoblast cells form an epithelial arrangement with tight junctions.

Carnegie stage 4: Attaching blastocyst
5-6 days after fertilization, 0.1-0.2 mm in diameter

This stage is characterized by the attached blastocyst, which corresponds to the onset of implantation. Attachment of the embryo occurs only once the endometrium has entered the secretory phase. At the site of attachment, the trophoblast cells are transformed into a

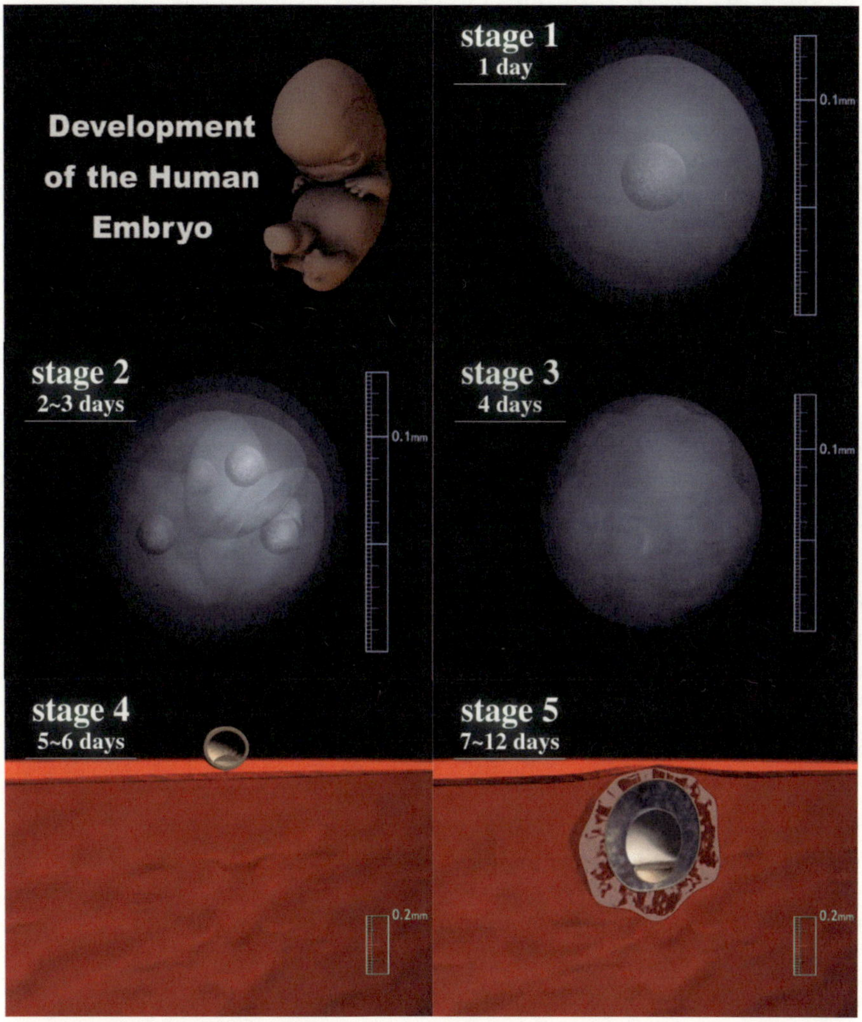

Fig. 3. Computer graphics illustrating embryonic human development: Carnegie stage 1-5.

syncytium and penetrate into the endometrial epithelium.

Carnegie stage 4: Attaching blastocyst
5-6 days after fertilization, 0.1-0.2 mm in diameter

This stage is characterized by the attached blastocyst, which corresponds to the onset of implantation. Attachment of the embryo occurs only once the endometrium has entered the secretory phase. At the site of attachment, the trophoblast cells are transformed into a syncytium and penetrate into the endometrial epithelium.

Carnegie stage 5: Implanted but previllous
7-12 days after fertilization, 0.1-0.2 mm in diameter

The blastocyst penetrates into the endometrium. The trophoblast grows rapidly but is previllous, i.e., it does not yet show definite chorionic villi. This stage is sub-divided into 3 stages according to the differentiation status of the trophoblast: solid trophoblast (stage 5a), lacunar trophoblast (5b), and perfusion of lacunae with maternal blood (5c).

Carnegie stage 6: Chorionic villi and primitive streak
13 days after fertilization, 0.2 mm in size

Chorionic villi appear and begin to branch. Trophoblastic lacunae coalesce to form the intervillous space (6a). The extra-embryonic mesoderm arises and the chorionic cavity is formed. The yolk sac is now called the secondary (definitive) yolk sac. The primitive streak appears later during this stage (6b, "stage 6" in Fig. 2).

Carnegie stage 7: Notochordal process
16 days after fertilization, 0.4 mm in length (embryonic disc)

The notochordal process develops in the mesodermal layer rostral to the primitive node. The length of the notochordal process varies from 0.03 to about 0.3 mm. The embryonic mesoderm spreads laterally and rostrally from the primitive streak. The embryonic disc grows cranially and the amniotic cavity expands over the yolk sac.

Carnegie stage 8 : Primitive pit, neuenteric canal
18 days after fertilization, 1.0 mm in CRL (crown-rump length)

This stage is characterized by the formation of the primitive pit, the notochordal canal and the neurenteric canal. Somites are not yet visible (presomitic stage). The embryonic disc is pyriform, tapering caudally. The notochordal canal is marked by the cavity extending from the primitive pit into the notochordal process. The floor of the canal soon disappears to form a passage between the amniotic cavity and the yolk sac (neurenteric canal).

Carnegie stage 9: 1-3 pairs of somites
20 days after fertilization, 1.5 mm in CRL

The neural groove and the first somites appear, and one to three pairs of somites can be observed. The embryonic disc resembles a shoe-sole, with the broad neural plate positioned into the cranial region. The neural groove appears during this stage and subsequently deepens. The paraxial mesoderm becomes segmented to form somites.

Carnegie stage 10: Neural folds begin to fuse, 4-12 pairs of somites
22 days after fertilization, 1.8 mm in CRL

The neural groove deepens and the neural folds begin to fuse to form the neural tube. The fusion of neural folds extends bidirectionally. The optic sulcus and branchial arch 1 (i.e., pharyngeal arch) begin to be visible. The cardiac loop starts to appear.

Carnegie stage 11: Anterior neuropore closes
24 days after fertilization, 2.5-3 mm in CRL

The human embryo now has 13-20 pairs of somites. The anterior neuropore is now closing up. Optic evagination is produced at the optic sulcus and the optic ventricle is continuous with that of the forebrain. The sinus venosus develops in the cardiac loop. The

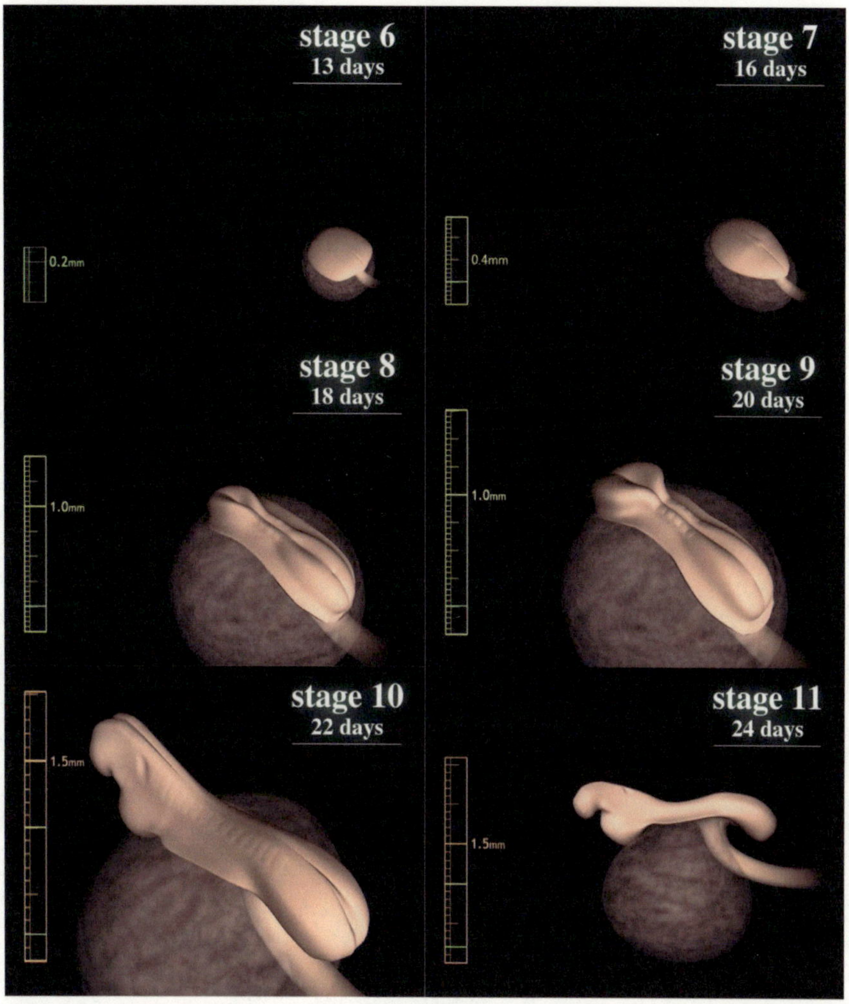

Fig. 4. Computer graphics illustrating human embryonic development: Carnegie stage 6-11.

(buccopharyngeal) membrane is ruptured. The otic vesicle is now formed.

Carnegie stage 12: Posterior (caudal) neuropore closes, 3-4 branchial arches, upper limb buds
28 days after fertilization, 4 mm in CRL

The posterior (caudal) neuropore is starting to close or is closed. Three branchial arches are present. Upper limb buds are distinct. The embryo now has 21-29 pairs of somites. The embryonic axis is curved as a result of the rounding out or the folding of the embryo. Internally, the lung bud appears and the interventricular septum has begun its formation in the heart.

Carnegie stage 13: Four limb buds, optic vesicle
32 days after fertilization, 5 mm in CRL

Two upper and two lower limb buds are visible. The optic vesicle can be easily recognized and the lens placode begins to differentiate. The embryo now has more than 30 pairs of somites, but the number of somites becomes increasingly difficult to determine and is no longer used in staging.

Carnegie stage 14: Lens pit and optic cup
34 days after fertilization, 6 mm in CRL

The lens pit invaginates into the optic cup but is not yet closed. The endolymphatic appendage emerging from the otic vesicle is well defined. The upper limb buds elongate and become tapering. The cephalic and cervical flexures are prominent. Internally, the future cerebral hemispheres and cerebellar plates are visible. The dorsal and ventral pancreatic buds are noticeable. The ureteric bud develops and acquires a metanephrogenic blastemal cap.

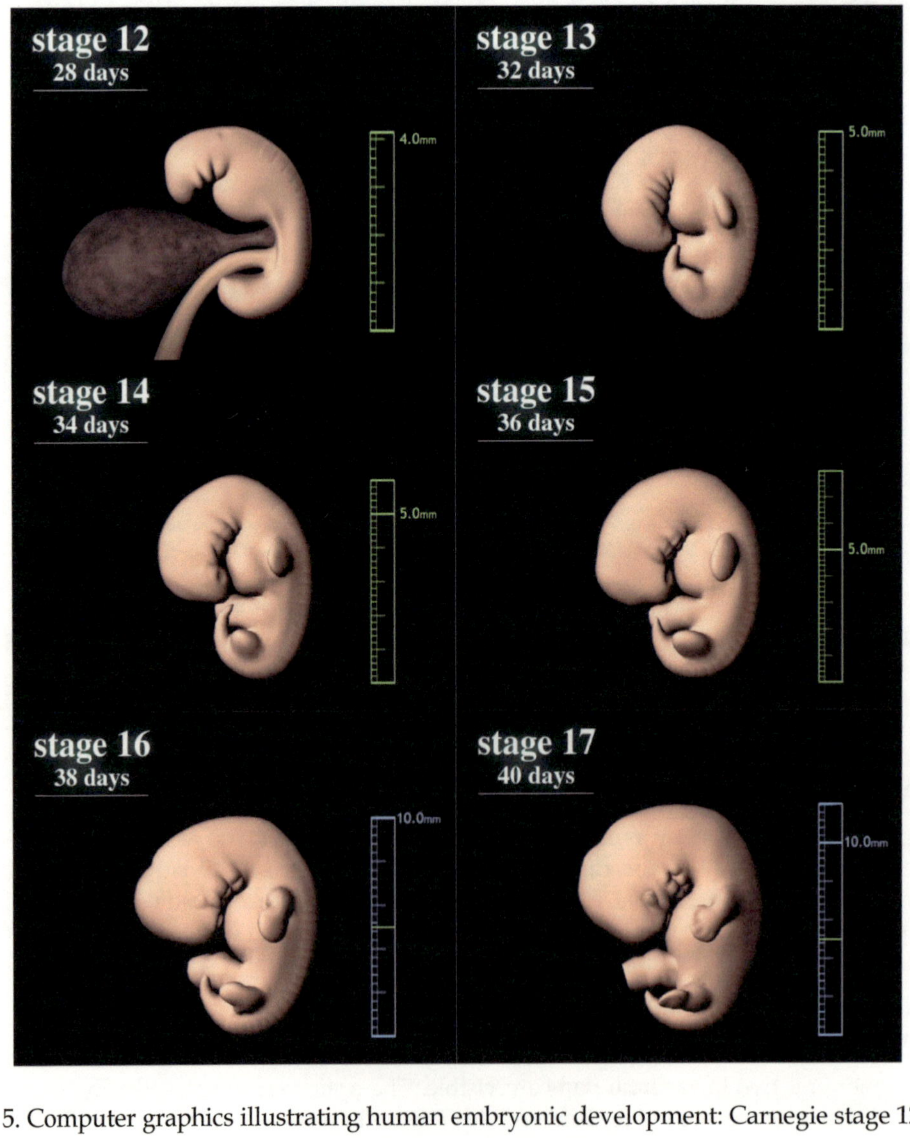

Fig. 5. Computer graphics illustrating human embryonic development: Carnegie stage 12-17.

Carnegie stage 15: Lens vesicles, nasal pit and hand plates
34 days after fertilization, 8 mm in CRL

Lens vesicles are closed and covered by the surface ectoderm. The nasal plate invaginates to form a nasal pit. Auricular hillocks arise. Hand plates are forming. The foramen secundum develops in the heart. Lung buds begin to branch into lobar buds. The primary urogenital sinus is formed.

Carnegie stage 16: Nasal pit faces ventrally, retinal pigment, foot plate
38 days after fertilization, 10 mm in CRL

Nasal pits deepen and come to face ventrally. Retinal pigment is visible externally. The hand plates are now distinct and the foot plate is emerging. The nasolacrimal groove has formed between the frontal and maxillary processes.

Carnegie stage 17: Head relatively larger, nasofrontal groove, finger rays
40 days after fertilization, 11 mm in CRL

The head is relatively larger than previously and the trunk has become straighter. The auricular hillocks and nasofrontal (nasolacrimal) grooves are distinct. The hand plates exhibit definite digital rays, and the foot has acquired a rounded digital plate.

Carnegie stage 18: Elbows, toe rays, eyelid folds, nipples
42 days after fertilization, 13 mm in CRL

The body shape is more cuboidal. Both cervical and lumbar flexures are denoted. The elbows are discernible and interdigital notches appear in the hand plates. Toe rays are observed in the foot plate. Eyelid folds appear. Auricular hillocks are being transformed into specific parts of the external ear. Ossification may begin in some skeletal structures.

Carnegie stage 19: Trunk elongation and straightening
44 days after fertilization, 16 mm in CRL

The trunk begins to elongate and straightens. Eyes and external ears gain definite shape. The eyes are positioned in the front of the face, owing to the growth of the brain. The upper and lower limbs are almost parallel, with pre-axial borders cranially and postaxial borders caudally. Intestines have developed and parts of them can be observed in normal umbilical cord (physiological umbilical hernia).

Carnegie stage 20: Longer upper limb bent at elbow
46 days after fertilization, cranio-rump length: 19 mm in CRL

The angle of cervical flexure becomes small, and the direction of the head goes up. Vascular plexus appears in the superficial tissues of the head. The coiled intestine observed in the umbilical cord has developed. Spontaneous movement begins at this stage. The upper limbs have increased in length and become bent at the elbows and hand joints. Fingers are curving slightly over the chest.

Carnegie stage 21: Fingers longer, hands approach each other
48 days after fertilization, cranio-rump length: 21 mm in CRL

The head becomes round. The superficial vascular plexus of the head has spread and surrounds the head. The tail becomes rudimentary. The hands are slightly flexed at the wrists and nearly come together over the cardiac prominence.

Carnegie stage 22: Eyelids and external ear more developed
50 days after fertilization, 23 mm in CRL

The vascular plexus of the head becomes distinct. The eyelids are thickening and encroaching into the eyes. The tragus and antitragus of the external ear are assuming a more definite form. The position of the external ears becomes higher on the head. The tail has almost disappeared.

Carnegie stage 23: End of embryonic period
52 days after fertilization, 30 mm in CRL

The head has rounded out and the trunk has adopted a more mature shape. The eyelids and ear auricles become definite. The limbs have increased in length and the forearm ascends to or above the level of the shoulder. The vascular plexus is approaching the vertex of the head. The tail has now disappeared. The external genitalia are relatively well developed but sex difference is not yet obvious externally.

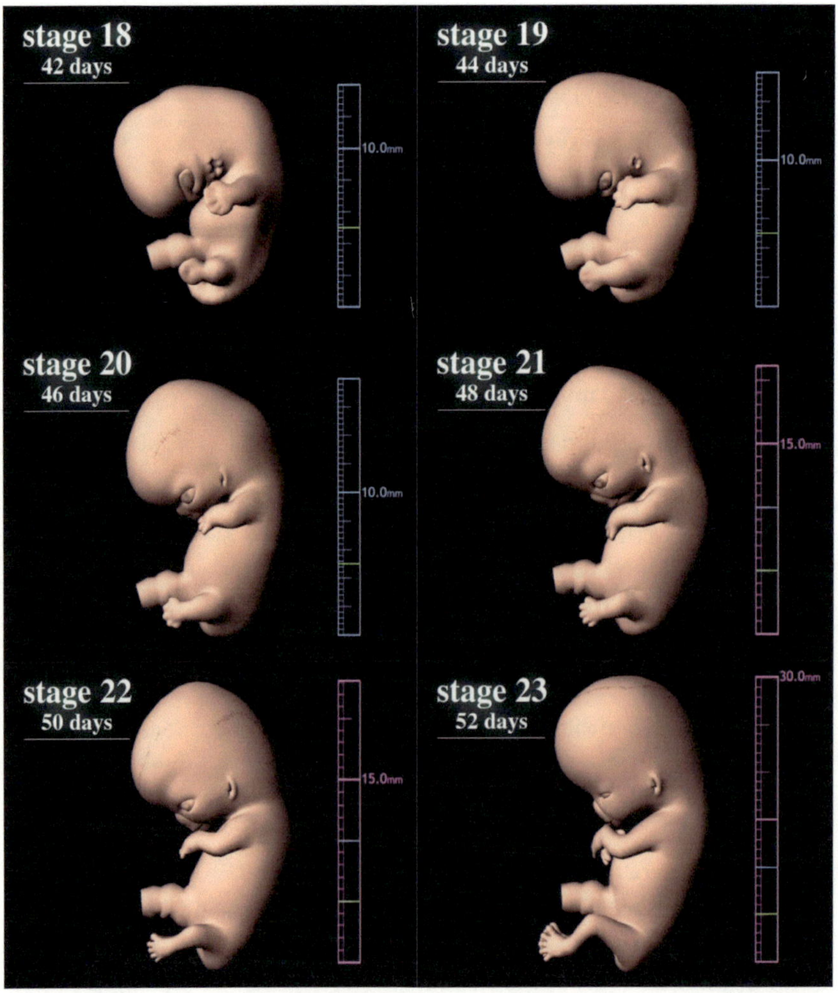

Fig. 6. Computer graphics illustrating human embryonic development: Carnegie stage 18-23.

2.2 The face

Three pharyngeal arches appear at Carnegie stage 12. The 1st pharyngeal gives rise to the maxillary and mandibular prominences (stage 13, Fig. 8), which will then constitute the lateral and caudal boundaries of the stomodeum (i.e., primitive oral cavity), respectively.

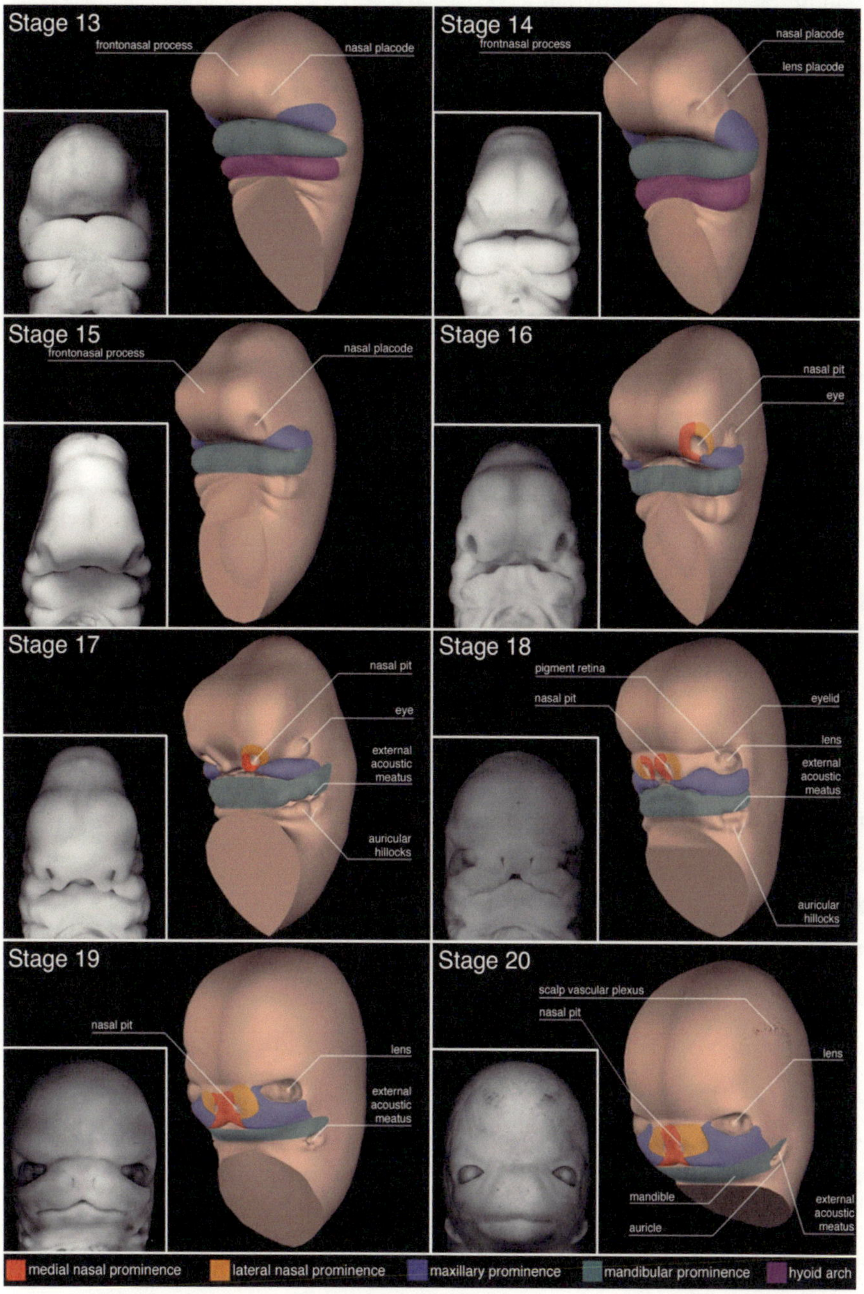

Fig. 7. Embryonic development of the face (stages 13-20).

The side and front of the neck arise from the 2nd pharyngeal arch, also known as the hyoid arch. The frontonasal prominence (FNP) grows to cover the ventral part of the forebrain (stage 13). It will form the forehead (frontal part of the FNP) and the primordial mouth and nose (nasal part of the FNP).

By the end of the 4th developmental week, nasal placodes (thickening of surface ectoderm to become peripheral neural tissue) develop on the frontolateral aspects of the FNP (stage 13). The mesenchyme swells around the nasal placodes resulting in medial and lateral nasal prominences (stage 16). The maxillary prominence will merge with the medial nasal prominences, and cause their fusion. The fused medial nasal prominences will form the midline of the nose and that of the upper lip, as well as the primary palate (stage 16-18). The nasolacrimal groove divides the lateral nasal prominence from the maxillary prominence (observed in stages 16, 17).

The 5th developmental week sees the formation of the primordial ear auricles around the first pharyngeal groove, at the interface between the mandibular prominences and the hyoid arches (stage 16). The auricular hillocks give rise to the auricle while the external acoustic meatus arises from the first pharyngeal groove. At the early period of ear development, the external ears are located in the neck region, and they ascend to the side of the head at the level of the eyes as the development of the mandible (compare Fig. 8 with stage 23 in Fig. 6).

The maxillary and lateral nasal prominences will fuse with the nasolacrimal groove during the 6th developmental week, and result in continuity between the nose and cheek (~stage 18).

The 7th developmental week is marked by the fusion of the two medial nasal prominences with the maxillary and lateral nasal prominences (stage 19~). The merge between the maxillary and medial nasal prominences creates continuity between the upper jaw and lip, and results in partition of the nasal cavity from the oral cavity.

2.3 Upper and lower extremities

The embryonic development of the limbs (O'Rahilly and Gardner, 1975) is illustrated here using computer graphics (Yamada et al., 2006).

Carnegie stage 12

The upper limb buds start to develop.

Carnegie stage 13

The upper limb buds appear in a definite manner, and the lower limb buds start to develop.

Carnegie stage 14

The upper limb buds grow and taper toward the tip, which will later form the hand plate. Innervation and blood supply begin at CS14 in the upper limbs. The development of the lower limb buds is delayed in respect to the upper limb buds.

Carnegie stage 15

The hand plates are distinct in the upper limb buds. In the lower limbs, the rostral half is rounded but the caudal half is tapered. Innervation begins in the lower limb buds.

Carnegie stage 16

Hand plates form a central, carpal part and a digital flange. Lower limb buds form a femoral part, a crural part and foot plate.

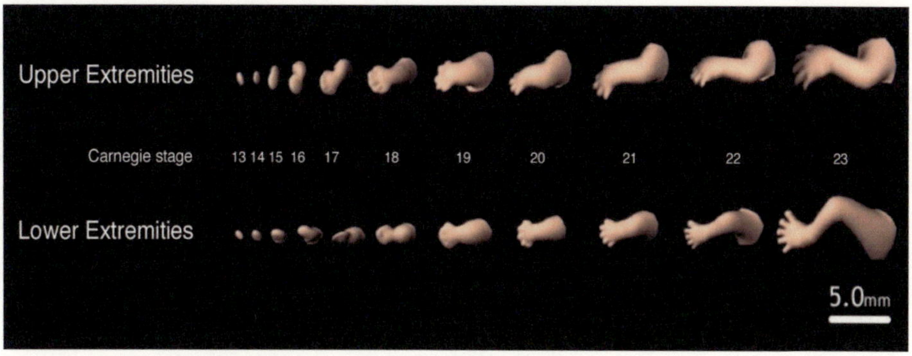

Fig. 8. Embryonic development of upper and lower limbs (CS13-CS23).

Carnegie stage 17

Finger rays appear in the hand plate, and the rim of the hand plate is crenated due to the presence of individual fingers in some advanced specimens. The lower limb buds have increased in size and a rounded digital plate is set off from the crurotarsal region.

Carnegie stage 18

The upper limbs have increased in length and become slightly bent at the elbow. Finger rays are distinct. Toe rays appear but the rim of the foot plate is not yet definitely notched in the lower limb bud.

Carnegie stage 19

The upper limbs rotate medially and seem to hold the chest. Apoptosis occurs in the mesenchymal tissues of interdigital areas, and creates deeper interdigital notches. Toe rays are prominent and interdigital notches appear in the foot plate. Knees and ankles start to appear.

Carnegie stage 20

The upper limbs are bent at the elbow and hand joints, resulting in a pronated position. The lower limbs are also bent at the knee joints. Notches are present between the toe rays in the foot plate.

Carnegie stage 21

Elbows in the upper limbs and knees in the lower limbs now become distinct. Hands cross each other in front of the chest. Fingers are longer and distal phalangeal portions are slightly swollen, indicating the beginning of palmar pads. The feet are also approaching each other.

Carnegie stage 22

Hands extend in front of the body and the fingers of one hand may overlap those of the other. Feet approach each other, but toe digits are still webbed.

Carnegie stage 23

Upper and lower limbs are well formed. They have lengthened and are bent at joints. Fingers get longer and toes are no longer webbed, all digits are now separate and distinct.

3. Conclusion

Large-scale human embryo collections started in the early 20th century and contributed to tremendous progress in human embryology. These compendiums of embryonic specimens are still widely used today, and are exploited through modern technologies such as imaging techniques and computer sciences. Using computer graphics prepared from specimens housed at the Kyoto Collection of Human Embryos, here we provided a clear overview of human embryonic development, with a special emphasis on the limbs and the face.

4. Acknowledgments

We are deeply grateful to Ms. Elizabeth Lockett at the National Museum of Health and Medicine, Washington D.C., for providing information on the Carnegie Collection; Dr. Sumiko Kimura for assistance and guidance in the experiments; Ms. Chigako Uwabe at the Congenital Anomaly Research Center at Kyoto University Graduate School of Medicine for technical assistance; Prof. Michihiko Minoh, Dr. Takuya Funatomi, Dr. Tamaki Motoki, Ms. Mikiko Takahashi, and Mr. Yutaka Minekura at the Academic Center for Computing and Media Studies at Kyoto University, for generating the computer graphics of human embryos; and Prof. Kohei Shiota, Vice President of Kyoto University for his support and guidance on the project. Part of this research was financially supported by Grants #228073, #238058, #21790180 and #22591199 from the Japan Society for the Promotion of Science (JSPS) and the Japan Science and Technology (JST) institute for Bioinformatics Research and Development (BIRD). The studies presented in this chapter were approved by the Medical Ethics Committee at Kyoto University Graduate School of Medicine (Kyoto, Japan).

5. References

Brown, D. D. 1987. The Department of Embryology of the Carnegie Institution of Washington. *BioEssays : news and reviews in molecular, cellular and developmental biology,* 6, 92-6.

Haishi, T., Uematsu, T., Matsuda, Y. & Kose, K. 2001. Development of a 1.0 T MR microscope using a Nd-Fe-B permanent magnet. *Magnetic resonance imaging*. 19, 875-80.

Hirose, A., Nakashima, T., Yamada, S., Uwabe, C., Kose, K. & Takakuwa, T. 2012. Embryonic liver morphology and morphometry by magnetic resonance microscopic imaging. *Anatomical record: advances in integrative anatomy and evolutionary biology*. 2011. 295, 51-59.

Hopwood, N. 2007. A history of normal plates, tables and stages in vertebrate embryology. *The International journal of developmental biology,* 51, 1-26.

Iffy, L., Shepard, T. H., Jakobovits, A., Lemire, R. J. & Kerner, P. 1967. The rate of growth in young human embryos of Streeter's horizons. 13 to 23. *Acta anatomica,* 66, 178-86.

Jirásek, J. E. 1971. *Development of the genital system and male pseudohermaphroditism,* Baltimore, Johns Hopkins Press.

Kameda, T., Yamada, S., Uwabe, C., Shiota, K. & Suganuma, N. 2012. Digitization of clinical and epidemiological data from the Kyoto Collection of Human Embryos: maternal risk factors and embryonic malformations. *Congenital Anomalies.* doi: 10.1111/j.1741-4520.2011.00349.x

Mall, F. P. 1914. On stages in the development of human embryos from 2 to 25mm long. *ANATOMISCHER ANZEIGER,* 46, 78-84.

Matsuda, Y., Ono, S., Otake, Y., Handa, S., Kose, K., Haishi, T., Yamada, S., Uwabe, C. & Shiota, K. 2007. Imaging of a large collection of human embryo using a super-parallel MR microscope. *Magnetic resonance in medical sciences: MRMS: an official journal of Japan Society of Magnetic Resonance in Medicine.* 6, 139-46.

Matsuda, Y., Utsuzawa, S., Kurimoto, T., Haishi, T., Yamazaki, Y., Kose, K., Anno, I. & Marutani, M. 2003. Super-parallel MR microscope. *Magnetic resonance in medicine : official journal of the Society of Magnetic Resonance in Medicine / Society of Magnetic Resonance in Medicine.* 50, 183-9.

Matsunaga, E. & Shiota, K. 1977. Holoprosencephaly in human embryos: epidemiologic studies of 150 cases. *Teratology,* 16, 261-72.

Nishimura, H. 1974. Detection of early developmental anomalies in human abortuses. *In:* Gianantonio, C. A., Berri, G. G. (ed.) *Pediatria XIV.* Buenos Aires: Editorial Medica Panamericana.

Nishimura, H. 1975. Prenatal versus postnatal malformations based on the Japanese experience on induced abortions in the human being. . *In:* BLANDEU, R. (ed.) *Aging Gamates.* Basel: S. Karger AG.

Nishimura, H. 1983. Introduction. *In:* Nishimura, H. (ed.) *Atlas of Human Prenatal Histology.* Tokyo: Igaku-shoin.

Nishimura, H., Takano, K., Tanimura, T. & Yasuda, M. 1968. Normal and abnormal development of human embryos: first report of the analysis of 1,213 intact embryos. *Teratology,* 1, 281-90.

Nishimura, H., Tanimura, T., Semba, R. & Uwabe, C. 1974. Normal development of early human embryos: observation of 90 specimens at Carnegie stages 7 to 13. *Teratology,* 10, 1-5.

O'Rahilly, R. 1988. One Hundred Years of Human Embryology. *In:* KALTER, H. (ed.) *Issues and Reviews in Terratology* New York: Plenum Press.

O'Rahilly, R. & Gardner, E. 1975. The timing and sequence of events in the development of the limbs in the human embryo. *Anatomy and embryology.* 148, 1-23.

O'Rahilly, R. & Müller, F. 1987. *Developmental stages in human embryos: including a revision of Streeter's "horizons" and a survey of the Carnegie Collection.,* Washington, DC, Carnegie Institution of Washington Publication.

Olivier, G. & Pineau, H. 1962. Horizons de Streeter et age embryonnaire. *Bulletin de l'Association des anatomistes.* 47, 573-576.

Shiota, K. 1991. Development and intrauterine fate of normal and abnormal human conceptuses. *Congenit Anom Kyoto,* 31, 67-80.

Streeter, G. L. 1942. Developmental horizons in human embryos. Description of age group XI, 13 to 20 somites, and age group XII, 21 to 29 somites. *Carnegie Institution of Washington publication 541, Contributions to Embryology,* 30, 211-245.

Streeter, G. L. 1945. Developmental horizons in human embryos. Description of age group XIII, embryos about 4 or 5 millimeters long, abd age group XIV, period of indentation of the lens vesicle. *Carnegie Institution of Washington publication 557, Contributions to Embryology,* 31, 27-63.

Streeter, G. L. 1948. Developmental horizons in human embryos. Description of age groups XV, XVI, XVII, and XVIII, being the third issue of a survey of the Carnegie Collection. *Carnegie Institution of Washington publication 575, Contributions to Embryology,* 32, 133-203.

Streeter, G. L. 1951. Developmental horizons in human embryos. Description of age groups XIX, XX, XXI, XXII, and XXIII, being the fifth issue of a survey of the Carnegie Collection (prepared for publication by C. H. Heuser and G. W. Corner). *Carnegie Institution of Washington publication 592, Contributions to Embryology,* 34, 165-196.

Yamada, S. 2006. Embryonic holoprosencephaly: pathology and phenotypic variability. *Congenital anomalies,* 46, 164-71.

Yamada, S., Samtani, R. R., Lee, E. S., Lockett, E., Uwabe, C., Shiota, K., Anderson, S. A. & Lo, C. W. 2010. Developmental atlas of the early first trimester human embryo. *Developmental dynamics : an official publication of the American Association of Anatomists,* 239, 1585-95.

Yamada, S., Uwabe, C., Fujii, S. & Shiota, K. 2004. Phenotypic variability in human embryonic holoprosencephaly in the Kyoto Collection. *Birth defects research. Part A, Clinical and molecular teratology.* 70, 495-508.

Yamada, S., Uwabe, C., Nakatsu-Komatsu, T., Minekura, Y., Iwakura, M., Motoki, T., Nishimiya, K., Iiyama, M., Kakusho, K., Minoh, M., Mizuta, S., Matsuda, T., Matsuda, Y., Haishi, T., Kose, K., Fujii, S. & Shiota, K. 2006. Graphic and movie illustrations of human prenatal development and their application to embryological education based on the human embryo specimens in the Kyoto collection. *Developmental dynamics : an official publication of the American Association of Anatomists,* 235, 468-77.

Yoneyama, A., Yamada, S. & Takeda, T. 2011. Fine Biomedical Imaging Using X-Ray Phase-Sensitive Technique. *In:* Gargiulo, D. G., Mcewan, A. (ed.) *Advanced Biomedical Engineering.* InTech. p107-128.

2

Presenting Human Embryology in an International Open-Access Reference Centre (HERC)

Beate Brand-Saberi[1], Edgar Wingender[2], Otto Rienhoff[2] and Christoph Viebahn[2]
[1]Ruhr-Universität Bochum,
[2]Georg-August-Universität Göttingen,
Germany

1. Introduction

Specimens from early human embryonic development largely originate from chance findings in material collected for pathological analysis following spontaneous or induced abortions, and minimally invasive gynecological surgery for termination of pregnancy (suction curettage) emerging in the early 1990s has now made it almost impossible to procure new intact specimens. Although the absolute number of specimens collected world-wide may be quite high due to the intrinsic fascination held by human embryos, few concerted long-term projects have managed to organise the complex and labour-intensive logistics of acquiring, processing and safely storing specimens for morphological (i.e. histological) analysis. As a result, only four centres world-wide house collections with an appreciable number of scientifically useful specimens.

2. Major embryo collections of the world

2.1 Washington D.C. (USA)

The Carnegie Collection of Human Embryos in Washington D.C. (USA) is the largest collection of embryos (some 10 000) cut into serial histological sections. Because many of these specimens stem from the time before optimal histological fixation protocols were available, only relatively few of them are suitable for high-resolution histological analysis. Nevertheless, this collection formed the basis for the definition of the 23 stages of human development during the first 8 weeks (O'Rahilly and Müller, 1987), which serves as the international standard. For further information on the Carnegie Collection see http://nmhm.washingtondc.museum/collections/hdac/index.htm in this book.

2.2 Kyoto (Japan)

The Congenital Anomaly Research Centre at Kyoto University (Japan) is at present the largest human embryology collection with some 40 000 embryos and fetuses. Emphasis here lies on nuclear magnetic resonance (NMR) analysis of intact specimens; however, 1,000 specimens of this collection are serially sectioned, with one half of them being diagnosed as normal and the other half as abnormal. Further information on the Kyoto Collection may be found in Yamada et al. (2010) and in the chapter by Yamada et al. in this book.

2.3 Göttingen (Germany)

The embryo collection at the centre of Anatomy, Göttingen University (Germany), is unique as it has probably the largest number of excellently preserved specimens of the latter half of the embryonic period (weeks 5 to 8 post conception) world-wide; this was achieved by a combination of a special fixation procedure adjusted by Erich Blechschmidt (1904-1992) to the then "state-of-the-art" gynecological practice (mechanical curettage or hysterectomy) for gynecological operations including termination of pregnancy. As a result, the quality of paraffin histological sections of the more than 120 embryos comprising this collection is unsurpassed and reveals valuable morphological detail of organ development in early human development (cf. Fig. 1). Unfortunately, microscopical glass slides used to hold histological sections are delicate and in constant danger of destruction during use; even under optimal storage conditions they have a finite useful life (in the order of decades) due to gradual deterioration such as evaporation of cover glass glue and bleaching of histological stains. Photomicrographs of individual histological sections from several specimens were published in Blechschmidt's embryology textbook (Blechschmidt, 1960) but the only chance to preserve for posterity morphological information contained in these specimens consisted, at that time, in building large-scale polymer plastic reconstruction models (cf. Fig. 2C) from camera-lucida drawings at an intermediate magnification of regularly spaced histological sections (Blechschmidt 1954). Unique in his approach was the strategy that using the same series of serial sections several times over, Blechschmidt made reconstructions of the surface anatomy and the morphology of several organ systems of the same embryo, thereby

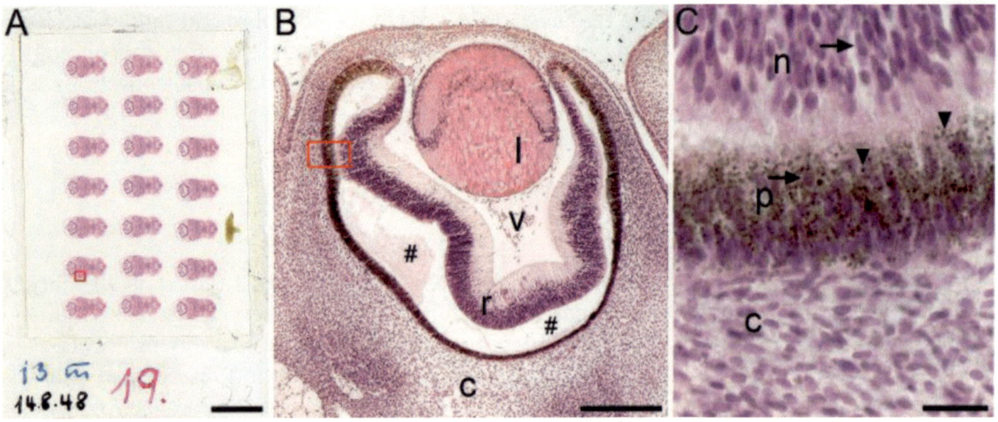

Fig. 1. **A:** Microscopical glass slide with three rows of seven hematoxylin-eosin stained transverse paraffin sections each from a 13-mm human embryo (stage 18) and original inscriptions of specimen details and section number. **B:** Magnification of area marked with the red box in A showing anlage of the eye bulb with lens (l), vitreous body (v), neural layer of the immature retina (r), choriocapillaris layer (c) and typical shrinkage artefacts (#) between the neural (inner) and pigmented (outer) layers of the retina. **C:** Highest magnification of choriocapillaris (c) and neural (n) and pigmented (p) layers of the retina in the area marked with the red box in B showing cellular details such as nuclei (arrows) and pigment granules (arrowheads). Magnification bars: 10 mm (A), 0.2 mm (B), 0.02 mm (C).

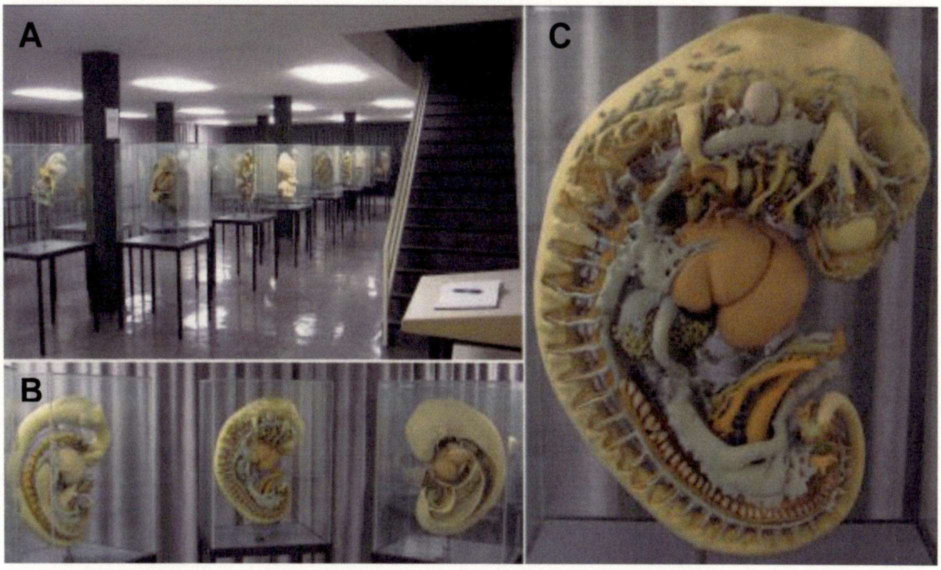

Fig. 2. Views of the large-scale reconstruction models of the "Humanembryologische Dokumentationssammlung Blechschmidt" in the exhibition hall of the Centre of Anatomy in Göttingen (**A**), a selection of three different models reconstructed from the same series of serial sections from a 4.2-mm embryo (**B**) and a close-up (**C**) of one of these models highlighting, amongst other features, the developing arterial and venous vascular systems (orange and blue, respectively), digestive system (green) and nervous system (beige).

enabling direct comparison of topographical characteristics and their dynamic changes during development, even though the cellular detail detectable at high magnification (cf. Fig. 1C) remained unexplored with this method. However, over the course of several decades (from 1946 to 1979) more than 64 models were created, which, to this day, form the basis of the "Humanembryologische Dokumentationssammlung Blechschmidt", a permanent exhibition housed at the Centre of Anatomy of Göttingen University (Fig. 2).

Detailed documentation on individual specimens of the Blechschmidt Collection is sparse. Collectively these specimens are known to be chance findings from pathological material obtained after gynecological operations including legal terminations of pregnancies for medical indications, but there is a catalogue of technical entries on both the histological sections and the large-scale reconstructions. Some of the specimens are depicted as colour drawings in Blechschmidt (1960).

2.4 Bochum (Germany)

Principles for high-quality tissue preservation similar to those successfully practised in Göttingen were applied by Klaus V. Hinrichsen, a pupil of Blechschmidt, after he took the chair of Anatomy and Embryology at the Ruhr University Bochum in 1970. As a result of improved fixative solutions for electron microscopy developed since the start of Blechschmidt's project, many excellent specimens, some of them suitable for subcellular analysis previously unknown from human specimens (cf. Figs. 1 and 3), were collected by Hinrichsen's team between 1969 and 1994 and are now housed in the Department of Anatomy and Molecular Embryology at the Ruhr-Universität Bochum, Germany. Details of many of these specimens in the Hinrichsen Collection (total number n = 70) were published in Hinrichsen's textbook on human embryology (Hinrichsen, 1990) and in many original publications (e. g. Hinrichsen et al. 1994) but reconstructions have not been attempted from these specimens and many specimens have likewise remained unexplored, to date.

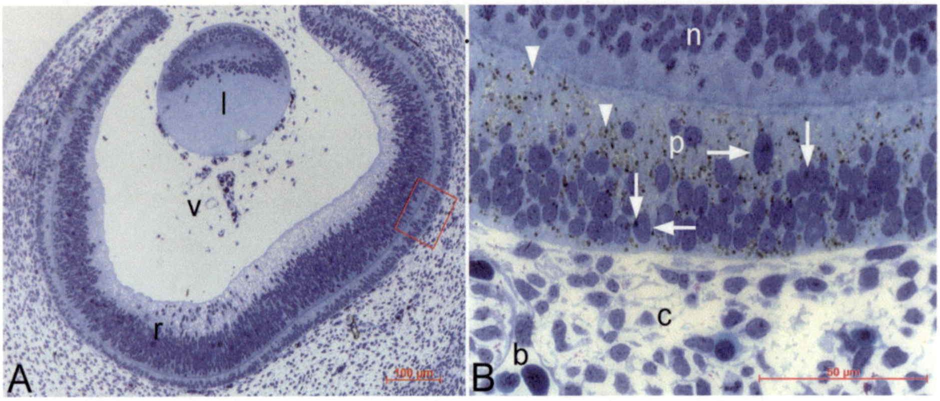

Fig. 3. Semithin plastic section of the eye anlage of a stage 18 embryo. **A** Survey photograph showing lens (l), vitreous body (v), retina (r) and surrounding connective tissue of the eye bulb. **B** Higher magnification taken from border between retina and choriocapillaris (c) layer (similar area marked with red box in A) with blood vessels (b) and the pigmented (p) and nervous (n) layers of the immature retina. Visible subcellular details include dark pigment granules (arrowheads) in the cytoplasm in the pigment layer (cf. Fig. 1C); within the cell nuclei nucleoli (vertical arrows) and the nuclear lamina (horizontal arrows) can be distinguished. Magnification bars: 0.1 mm (A), 0.05 mm (B).

Derivation of the Bochum specimens was in the tradition of the Blechschmidt collection, i.e. they were chance findings in the pathological material derived from legal abortions, as well as from spontaneous abortions. Documentation includes hospital names and dates, but further specimen details are missing. The approval of the ethics committee of Bochum University was recently obtained for the use of specimens from the Hinrichsen collection in medical dissertations (Reg. No. 3791-10).

3. Current methods for digitisation of microscopical specimens

3.1 Digitisation of sectional embryonic morphology

With the advent of digital microphotography serial sections of human embryos from the Carnegie Collection at Washington DC were scanned at high resolution at Louisiana State University Health Center in New Orleans (USA) as part of the Virtual Human Embryo (VHE) project funded by the National Institutes of Health, Maryland, USA. Because the stitching of neighbouring high-magnification microphotographs had to be carried out manually after the scanning was complete, this initial project ran for many years and a complete set of one specimen each for the first 17 Carnegie stages of the first 5 weeks of prenatal development is now available in DVD format (http://virtualhumanembryo.lsuhsc.edu/). The remaining stages up to stage 22 are due to be completed by April 2012 (R. Gasser, pers. inf.). Technological advances during the close of the VHE project brought about a major breakthrough in automatic scanning of microscopical slides for seamless virtual microscopy, 3D-construction and on-line usage which, however, could not yet be used for the VHE project.

In their clinically oriented approach, the Congenital Anomaly Research Centre at Kyoto University (Japan) created a web-accessible annotated 3-D Human Embryo Atlas using their extensive data base of nuclear magnetic resonance (NMR) and episcopic fluorescence capture (EFIC) images of first trimester human embryos (Yamada et al. 2010; http://apps.devbio.pitt.edu/HumanAtlas).

3.2 Virtual microscopy

Virtual microscopy uses digitally stored histological slides previously scanned at high resolution and stored in an open format, to browse through all parts of the histological specimen and zoom in *ad libitum* to any part of the section at the highest light-microscopical resolution, in a manner close to conventional (physical) microscopy. Powerful and versatile light microscopy scanning systems are presently produced by a few leading manufacturers only (Olympus and Zeiss/Metasystems) and consist of a light microscope, digital camera, motorised scanning microscope table, a computer workstation and software for scanning, archiving and viewing whole histological slides. Virtual microscopy includes visualisation of the specimens at continuous intervals of magnification (up to 40x) and fine focusing of the specimen along the z-axis at a given magnification (Fig. 4). Initial tests with the Olympus system carried out on a microscopic slide containing 3 rows of 7 histological sections each from a 13-mm human embryo from the Blechschmidt collection (cf. Fig. 1) provided the proof of principle for scanning serial sections mounted on over-sized glass slides and, most importantly, gave an approximation for the scanning time of about 20 min when using the 40x lens on an individual histological section with a tissue surface of about 2 cm^2 (cf. Fig. 4).

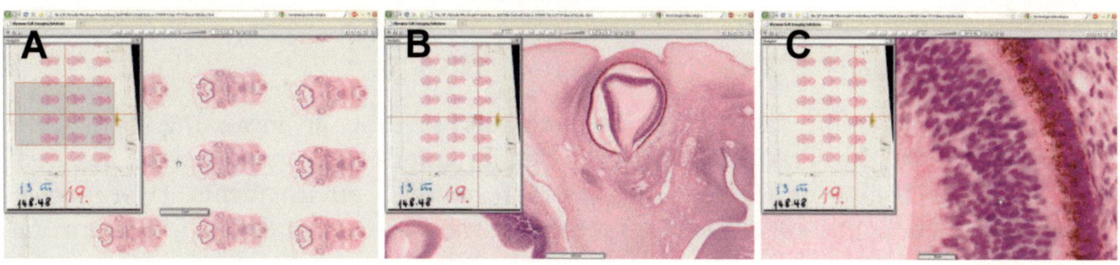

Fig. 4. Screen shots of the Olympus virtual microscopy viewer applied to the slide shown in Fig. 1 containing the developing eye ball at stage 18 at low (0.2x, **A**), middle (2.5x, **B**) and maximal (40x, **C**) digital zoom level. The high zoom level (**C**) shows subcellular detail such as position of cell nuclei and pigment granules (brown) in the nervous and pigmented layers of the immature retina, respectively.

Virtual microscopy - with or without annotation - is widely used for teaching normal (http://www.mikroskopie-uds.de, http://mirax.net-base.de/Home.uni-ulm.0.html) and pathological anatomy (http://patho.med.uni-magdeburg.de/Virtuelle_Pathologie/goea.shtml). Solutions suitable for embryological research purposes are only beginning to be established but will have to connect to existing digital atlases containing conventional images (of defined but fixed magnification) of human development (i.e. NMR and EFIC data at the Kyoto collection: http://apps.devbio.pitt.edu/HumanAtlas) or of various animal model organisms for developmental biology (mouse, chick, frog, zebrafish, fruit fly): http://www.sdbonline.org/index.php?option=content&task=view&id=17&Itemid=22).

3.3 Annotation

Prerequisites for teaching and, most importantly, for reconstruction are annotation systems for individual structures and organ systems within a given histological section. Due to the high-quality conservation methods used by Blechschmidt and Hinrichsen, the cellular structure in the tissue sections is generally so well preserved that annotating substructures of embryos and cells will be possible at different high-resolution levels.

However, annotation may create problems in case of ambiguous terminology or unforeseen tissue artefacts which may occur during cutting and staining of histological sections. The former problem can be minimised (1) by closely adhering to the Terminologia Embryologica (TE) which has been completed in 2010 by an international committee of embryologists (FIPAT), and (2) by use of the ontology databases (s. Burger et al. 2008). In these databases material entities and immaterial concepts of a knowledge domain are interconnected with a set of specified relationships (e.g. "partOf" or "developsInto"), which makes an automatic interpretation of entities possible and embeds them into a semantic web. For the HERC project the "Cytomer" database (Michael et al. 2005) will be used which is the only known ontology of anatomical entities directly connected to (Carnegie) stage-related information such as precursor structures ("anlagen") and germ layer origin of tissues: the entity 'heart', for example, is defined as (1) being an organ, (2) being part of the cardiovascular system, (3) developing from the heart tube and (4) having parts such as the heart valves. This information will then be linked to the annotated structures in serial sections and whole embryos. If earmarked with persistent or unique object identifiers (PID and UOI, respectively) such metadata enables multiple search and filtering functions and facilitates the integration of other resources, such as specimens and structures defined in other embryo collections and anatomical atlases, and in databases for molecular biology (e.g. UniProt, GenBank) and for scientific publications (e.g. PubMed).

3.4 Metadata handling

Handling of the scientific data created by annotation presents an increasing challenge to data management. The latest tendencies in scientific information management, therefore, deal with establishing well integrated virtual research environments (VRE) across organizational boundaries of academic institutions. The Department of Medical Informatics of Göttingen University has accumulated ample experience in the BMBF joint project WissGrid with regard to VREs being built on a distributed IT infrastructure. This experience will serve to integrate and optimise the software used in the project presented here. WissGrid is linking knowledge of several key research partners (e.g. State and University Library Göttingen and e.g. the Astronomy Center in Potsdam). Therefore image-handling as well as annotation have formed part of BMBF funded research in the Department. The results of WissGrid were discussed with the DFG in September 2010; the recommendations from those discussions will be the basis of the work programme for this project.

3.5 Longterm archiving

Preserving research data is paramount for all sciences (cf. Vorschläge zur Sicherung guter wissenschaftlicher Praxis, DFG, 1998-2010). The Dept. of Medical Informatics has been constantly involved in several projects which foster this goal: A research oriented web based image database (Chili PACS) has been hosted since 2005 (this database contains data of 8 projects including the national competence networks for congenital heart defects, dementia, and multiple sclerosis). Digital preservation has also been established within the DFG joint project KoLaWiss from 2008 to 2009, and in the BMBF joint project WissGrid generic biomedical requirements are investigated with regard to digital preservation. Finally, the department is a leading partner in the digital preservation related DFG joint project LABIMI/F, expected to start in March 2011.

WissGrid addresses bitstream preservation and generic technical aspects of content preservation within the world-wide available and standardized Grid Computing infrastructure. Additional biomedicine related aspects of digital preservation will be investigated in the DFG joint project LABIMI/F which can also deal with data from magnetic resonance imaging (Kyoto website) and other research oriented databases (Edinburgh mouse atlas: http://genex.hgu.mrc.ac.uk/) and can therefore intersect with the present project on the generic level of digital preservation of digital image data. The Open Archival Information System (OAIS) provides a generic digital preservation approach (CCSDS, Consultative Committee for Space Data Systems: http://public.ccsds.org/publications/archive/650x0b1.pdf). Against this background Göttingen provides an ideal research environment for the digital preservation envisaged here due to a number of highest-level cooperative IT projects: - **GoeGrid:** interdisciplinary cooperation of grid computing communities: http://goegrid.de. - **GWDG:** experienced IT service provider for bitstream preservation: http://www.gwdg.de /index.php?id=898. - **SUB:** strong experience in digital preservation and leader of the TextGrid joint project: http: //rdd.sub.uni-goettingen.de.

4. The project

4.1 General aims

Bringing together four partners from two universities and with a view to providing the basis for an international human embryonic reference centre (HERC), this pilot project aims at developing methods and standards for the preservation and open-access presentation of microscopic preparations of early human development. Cutting-edge computer technology in image acquisition, digital annotation and cross-border information management will be developed and applied to selected specimens from two large collections of irreplaceable human embryonic specimens. Strategic long-term commitment to follow the first project period in both Universities will eventually enable the complete digitisation and open-access provision of the two collections as an indispensable step to secure this unique resource for scientific use.

Separable goals are as follows:

1. creating a virtual research environment (VRE) across organizational boundaries of the academic institutions involved.
2. implementing a system of high-resolution digitisation of histological serial sections of human embryology taken from representative organogenesis stages of development (Carnegie stages 12 to 23).
3. development of an ontology based annotation client optimised for a high number of related histological sections.
4. annotation of embryos, relevant structures and landmarks with persistent identifiers (PIDs) using international terminology standards (e.g. the TE) and the Cytomer ontology.

5. use of PIDs defined in the annotation process (goal 3) for complex cross-linking to similar entities in neighbouring histological sections, different specimens, developmental stages and research databases.
6. close cooperation with databases of (1) The Human Developmental Anatomy Collection (Carnegie Collection) at the National Museum of Health and Medicine at Washington DC, USA and (2) The Congenital Anomaly Research Center in Kyoto, Japan.
7. establishing a platform for intelligent search functions for PIDs.
8. development and implementation of hardware and software for mass data handling and long-term archiving.
9. open access presentation at the official website of Göttingen University.

Future perspectives consist in (1) detailed comparison of individual variations between embryos of the same stage digitised in the two other human embryology centres (Washington DC and Kyoto), (2) cross-referencing with gene expression databases such as Mouse Genome Informatics of The Jackson Laboratory, Bar Harbor, ME, (USA), and (3) 3D-reconstruction of whole embryos complete with annotation and open-access presentation.

4.2 The schedule

The complex aims set out in this enterprise can only be met if a plausible time schedule is followed so that initial technical problems can be solved and methods come to fruition in the long term and for further projects on a similar line. The 2-year time frame shown at the end of this chapter (s. Table 3) is based deliberately on a set of 4 defined work packages (WP1 – WP4) and a subset of 2 – 5 milestones (M) using a given number of specimens from which extrapolation may be deduced for other specimens, collections and cooperative set-ups.

4.2.1 Digitisation (WP1)

Göttingen. Digitisation of histological sections requires dedicated scanning software. A virtual microscopy system provided either by Olympus or Zeiss/Metasystems will be installed in a room close to the safe store of the microscopical slide collection in the Centre of Anatomy. After capture files will be transferred for further use and backup storage to the two servers housed in different departments.

Stage	Embryo no.	embryo size (greatest length)	approx. no. of sections à 10μm
11 (13 somites)	HERC11-1	3.1 mm	310
12 (23 somites)	HERC12-1	2.5 mm	250
12 (27 somites)	HERC12-2	3.4 mm	340
13 (30 somites)	HERC13-1	4.2 mm	420
14	HERC14-1	6.3 mm	630
15	HERC15-1	7.5 mm	750
16	HERC16-1	10.0 mm	1000
17	HERC17-1	13.5 mm	1350
19	HERC19-1	17.5 mm	1750
		total:	6800

Table 1. List of 9 representative embryos from the Blechschmidt Collection.

Paraffin sections:

Stage	Embryo no.	embryo size (gr. length)	plane	approx. no. sections à 10μm
19	HERC19-2	19 mm	sag.	800
20	HERC20-1	21 mm	sag.	800
22	HERC22-1	26 mm	transv.	1600
23	HERC23-1	29 mm	front.	1500
			total:	4700
Semithin sections:				
1. Heart				
Stage 13	HERC13-2	5.5 mm	front.	400
2. Eye				
Stage 18	HERC18-1	16 mm	sag.	600
Stage 18	HERC18-2	15.5 mm	sag.	300
			total:	1300

Table 2. List of representative embryos of the Hinrichsen Collection.

An initial six-week training phase will be arranged to develop time-efficient handling of the virtual slide system and the data management. This training period will also be used to establish an efficient work-flow within the local network of project partners. Subsequently, the whole series of histological sections from nine embryos chosen for their excellent tissue preservation (Table 1) will be scanned continuously over the two-year period of the project. Preliminary tests using the Olympus virtual slide system VS110-S5-E showed that the scanning time in one z-layer per average histological section of the collection is about 20 minutes. Following an estimation of the number of histological sections per embryo at different stages (s. Table 1) and taking the variable surface area of sections in different parts of the embryo and at different stages of development into account, a minimum of time needed for scanning all histological sections of the nine selected embryos, some of them at several z-layers per section, is calculated as follows: 6800 sections : 3 = 2268 hours; using a working time of 20 h per week for a 0,5 - technician position this results in just over 110 working weeks pure scanning time, which can be accommodated in a project period of two years.

Scanning will start with the youngest embryo (No. HERC11-1, stage 11, 3.1 mm, 13 somites) and will end with the embryo of the most advanced stage (No. HERC19-1, stage 19, 17.5 mm). This approach will optimize the efficiency of the annotation procedure (see 3.2.2) as work will proceed along the normal developmental time-line from simple to complex and more numerous morphological structures. Only continuous interactions between the departments involved will guarantee efficient and scientifically correct definition of annotations.

Bochum. After installing a virtual microscopy system with the same manufacturer's specifications as in Göttingen, four complete series of embryos of the Hinrichsen Collection ranging between 5 and 29 mm (Table 2) will be scanned with a view to comparing digitisation conditions and requirements on the basis of different sectional planes (sagittal, frontal and horizontal), and three alternating staining procedures: Trichrome, Hematoxylin-Eosin and Azan. In addition, semithin (1 μm thick) sections of one embryonic heart specimen and of two embryonic eye specimens (Fig. 3) will be digitised.

Scanning time for these paraffin sections is as calculated above for the Blechschmidt specimens. Scanning times for single organ anlagen such as heart and eye are expected to be similar to those for scanning complete embryonic cross sections. For 6000 sections 2000 hours will be needed; at 20 h per week of a 0.5 technician's position this results in about 100 weeks' pure scanning time spread over a two-year project period.

4.2.2 Annotation (WP2)

Development of annotation tools and the annotation itself will be carried out as a basis for a virtual research environment (VRE) about to be established. An annotation format and a procedure for data exchange will be defined. A software engine will be built to dynamically operate on the extracted slides and sections, to allow an on-the-flight visualisation of the observed image part without loading every single image. This requires stream loading processes in order to transfer only the involved tiles which increased performance for optimal usability. During the project the annotation client will be constantly enhanced based on the outcomes of the semi-automatic image processing (s. below).

The annotation client will expand on features implemented in existing tools for annotation of teaching material (e.g. the Netbase solution for MyMicroscope: http://mirax.net-base.de/UK-Ulm.411.0.html) to meet the requirements of the present project:

- definition of persistent identifiers (PIDs) and unique object identifiers (UOIs)
- semi-automatic edge detection (segmentation) in preparation for manual annotation
- continuous access to changes in annotation with respect to advances in knowledge
- solutions for concurrent annotations in cases of conflicting terminology
- persistent annotation while focussing through Z-stacks of the same histological section,
- fast search through sections of the same embryo along contours of a defined structure (individual organ anlagen)
- intelligent searches for specimens, sections, defined edges, terminology, items defined in ontology databases (e.g. Cytomer ontology)
- crosslinking to international databases in prospect of 3-D reconstructions.

Systematic annotation will start at a basic level, i.e. with the technical details of each specimen, to render scanned images efficiently accessible and to uniquely identify each data point defined thereafter. This content-based metadata will already be defined with a view to being interlinked with other information available on the world wide web, such as the data provided by cooperation partners at Washington DC and Kyoto.

At the next level, annotations which guide the user to specific points of interest or explain basic facts will be assigned using arrows and (pop-up) labels to important morphological structures. A standardised vocabulary derived from the terminologia embryologica (TE) will help to name structures in a stereotype, unambiguous way. Frequent reconciliation with partner departments will help to increase annotation quality. As with the technical data of each specimen morphology-related annotation data will be stored alongside the images to render specific structures retrievable from the archive. To optimize and accelerate the annotation process images will be processed by application of an edge detection algorithm (segmentation) for the embryonic structures within neighbouring sections to be developed as part of this project. Adjacent sections will then inherit annotation from each other in a semi-automatic manner.

Annotation information for certain structures and organs (e.g. the eye anlage) will be linked in multiple ways to the same morphological entity (1) in different sections, (2) in different embryos of the same stage, (3) in embryos of the same stage but fixed or stained with alternative methods (e.g. embryos sectioned at 1 and 10μm, Kyoto embryos analysed by NMR), (4) in embryos of different stages, (5) in embryos from different collections, etc.. Multiple search and filtering functions will be implemented to integrate other resources, embryonic collections or other anatomical data, based on their distinct annotation.

In a further phase of annotation terms from the Cytomer ontology will be linked to structures visible and annotated in the individual sections; depending on the resolution available in individual embryos (e.g. in embryos sectioned at 1μm), the annotation client will consider subcellular structures also.

A final version of the annotation client will enable the annotator to trace individual structures with a polygon line instead of the simple arrows used as the standard method. Semi-automatic edge detection for images will be included to suggest borders of anatomical structures to the annotator in an editable manner. The confirmed or corrected structures are returned to support the image processing of the adjacent sections. To foster consistent annotation among human embryology centres world-wide the client will finally be made available to the international partners in Washington DC and Kyoto and to future partners providing relevant data.

4.2.3 Data handling (WP3 and WP4)

Data handling in this project contains at least two aspects, i.e. data presentation and data preservation, which will be dealt with separately below:

Data presentation (WP3). After the first scan is complete, image files - containing all layers and sections - will be disassembled into genuine sections of the defined graphics format for digital preservation. The digital data originates in a free (Zeiss/Metasystems) or proprietary image format (VSI, Olympus) with about 1.7 terabyte per embryo (each image file scales at about one gigabyte). The images are named and stored in a unique and structured way in a file system, compressed if applicable, and managed by a database that is assembled after the export process by the Olympus or Zeiss/Metasystems scanning system. This process will be repeated for each scan over the project period. This aims to implement a solution which guarantees that it will be possible to access all relevant information of the unique embryology collection presented in HERC, once it has been transformed into digital image data.

In close cooperation between partner departments, the portal will integrate the ability to segment the image data as well as edit and adjust the intellectual metadata. This will significantly influence the development of the annotation tool itself. In order to facilitate the annotation process, a semi-automatic segmentation algorithm will be developed to find structural borders in the embryonic section. This will significantly improve the annotation process - if segments can be re-identified in neighboring layers, the annotation can also be re-used. A suitable segmentation algorithm as well as the software engine for segmentation will have to be developed: The algorithm will comprise colour level windowing followed by edge detection, thus giving isolated objects for annotation. Finally, the annotated slides will be disseminated in an online open-access portal for other researchers and student teaching (s. below). Depending on the quality of the image sections (fragments, contrast, noise etc.) the segmentation solution may later be utilized to generate a 3-D-reconstruction of the whole embryo to be displayed in the web based portal.

The visualisation component has to consider performance issues due to the large data size for both the VRE as well as the open access microscopy. Therefore, the computational and major data analysis has to be performed server-sided. Users will be provided with optimized data streams to their client computers. The internet portal for the embryo collection data will implement the working environment for the anatomy and molecular biology researchers and it will combine the annotation tools in combination with a visualisation component. The portal will thus have two areas of application: a) virtual research environment, and b) open access microscopy.

The VRE part will use a role-based access in order to ensure data protection. In this area researchers will have full or limited access to the research data and will be able to create their own annotation information sets. In this context the established national Public Key Infrastructure (PKI) of the local D-Grid infrastructure will be able to support the cross-institutional integration of the VRE. The open access portal will be available to national as well as international users but limited to read-only access. Primary aim of the portal is to offer an initial working solution with the possibility of later extension. A dedicated visualisation related infrastructure for a portal prototype with high performance computational capabilities will be provided. This will allow world-wide provision of the embryo collection data backed up by profound data preservation in combination with the digital preservation concept to be developed (s. below).

Digital preservation (WP4). The Open Archival Information System (OAIS) provides a generic digital preservation approach. This includes the three primary layers of digital preservation: a) bitstream preservation - digital layer, b) content preservation - logical layer, and c) data curation - intellectual / conceptual layer. Besides aspects of preservation, possible threats to the digital images will be considered in a bottom-up approach based on digital preservation best practises (Rosenthal et al. 2005).

The major data structure of the digital embryology collection is presently determined by digital images and related annotation data. According to digital preservation best practices, it is vital to convert any proprietary data into a standardized and open format. Thus, an image data format needs to be specified as well as the process of format and technical metadata conversion. In addition to the content preservation mechanisms it is necessary to define a concept for data curation. While content preservation deals with technical metadata and data format specifications, data curation is necessary to provide researchers with profession-related metadata - intellectual metadata - of the digital content. In that context, a persistent identifier (PID) for digitized embryonic data will be defined together within the departmental consortium to ensure non-ambiguous data access. A digital object identifier (DOI) related solution, as established for geo science data (http://www.tib-hannover.de/de/spezialsammlungen/forschungsdaten) is a possible solution. Furthermore, until released for publication, intellectual property rights (IPR) potentially apply to images in combination with intellectual metadata. Therefore, it is necessary to consider data protection aspects in the VRE.

Because the digital preservation infrastructure to be implemented relies on profession related requirements, three workshops will be organised in the first 6 months of the project period: A first workshop with experts from the areas of molecular biology, anatomy and embryology, bioinformatics as well as digital imaging will be organized to define basic requirements and standards for digitisation and annotation. In a second workshop the digital preservation related aspects and requirements will be investigated with the help of experts from the area of digital preservation. Relevant frameworks such as the FedoraCommons repository (http://fedora-commons.org) will be discussed and a first recommendation derived. Furthermore, by including international experts in both workshops, aspects of information interchange and metadata standardisation will be addressed. In that context it will also be possible to address the aspect of financial necessities, software sustainability and further preservation threats based on a broad perspective. A third workshop with experts from both groups will pool the facts from the previous workshops, international cooperation and produce recommendations for the digital preservation concept. Based on the feedback of the first two workshops potential digital preservation frameworks will be investigated. The results of the primary investigation will be used to propose a selection of relevant frameworks within the third workshop in the course of which a selection recommendation will be determined.

Based on the clarification of the profession related requirements in the workshops a first prototype will be developed on a Grid Computing cluster located at the Göttingen University. This prototype will implement a metadata and image data preservation concept in a provided test environment. The prototype will be validated on the basis of a developed parameter set within the project. This will also include the international access perspective of the digital preservation infrastructure as well as the definition of a profound persistent identifier definition.

The final stage of development of the digital preservation infrastructure will be achieved as an operational implementation. The operational implementation will be available for the designated laboratory environment in Bochum and Göttingen as a proof of concept. An expansion to further users and the transfer to production environments are not part of the development, but it will be possible to achieve this by application of the concept to those areas.

4.2.4 Time frame

To arrive at a manageable time frame for this project the four work packages defined in this chapter are subdivided further into two to five milestones (M1.1, M1.2, M2.1, ..., M3.1, etc.; s. Table 3). The time needed (in the order of months) for each milestone is meant to be an approximation which may have to be adjusted as the project proceeds. The closest correlation exists, of course, with the time periods calculated in connection with the digitisation process (s. 4.2.1).

Work package / Month	1	2	3	4	5	6	7	8	9	10	11	12	13	14	15	16	17	18	19	20	21	22	23	24
WP0 - Coordination																								
WP1 - Digitisation						M1.1																		M1.2
WP2 - Annotation																								
WP2.1 - Requirements		M2.1																						
WP2.2 - Implementation												M2.2						M2.3						M2.4
WP2.3 - Data Interchange																								M2.5
WP3 - Data Presentation																								
WP3.1 - Requirements	M3.1																							
WP3.2 - Viewer Prototype						M3.2																		
WP3.3 - Segmentation engine																M3.3								M3.4
WP4 - Digital Preservation																								
WP4.1 - Requirements		M4.1	M4.2		M4.3																			
WP4.2 - Prototype												M4.4												
WP4.3 - Production System																								M4.5

Table 3. Time schedule for work packages (WP) and milestones (M).

5. Conclusion

Open access to digitised, annotated and extensively cross-linked high-resolution microscopy of irreplaceable specimens of human embryonic development can be expected to be widely used in the international biomedical scientific community. Preservation and presentation of this data will help to reduce vexing uncertainties about methodological artifacts and inter-individual variations during normal and abnormal human development, which still represent a serious hindrance for determining the significance of morphological and molecular results obtained in animal models for the human condition. After standards and procedures are established by this pilot project, the database is likely to expand quickly to become an internationally recognised reference centre, through the long-standing commitment of the cooperation partners and through cooperation with other centres with a research interest in human development and disease.

6. Acknowledgment

The authors wish to thank Hans-Georg Sydow for his excellent help with the graphics work.

7. References

Blechschmidt E. (1954) [Reconstruction method by using synthetic substances; a process for investigation and demonstration of developmental movements.]. *Z Anat Entwicklungsgesch.* 118(2):170-4

Blechschmidt E (1960) The stages of human development before birth. Karger, Basel, 684 pp.

Burger A, Davidson D, Baldock R (2008) Anatomy Ontologies for Bioinformatics. Springer, 356 pp.

Consultative Committee for Space Data Systems (2002). Reference Model for an Open Archival Information System (OAIS). *Blue Book 1.* CCSDS Secretariat, Washington D.C. (USA), http://public.ccsds.org/publications/archive/650x0b1.pdf

Hinrichsen VK (1990) Humanembryologie. Springer, Berlin, 909 pp.

Hinrichsen, K.V., Jacob, H.J., Jacob, M. Brand-Saberi, B., Christ, B., Grim, M. (1994). Principles of foot ontogenesis. *Ann. Anat.* 176:121-130.

Michael H, Chen X, Fricke E, Haubrock M, Ricanek R, Wingender E (2005) Deriving an ontology for human gene expression sources from the CYTOMER database on human organs and cell types. In silico biology 5(1):61-6

O'Rahilly R and Müller F (1987) Developmental stages in human embryos. *Carnegie Inst Washington Publication* 637.

Rosenthal DSH, Robertson TS, Lipkis T, Reich V, Morabito S. (2005) Requirements for Digital Preservation Systems: A Bottom-Up Approach. *D-Lib Magazine,* http://arxiv.org/abs/cs/0509018.

Yamada S., Samtani R. R., Lee E. S., Lockett E., Uwabe C., Shiota K., Anderson S. A., Lo C. W. (2010) Developmental atlas of the early first trimester human embryo. *Dev Dyn.* 239(6):1585-95.

Part 2

Implantation

3

Optimal Environment for the Implantation of Human Embryo

Paweł Kuć
Medical University of Białystok, Department of Perinatology
Centre for Reproductive Medicine KRIOBANK, Białystok,
Poland

1. Introduction

The molecular basis of embryo-maternal relationship, that leads to proper implantation into a receptive maternal endometrium to successfully establish a pregnancy, is still not fully understood. The human endometrium undergoes morphological and hormonal changes during the menstrual cycle in preparation for successful embryo implantation, or menstrual shedding in the absence of implantation. The success of implantation process depends on a receptive endometrium, a blastocyst quality as well as embryo-endometrial interface synchronization. Only 5% of collected oocytes and only 20-25% of transferred embryos can lead to a birth of a healthy newborn.

How can we improve implantation rate following infertility treatment? Two main hypotheses can be put forward as a solution:

1. Patient-determined embryo quality,
2. Endometrial quality: patient-determined or a results of a synchronous steroid hormone preparation.

The discussion on these hypotheses will be presented in the following issues of this chapter.

2. Embryo quality

Since the in vitro fertilization (IVF) procedure was involved to Assisted Reproductive Technology (ART), there are lots of efforts trying to improve the IVF outcomes. At the beginning, the higher pregnancy rates observed in IVF cycles than in natural, were obtained by stimulating the growth of more than only one follicle as well as by transferring to the uterus excessive numbers of embryos. It has been led to negative side effect as multiple pregnancy, which is nowadays considered as a complication of infertility treatment. The quality of embryos seems to be the basic determinants of success for embryo implantation in the natural as well as in the stimulated cycles. The most important challenge in ART nowadays is the ability to identify the embryos with the greatest development potential. These embryos should be selected and transferred to the uterus.

Some studies have supported the idea that only embryo quality is the best predictive factor for pregnancy in IVF cycles (Brezinova et al.,2009; Fauque et al.,2007), significantly better than the assessment of endometrial features (Terriou et al.,2007; Terriou et al.,2001; Zhang et al.,2005). Some of them present results showing the relations between endometrial features and IVF outcomes analysed at different stages of embryo development.

There are lots of methods for evaluating embryo implantation potential and correlations between characteristics of follicles, the oocytes, the zygotes, the early cleavage embryos, the morulas and blastocysts. The ideal method for embryo selection should be non-invasive, easy to assess, standardized, with correlation to pregnancy outcomes.

The studies concerning the determination of new methods for assessing embryos using metabolomics, proteonomics and genomics are still pending, and their results are not yet clinically applicable. Most laboratories still use morphological criteria for embryo assessment. The assessment of embryo morphology is the most important part of many embryo scoring systems. Morphological characteristics provide a lot of information about regular or irregular embryo development, but also present many limitations. They cannot detect genetic disorders of gametes or embryos, and either predict normal pregnancy outcome.

In natural cycles fertilization of oocyte and early cleavage embryo development have place in fallopian tube and then blastocyst is transferred to the uterus where it is implanted in uterine endometrium. In the IVF cycles the early embryo development from zygote to blastocyst can be observed in lab conditions, where the analysis of morphological characteristic is allowed.

2.1 Zygote scoring systems

The most important predicting factor of normal embryo development in the zygote stage is the visualization of two pronuclei (PNs), one from sperm cell and one from oocyte. It should occur between 16 and 19 hour after fertilization. In the past, 5 grade zygote scoring system presented by Scott et al. (Scott et al.,2000) was based on five zygote features: PNs size, the nuclear alignment, the nucleolar alignment and the distributions, and the position. Grade 1 was described as equal number of nucleoli aligned at the pronuclear junction. Grade 2 - as an equal number of nucleoli in equal size in the same nuclei, and one of nuclei having alignment at the pronuclear junction, and the second one with scattered nucleoli. Grade 3 was described as equal numbers of nucleoli in equal size equally scattered in the two nuclei. Grade 4 – unequal numbers of nucleoli and/or unequal size. Grade 5 – with not aligned pronuclei, in different size, and not placed in the central part of zygote. This system was then modified by author to the 4 grades Z score system. The following parameters which were assessed: PNs size and alignment, aligment of nucleoli within the PNs and cytoplasmic morphology. The total number of points which could be achieved was ranged between 3 and 35. Embryos with more than 15 points were classified as embryos with the highest implantation potential, and presented about 70% pregnancy rate (Scott et al.,2000; Scott & Smith,1998).

The last modification of Z score system was proposed in 2003 by Scott (Scott,2003). The scoring system was based on the zygotes features that can be observed at the time of fertilization. The last version has been commonly used by many labs. In comparison to the previous version the presence of halo was associated with better morphology of embryos assessed in the 3rd and the 5th day of their development. Zygotes assessed as Z1 and Z2 had the highest implantation rate. The Z1 and Z2 zygotes presented significantly higher number of good quality blastocysts on the 5th day after fertilization. All pregnancies from day 5 transfers resulted from the transfer of blastocysts that originated from Z1 or Z2 zygotes. Figure 1 shows comparison the 5 grade score with Z zygote scoring system.

5-grade score system	Z score	Pronuclear morphology	Representative embryo images
Grade 1	Z1		
Grade 2	Z2		
Grade 3	Z3		
Grade 4	Z3		
Grade 4	Z3		
Grade 4	Z3		
Grade 5	Z3		
Grade 5	Z4		
Grade 5	Z4		

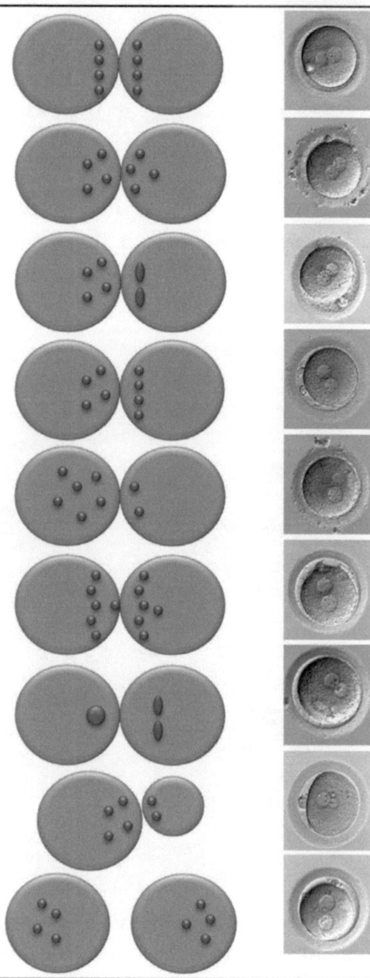

Fig. 1. The 5 grade score and Z zygote scoring systems.

There are some studies that evaluate the usefulness of cumulative zygote scoring systems on embryo implantation. Ludwig et al. (Ludwig et al.,2000) presented modified Scott's Z score system, where the threshold for positive IVF results was 13 points. Embryos presented less than 13 points according to the Z score system presented negative implantation results in 92%. Zollner et al. (Zollner et al.,2002) created the cumulative zygote scoring system similar to the Z score system. The following features of zygote were used to evaluate zygote quality:

number, the position and size of pronuclei, the alignment and the number of nucleoli in each pronuclei, halo effect, morphology of vacuoles and structure of cytoplasm. The zygotes with more than 15 points were associated with higher quality of blastocyst in the 5th day of embryo development.

Another zygote scoring system was proposed by Tesarik and Greco (Tesarik & Greco,1999). They created the system based on the assessment of the number and distribution of each PN. The system divide embryos into 2 groups: pattern 0 and non pattern 0. Its allows efficient prediction of implantation rate using static, single observation of zygote's state. Authors reported 30% implantation rate among pattern 0 embryos, and 11% among non pattern 0 embryos.

The assessment of zygote morphology at 16 and 19 hour after fertilization seems to be helpful in selection of the embryos with the highest potential for implantation. The evaluation of zygote morphology seems to be helpful in countries with internal law regulations imposing embryo selection at the PNs stage. This scoring systems can be used in patients who would have benefited from the 5th day embryo transfer (ET), especially in countries where the high costs of ART techniques exist parallel with the poor, not optimal embryo culture systems.

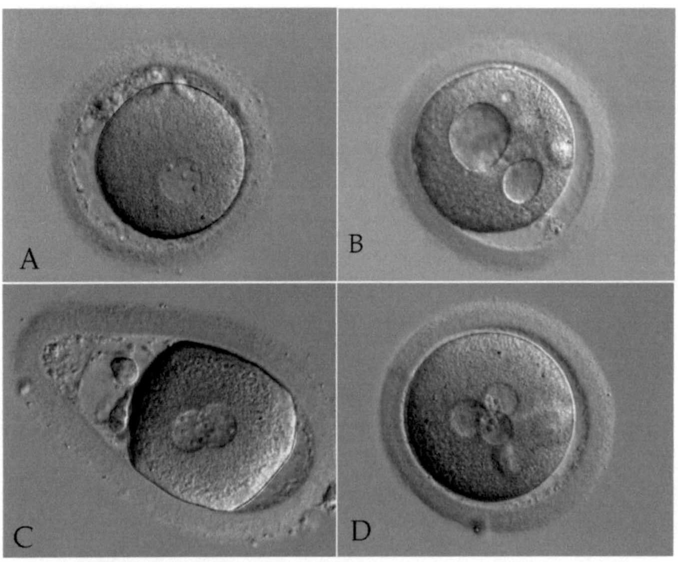

Fig. 2. Abnormalities of zygote stage embryos: A – mononucleation (1PN); B – vacuoles in cytoplasm; C – dysmorphic zygote (2PNs); D – multinucleation (3PNs).

2.2 Cleavage embryos scoring systems

Twenty five hours after the fertilization embryos reach 2-cell stage of their development. There are very few studies focusing on this stage and on its impact on the positive implantation. Most of them (Ciray,2007; Ciray et al.,2004) presented the conclusions that assessment of 2-cell embryo stage together with the subsequent stages of embryo development can present additive positive value in embryo reproductive potential and implantation rate.

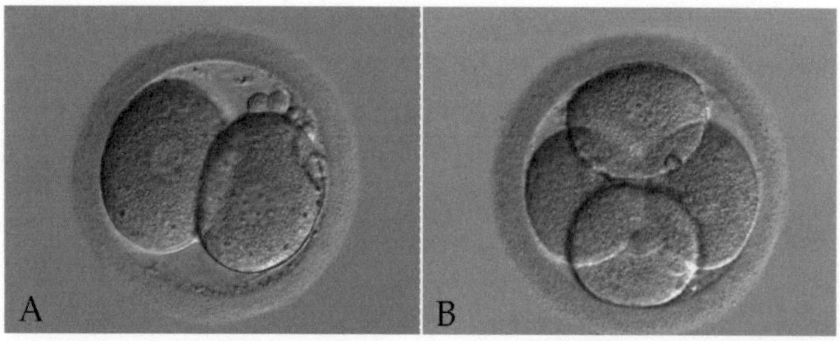

Fig. 3. Good quality early cleavage embryos: A - 2 blastomer stage; B - 4 blastomer stage.

The perfect 4-cell embryo should have equal size of regular symmetrical blastomers with minimal fragmentation (Giorgetti et al.,2007; Terriou et al.,2007). Nowadays, the nucleation of blastomers has important value in selection of abnormal embryos. Multinucleated blastomers are associated with lower implantation rate due to the high risk of chromosomal abnormalities. Mononucleation of all 4 blastomers is associated with higher embryo reproductive potential (Saldeen & Sundstrom,2005).

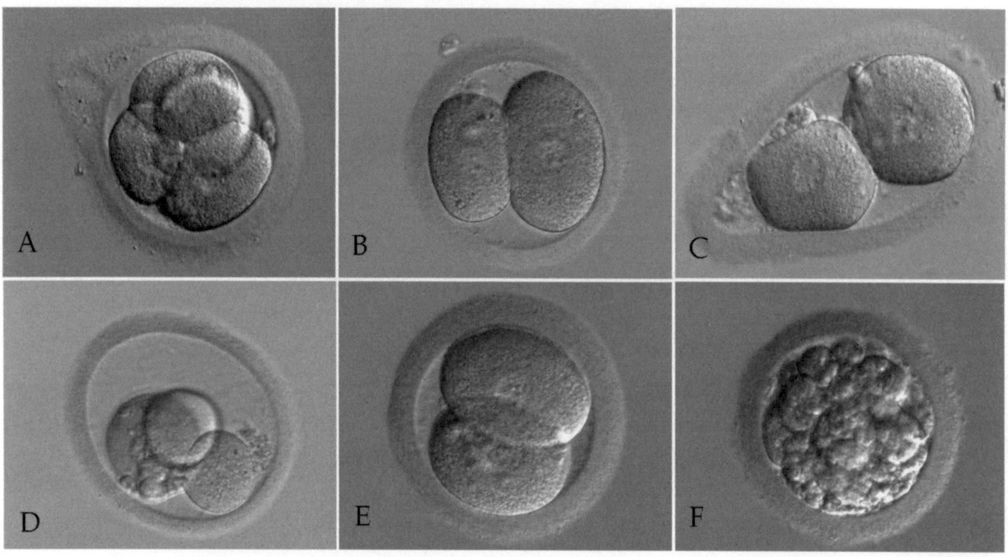

Fig. 4. Abnormalities of early cleavage embryos: A – defect of zona pellucida; B - irregular size of blastomers; C – dysmorphic 2 blastomer embryo; D – shrink blastomers; E – thick zona pellucida; F – total cytoplasm defragmentation.

On the third day after fertilization 8-cell stage of embryo development should be confirmed. The assessment of three day embryo includes the number of cells, the symmetry of blastomers, the degree of fragmentation, and eventually the early embryo compaction. Many studies confirmed the relationship between the number of blastomers observed on the third day after fertilization and implantation rate following transfer taking place on this day. Some authors suggest that embryos having exactly 8 blastomers on the third day present the highest reproductive potential. These embryos have the highest implantation rate (Racowsky et al.,2003).

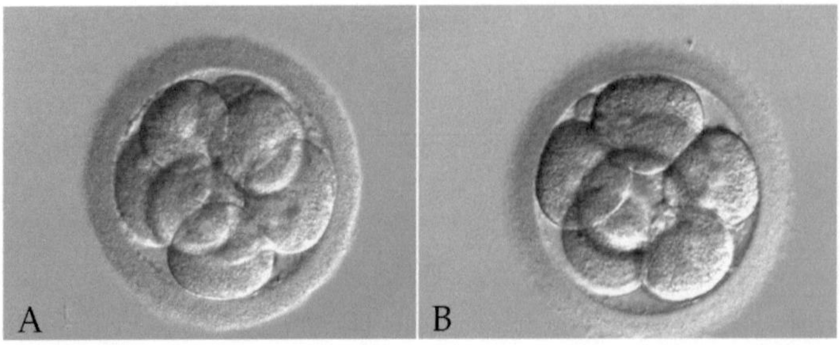

Fig. 5. Good quality cleavage stage: A - 8 blastomer stage; B – 6 blastomer stage.

Another study showed that at least 8 or more blastomers observed in the third day of embryo development were associated with higher implantation rate in comparison to less than 8 cells (Carrillo et al.,1998). Other authors maintained that 7 to 9 blastomers observed on the third day was connected with the highest implantation potential (Alikani et al.,2000).

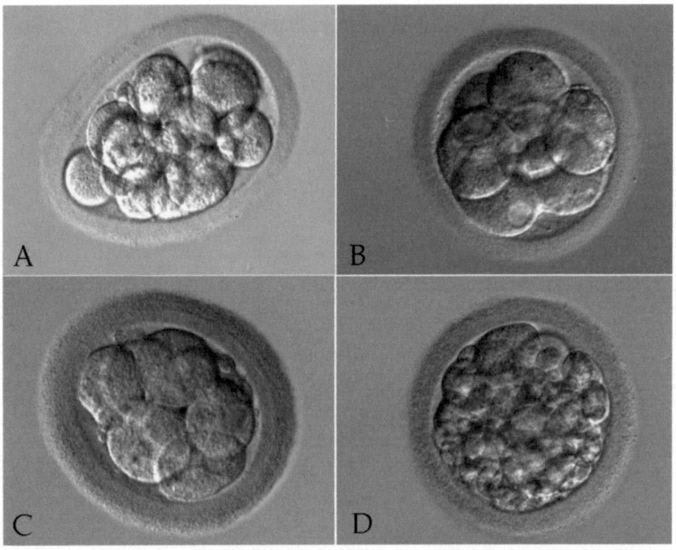

Fig. 6. Abnormalities of cleavage embryos: A – dysmorphic embryo; B – vacuole into one of blastomers; C – thick zona pellucida; D - total cytoplasm defragmentation.

The percentage of fragmentation is still under discussion by many authors. The minimal fragmentation and symmetry of blastomers positively correlate with implantation rate similar to the 4-cell stage embryos. There are few studies that present that the early visualization of embryo compaction on the third day of embryo development is a positive prognostic factor for further embryo implantation. In at least 8-blastomer embryos with minimal fragmentation, early compaction was associated with higher implantation rate (Skiadas et al.,2006). Desai et al. (Desai et al.,2000) suggested that to assess reproductive potential of 3 day embryo, the following features should be taken under consideration: number, size and the symmetry of blastomers; compaction; the grade of fragmentation; vacuoles in cytoplasm; blastomer expansion. The evaluation of this characteristics was connected with more than 80% sensitivity in prediction of positive implantation.

2.3 Blastocyst scoring systems

The progress in ART techniques, especially in culture media and metabolimics, allow longer incubation of embryos in lab conditions and their development to blastocyst stage. The transfer of blastocyst imitates the natural conception cycles, where such "embryo-uterine dialogue" is responsible for creation of a new life. Similar to the cleavage stage embryos, embryo morphological features are very important in assessment of blastocyst quality and its reproductive potential. Most of blastocyst scoring systems are based on evaluation embryo morphology and are focused on: blastocyst development stage - expansion and hatching status, inner cell mass (ICM) quality; trophoectoderm (TE) quality. The blastocyst stage is usually reached on the fifth day of embryo development. One of the most common used blastocyst scoring system was proposed by Gardner (Gardner et al.,2000).

Blastocysts are named using numerical score from 1 to 6 according to their expansion and hatching status:

1. Early blastocyst, blastocoel cavity less than half the volume of the embryo
2. Blastocoel cavity more than half the volume of the embryo
3. Full blastocyst, cavity completely fills the embryo
4. Expanded blastocyst, cavity larger than the embryo, with thinning of the zona
5. Hatching blastocyst, the trophoectoderm has started to harniate through the zona
6. Hatched blastocyst, has completely escaped from the zona

The blastocyst are also assessed according to ICM quality:

a. Many cells, tightly packed
b. Several cells, loosely grouped
c. Very few cells

As well as according to TE quality:

a. Many cells, forming a cohesive layer
b. Few cells, forming a loose epithelium
c. Very few large cells

Blastocysts are given a quality grade for each of the 3 components and the score is expressed with the expansion grade listed first, the inner cell mass grade listed second and the trophectoderm grade third. For example, a blastocyst quality grade of 4AA means that the blastocoel cavity is expanding and the zona is thinning (grade 4), it has many tightly packed cells in the inner cell mass (grade A), and has a trophectoderm can be seen to be composed of numerous cells (grade A).

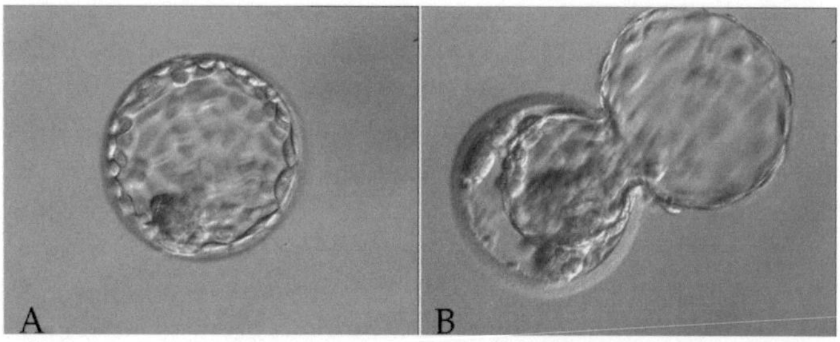

Fig. 7. Good quality blastocysts: A - good quality expanded blastocyst (4AA); B – hatching blastocyst (5AA).

Another scoring system was proposed by Dokras et al. (Dokras et al.,1993). The blastocyst grading according to following schema is presented as: grade 1 blastocysts with early cavitation resulting in the formation of an eccentric and then expanded cavity lined by a distinct ICM region and TE layer; grade 2 blastocyst exhibited a transitional phase where single or multiple vacuoles were seen that over subsequent days developed into the typical blastocyst appearance of the grade 1 blastocysts; grade 3 - blastocysts with several degenerative foci in the ICM with necrotic cells. The Dokras system is mainly based on embryo developmental potential and expansion of the blastoceol cavity. The Gardner's system is more detailed than Dokras system, taking into account the appearance of ICM and TE quality. Balaban et al. (Balaban et al., 2006) in randomized trial compared both scoring systems, and observed the better outcome in the Gardner system, where higher implantation rates were observed. Gardner's system offers higher selective criteria for the blastocysts, which in turn is reflected in the clinical outcome following embryo transfer.

Rehman et al. (Rehman et al., 2007) presented a numerical blastocyst-morphology grading system (blastocyst quality score BQS). This system correlate with criteria established by Gardner. BQS is defined as the product of degree of expansion and hatching status and ICM and TE grades, where letter grade A is given the value 3, grade B –value 2, and grade C – value 1. For example BQS calculation for a 4AB blastocyst is 4x3x2, with a BQS of 24 points. The authors calculate each Gardner's scale score with BQS. Authors tried to present a possible correlation between BQS and number of cells in the blastocysts, but they did not present the number of cells in studied blastocysts. Although Gardner's blastocyst morphology grading system is clinically useful scheme and has been shown to predict implantation rates, there are several limitations associated with the use of BQS in clinical practice.

In the literature, there are few studies investigating the usefulness of cumulative, combined multiday embryo scoring systems in evaluation the embryo reproductive potential. The investigators tried to combine morphological characteristics of zygotes, cleavage stage embryos and blastocysts to improve the embryo selection process. Available data suggests that combined mulitiday embryo assessment provides many usefulness information about embryo development, than a single day scoring systems. However, there is no ideal multiday system which could be implemented to clinical practice nowadays. There have been still undetectable critical time points of embryo development which could provide accurate information about the ideal time for successful embryo transfer.

More clinical trials are needed to find more accurate embryo selection parameters. Over the last few years, few continuous time lapse embryo monitoring systems were presented, as a device that can improve IVF outcomes by better embryo selection. Special incubators equipped with digital camera allows 24 hours observation of embryo incubation, from the conception till the time of transfer. Images of each embryo are automatically recorded at preset time intervals. Detailed information about timing of cell divisions and other critical events can provide future extensive documentation that embryologists can use to select a viable embryo for transfer during an IVF treatment. This method is reported as sufficiently safe. Constant embryo monitoring is performed inside incubators, so the embryos are never exposed to adverse growth conditions or temperatures. Images and detailed information about incubation conditions can be stored in patient data files for future reference. There is also an global idea for creation of the large database of embryo images (more than 20 million images) and a detailed analysis of the development pattern of embryos that successfully implanted and resulted in ongoing clinical pregnancies compared to embryos that failed to implant. The prospective clinical trials are required to analyze the obtained data, which can contribute to creation of novel embryo selection procedures, and thus improve IVF outcomes.

The optimum day for embryo transfer procedure seems to be established. Most of the recent studies suggest that the ideal time for embryo transfer is blastocyst stage in the fifth day. Prolonged embryo culture and the availability of blastocysts for transfer are associated with increased implantation rate and better neonatal outcomes compared with 2 or 3 day transfers of cleavage embryo stages (Blake et al.,2007; Kallen et al.,2010; Gardner et al.,2000; Papanikolaou et al.,2006). Taking under consideration the high implantation rate of blastocyst, a single embryo transfer can be offered for selected patients, which tends to reduce the number of multiple pregnancies (Kawachiya et al.,2011; Papanikolaou et al.,2010). The transfer only one blastocyst in the first attempt may lead to higher cumulative pregnancy rate by allowing transfer remaining frozen blastocyst in the next cycle. However, blastocyst transfer may not be ideal for all IVF patients, in all clinical situations. A Cochrane review of 16 trials on efficiency of blastocyst and day 3 embryo transfer, did not find the significant differences in pregnancy rate, miscarriages rate and multiple pregnancy. Some IVF canters still have problems with blastocyst culturing and/or freezing so the third day of transfer is an optimal solution in these cases. The problem of the optimal day of embryo transfer return back nowadays, and remains a significant element of discussion in many scientific societies working on reproductive medicine.

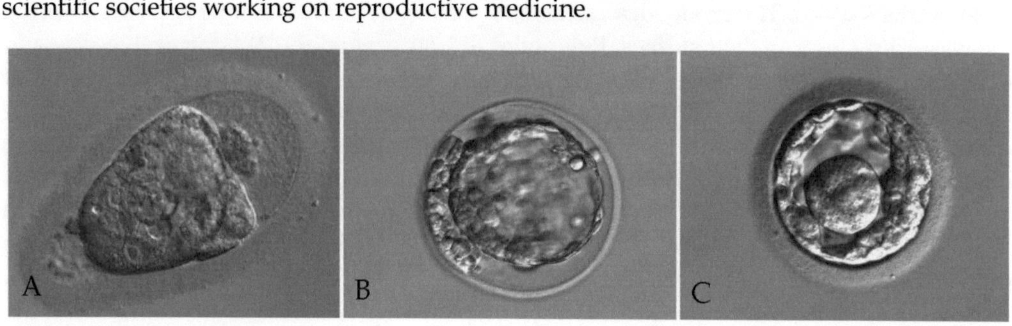

Fig. 8. Abnormalities of 5 day embryos: A – dysmorphic morula; B – degenerating blastocyst before hatching; C – remained undeveloped blastomer in blastocyst.

The assessment of just the embryo morphology cannot disclose, whether a particular embryo will be implanted or not, and it can not disclose all the information contained in the embryo. The most precise evaluation of the impact of embryo quality and endometrial features on the pregnancy rate should be carried out on patients with a single, high quality blastocyst transfer. The analysis of all the information obtained from the elective single embryo transfer procedures can help embryologist in the better embryo selection, leading to the improvement of implantation and pregnancy rates. The role of a single embryo transfer, the limitations of multiple embryo transfer, and the role of cryopreservation are still discussed nowadays.

3. Growth factors and endometrial receptivity

The estrogen dependent proliferative phase of the endometrium, which lasts from the menstrual bleeding until ovulation, is characterized by proliferation of endometrial glands and endometrial stromal tissues as well as neoangiogenesis of endometrial blood vessels. The progesterone dependent secretory phase, which starts after ovulation with a peak of luteinizing hormone (LH) and ends with menstrual bleeding, is accompanied by high secretory activity of endometrial glands, elongation and growth of spiral arteries as well as decidualization of endometrial stroma. These all mechanisms enable embryonic invasion during the implantation window. Growth factors, cytokines and chemokines play an important role in paracrine and autocrine actions to affect the histologic and biochemical changes in endometrium before and during the implantation process.

Communication between the embryonic and maternal tissues, while the embryo is transferred through the fallopian tube and in uterine cavity, seems to be an important factor in the successful embryo implantation. The embryo communicate with the maternal organism, by producing and secreting several cytokines, chemokines, growth factors during its development.

At the time of implantation, according to increase the production of prostaglandins (mainly prostaglandin E_2) in endometrium, the increase of capillary permeability in endometrial stroma is observed. By this time, secretory activity presents a peak, and endometrial cells becoming to be reach in lipids and glycogen. The window for endometrial receptivity is restricted to the 20th - 24th day in spontaneous 28-day regular cycle. Progesterone-induced formation of pinopodes (surface epithelial cells with smooth protrusions) appears on the endometrial surface. The pinopodes are able to absorb an intrauterine fluid trying to bring the blastocyst closer to their surface. Pinopodes appear around the 21st day of the cycle and exist only for a few days. After hatching the blastocyst from the zona pellucida, blastocyst adheres to the endometrial surface. During the last decade, the knowledge about communication between implanting blastocyst and maternal endometrium increased due to novel RNA and protein microarrays analyses. Without the presence of blastocyst, decidua synthesizes the factors that inhibiting the implantation process such: insulin-like growth factor binding protein-1 (IGFBP-1), tissue inhibitors of metalloproteinases (TIMPs). On the other site blastocyst promotes secretion the following factors counteracting maternal restraint mechanisms and promote embryo implantation into the endometrium: matrix metalloproteinases (MMPs), leukaemia inhibitory factor (LIF), epidermal growth factor (EGF), insulin like growth factor II (IGF II), and interleukins (IL) (Giudice,2003). Trophoblast penetrates the uterine epithelial basement membrane by with use of some proteolytic enzymes, and finally implant in the endometrial stroma. Matrix metalloproteinases (MMPs) are the most important enzymes taking part in endometrial tissue reconstitution during implantation. MMPs degrade the extracellular matrix components as collagens, proteoglycans, glycoproteins. Among all the metelloproteinases, MMP-2 and MMP-9 seems to play the most important role in the tissue remodeling that accompanies implantation and decidualization. MMP-2 may participate in the early phase of decidual remodelling as well as in neoangiogenesis. MMP-9 can coordinate trophoblast invasion into the endometrial layer. Changes in the expression of these two metelloproteinases during implantation can occur without direct signals from the blastocyst. Some investigators indicate that the expression of these two metelloproteinases might be induced by some cytokines or growth factors, such as vascular endothelial growth factor (VEGF), transforming growth factor (TGF), epidermal growth factor (EGF) as well as by their specific tissue inhibitors (TIMPs) (Zhang et al.,2005).

There are studies suggesting the role of VEGF in endometrial neoangiogenesis during embryo implantation. Angiogenesis is a key process in preparation of endometrium for implantation. VEGF is a specific mitogen for endothelial cells that exerts its functions through two receptor tyrosine kinases (Flt-1 and Flk-1/KDR). These receptors were found in epithelial cells and stroma of endometrium. Neuropilin-1 (NRP-1), another receptor for VEGF, was found overexpressed in endometrium in the proliferative phase, in comparison to secretory phase of the cycle. Charnock-Jones et al. (Charnock-Jones et al.,1994) demonstrated that mRNA VEGF receptor, Flt-1, was overeexpressed in the cytotrophoblast and also by the extravillous trophoblast in the maternal deciduas in early pregnancy. VEGF may induce vascular and endometrial cells proliferation and differentiation, as well as be involved in the invasion process of embryos implanting into the endometrium.

Cytokines/ Growth factors	Enzymes/Tissue mediators
VEGF - Vascular Endothelial Growth Factor	MMP-2 - Metalloproteinase-2
EGF - Epidermal Growth Factor	MMP-9 - Metalloproteinase-9
IGF I and II - Insulin-like Growth Factor I and II	TIMPs -Tissue Inhibitors of Metalloproteinases
FGF - Fibroblast Growth Factor	PGE$_2$ - Prostaglandin E$_2$
TGF α and β - Transforming Growth Factor α and β	
Il-1 - Interleukin 1	
Il-6 - Interleukin 6	
Il-11 - Interleukin 11	
LIF - Leukemia Inhibitory Factor	
TNF α - Tumor Necrosis Factor α	
IGFBP-1 - Insulin-like Growth Factor binding protein-1	
CSF-1 - Colony Stimulating Factor 1	

Table 1. Biochemical factors involved in the human embryo implantation.

Interleukins may also exert an influence on human embryo implantation. The increase of the expression of interleukin-1 in endothelial cells of uterine spiral vessels and endometrial stroma was observed before implantation. Decidualization of endometrial stromal cells in vitro is enhanced by interleukin 11. Interleukins can exert an influence on proper endometrial receptivity and could have an important impact on successful semi-allograft blastocyst implantation (Paiva et al.,2007; White et al., 2007). The expression of colony stimulating factor-1 and leukemia-inhibitory factor (LIF) were also found in human endometrium as well as in blastocyst structures. It suggest also their possible role in human embryo implantation (Simon et al.,1996).

Cytokines, chemokines, and growth factors have been still investigated in all tissues associated with implantation as well as in embryonic structures. These factors are the biochemical tools involved in the implantation process. Their cataloguing process is still pending, and their role in consecutive parts of embryo implantation process is still not completely understood. Table 1 presents the most important factors involved in the human embryo implantation.

4. The role of uterine contractility in embryo implantation

What could be the reason of recurrent implantation failure among especially young women undergoing IVF treatment, when good quality blastocysts are transferred, in patients with any uterine anatomical anomalies, and with any hormonal disorders? The ideal intrauterine conditions that enable implantation include appropriate endometrial status, sufficient endometrial blood perfusion and absence of excessive uterine contractions. The contractile activity of the pregnant and non-pregnant uterus plays an important role in the human reproduction. The stimulation of uterine contractions by estrogens during the follicular phase in the non-pregnant uterus, supports transport of spermatozoas from vagina to the Fallopian tubes. The absence of the uterine contractility, in response to rising progesterone serum level, provides an optimal environment for successful embryo implantation.

Embryo attachment to the endometrial layer and its invasion require the uterine quiescence for implantation (Bulletti & de Ziegler,2005,2006). Implantation failures in IVF cycles when good quality embryos are transferred, could be a results of increased uterine contractile activity during and after transfer procedure (Fanchin et al.,1998,2001). About 15% of embryos could be found in vagina after the transfer procedure, and only 45% of transferred embryos could be found in the uterus one hour after the transfer (Poindexter et al.,1986).

Implantation rate seems to be strictly dependent on the uterine activity during embryo transfer. The excessive uterine contractile activity during ET procedure is found in about 30% of IVF patients. Some investigators found almost 3 times higher clinical pregnancy rates in patients with uterine quiescence, than in women with excessive uterine activity (53% and 13%, respectively) (Ayoubi et al.,2003). Ayoubi et al. observed changes in uterine contractile activity appearing after ovulation in the spontaneous menstrual cycles and in stimulated IVF cycles. Uterine contractile frequency did not differ between studied groups of patients on the day of luteinizing hormone surge (5 uterine contractile per 1 minute) and hCG administration (5.3 uterine contractile per 1 min). In the normal regular menstrual cycle, the uterine quiescence is reached about 4 days after the peak of luteinizing hormone. Uterine contractile activity in IVF cycles remained elevated until the 4th day after hCG administration, despite of higher serum progesterone levels reached after additive oral or vaginal progesterone supplementation. The limit of uterine contractility after exposure to vaginal progesterone was established by Fanchin et al. study (Fanchin et al.,2001) and Bulletti et al study (Bulletti & de Ziegler,2006). Seven or less contractions detected during five minute intervals in ultrasound measurements were found as uterine quiescence. More than 7 contractions detected during five minute intervals were presented as increased uterine activity. This excessive uterine activity can be also amplify in stimulated cycles, by higher serum concentration of estrogens stimulating uterine contractility. In IVF patients uterine activity has declined on the 6th day after human chorionic gonadotropin (hCG) administration (Ayoubi et al.,2003). These findings can be explanation to improved implantation rate observed after blastocyst transfers. There are many studies confirming the highest implantation rate after the transfer of embryos in blastocyst stage (Fauque et al.,2007; Zander-Fox et al.,2011; Kallen et al.,2010; Gardner et al.,2000). If the uterine contractile frequency decreases at the time of blastocyst transfer in patients with excessively expressed uterine activity, the postponing of the embryo transfer procedure could be considered in these group of patients during IVF treatment.

The study by Fanchin et al. (Fanchin et al.,2001) showed the possible influence of decreased uterine contractility on the high blastocyst implantation rate. Investigators compared the frequency of uterine contractions on the day of hCG administration, on the fourth day after hCG and on the 7th days after hCG. The significant decrease in uterine contractions frequency was observed from the day of hCG administration (4.4 uterine contractions per 1 minute), by the 4th day after hCG (3.5 uterine contractions per 1 minute), to the 7th day after hCG (1.5 uterine contractions per 1 minute). The decrease of uterine activity was progressive, and reached the lowest frequency on the 7th day, at the time of blastocyst transfers. This uterine quiescence can be associated with the higher blastocyst implantation rate, in comparison to cleavage embryos. However, the most of embryos are still transferred on the 2nd or the 3rd day after fertilization, when the elevated uterine contractile activity is observed.

There is no still an ideal method for assessing the uterine activity of non-pregnant uterus. Cardiotocography, bioimpedance measurement or electromyography, or magnetic resonance scanning are restricted to evaluation of the activity of only pregnant uterus. Only few methods assessing the uterine activity in non-pregnant uterus were described in the literature (Kitlas et al.,2009; Rabotti et al.,2009; Kissler et al.,2004). One of the most sensitive method, but unfortunately invasive, is the measurement of changes in intrauterine pressure which reflect the uterine contractile activity.

Kissler et al. (Kissler et al.,2004) tried to evaluate the activity of non-pregnant uterus using hysterosalpingoscintigraphy (HSSG). This study was the first one to be designed to investigate utero-tubal transport function by HSSG and uterine contractility by intrauterine pressure (IUP) measurement. Investigators compared these parameters in 21 patients on the same day in the periovulatory phase. In HSSG, the transport function was visualized using 99m-technetium-marked albumin. In IUP measurement methods, the amplitude and frequency of uterine contractions per minute, as well as the basal pressure tone were assessed by an intrauterine catheter. In periovulatory phase, the mean value of uterine contractions was 3.4 contractions per minute, the mean amplitude was 12.0 mmHg and basal pressure was 70.7 mmHg. These two methods positively correlated with uterine activity. The IUP measurement using special catheter or hysterosalpingoscintigraphy are unfortunately invasive and with many limitations in clinical practice.

Kitlas et al. (Kitlas et al.,2009) tried to assess synchronization between contractions in different topographic regions of the uterus in patients with dysmenorrhea. The authors presented four different analytic methods to assess uterine signals: the cross-correlation function, the coherence function, the wavelet cross-correlation and the wavelet coherence. Spontaneous uterine activity was recorded directly by a dual micro-tip catheter consisted of two ultra-miniature pressure sensors. One sensor was placed in the fundus, the other one in the cervix. The study showed, that the analysis of synchronization of the uterine contractions signals may have a diagnostic value, but this method has never been used to assess uterine contractility before embryo transfer.

A promising technique for uterine contractile activity evaluation could be electrohysterography (EHG). The EHG measures the electrical activity from the abdominal surface, which triggers the contraction of the uterine muscle. Rabotti et al. studies (Rabotti et al.,2009) tried to compare electrohysterography with the measurement of intrauterine pressure in pregnant uterus. However, a quantitative estimation of the internal uterine pressure by EHG is not available for clinical practice in reproductive medicine, probably because of small size of non-pregnant uterus.

In humans, ethical issues do not allow to use any invasive assessment of uterine contractions such as intrauterine pressure measurements, during or after embryo transfer procedure. Consequently, the assessment of uterine activity should be non-invasive. Several methods involving transvaginal ultrasonography for assessing endometrial and myometrial layer movements have been already described.

The oldest method for assessing the ultrasound images, which can provide information about uterine activity, is the M-mode presentation ultrasound technique (Figure 9). This method allows the assessment of low-level image data and thus does not provide additional information about the object's shape or location. Application is limited by a number of conditions specific to medical imaging. The M-mode technique has a number of disadvantages. This method does not measure the movements of the whole uterus, only the upper and lower boundaries present within a user specified intersection. This lack of provision becomes significant in cases of exaggerated bowel or respiratory movement that may change the location of previously marked gaps in the uterus. The uterus can also move forward or backward in relation to the intersection that has been set. Since the method does not take into account the whole uterine shape into account, only the boundaries crossing the intersection are trackable which can make measurement difficult. Even in ideal conditions where the boundaries are clear and easy to track, accurate measurement can still be difficult to perform. Similarly, it is also difficult to interpret images where contractility is present, but not causing movements of boundaries and influencing only the texture of the endometrium. This technique also depends on proper visualization of the uterus which is highly variable and influenced by factors such as its retrovert position or filling of the urinary bladder.

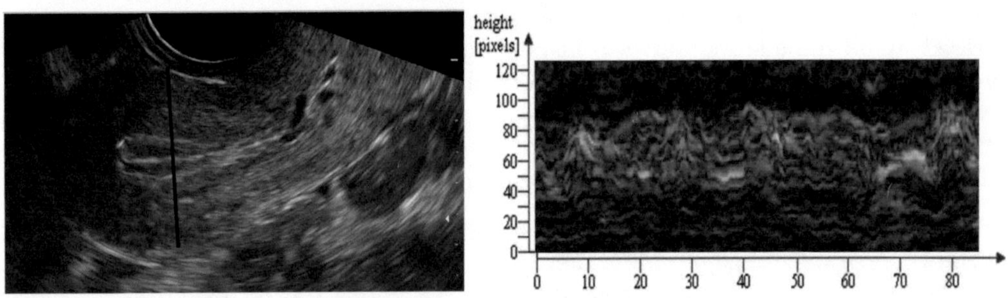

Fig. 9. M-mode ultrasound technique for assessing endometrial and myometrial movements.

Fanchin et al. (Fanchin et al.,1998) proposed a method based on analyzing of a line segment of the uterus and video sequence that shows two-dimensional plot using successive frames. The horizontal component represents line segment length and the vertical component time. Although the method is simple and easy to implement, the prototype clearly demonstrates drawbacks. In the presence of a slight increase in the amount of noise or movement of the uterus, the method is prone to generating mistakes and does not provide useful information about uterine contractility. The method was presented in 1998, and the authors did not analyzed any good quality film sequences, which are available now thanks to the progress in ultrasound imagining. The method was not found to be an accurate tool for the measurement of contractility of non-pregnant uterus.

There are also some possibilities of pharmacological treatment of excessive uterine activity in IVF patients. Oral or vaginal progesterone supplementation, even when acting on uterine receptivity, improving endometrial status, presents limited benefits for implantation rates in patients with excessive uterine activity. Studies assessing the effectiveness of prostaglandin synthesis inhibitors and β_2-adrenoreceptor agonists have shown a positive effect on pregnancy rates, but these drugs have failed to enter routine clinical use because of safety concerns.

In randomized control trial, Bernabeu et al. (Bernabeu et al.,2006) analyzed the influence of administration of indomethacin on implantation rate in oocyte donation recipients. Indomethacin is one of the non-steroid anti-inflammatory drugs (NSAIDs), which inhibit the prostaglandin synthesis. Prostaglandins are synthesized from arachidonic acid by cyclooxygenase (COX). Indomethacin blocks the COX enzyme, inhibits the production of prostaglandins and reduces or inhibits the uterine contractile activity. Prostaglandins are the most important factors stimulating the uterine contractions in non-pregnant uterus. Bernabeu et al. (Bernabeu et al., 2006). Oocyte donation is the best model to evaluate the determinants of implantation, because of the limitations concerned with the fertilized oocyte quality. In the studied group of patients the authors administered 100 mg of indomethacin rectally (in three doses every 12 hours) starting on the night prior to transfer. Implantation rate was 27.8% in the indomethacin group, and 26.4% in the placebo control group. The study did not show significant differences in implantation rate among studied groups of patients.

Moon et al. (Moon et al.,2004) examined the effect of other prostaglandin synthesis inhibitor piroxicam on implantation rate in IFV patients. In prospective, randomized double-blind, placebo controlled trial the authors compared the effect of piroxicam administered in the day of embryo transfer in patients undergoing fresh as well frozen IVF cycles, on implantation rate. The piroxicam was chosen from several different NSAIDs for its good pharmacological efficacy in clinical relief of primary dysmenorrhea. It is supposed that primary dysmenorrea is a disease associated with excessive uterine activity appearing during menstruation. In studied group of patients, the authors administered 10 mg of piroxicam 1-2 hours before embryo transfer. The study showed that piroxicam increased the implantation rate in both fresh and frozen cycles. In fresh cycles, the implantation rate in the piroxicam group was 18.7% vs. 8,6% in controlled placebo group. In frozen cycles, the implantation rate in patients received piroxicam was also higher than in control group, (9.4% and 2.3%, respectively). The investigators observed greater beneficial effect of piroxicam in patients under 40 years of age in both fresh and frozen IVF cycles. The results confirmed the effectiveness of piroxicam in priming the uterus for embryo implantation.

Pierzyński et al. (Pierzyński et al.,2007) presented a case report describing the first administration of atosiban (oxytocin and vasopressin V1 receptor antagonist) in IVF treatment. The authors used intravenous bolus dose of 6.75 mg of atosiban administered one hour before embryo transfer and continuing the intravenous infusion of atosiban solution up to 2 hours after the ET procedure. The total dose of administered drug was 37.5 mg. One hour before embryo transfer investigators assessed the patient's uterine activity using ultrasound, and detected mean 2.75 contractions per 1 minute during 4 minute ultrasound recording. Directly before embryo transfer, one hour after starting atosiban administration, the uterine contractility decreased to 1.75 contractions per 1 minute. Two good quality blastocyst were transferred to the uterus, without complications. Due to ethical reasons detecting the uterine contractility after 2 hours after ET, was not performed. The treatment resulted in twin pregnancy, delivered by caesarean section at the 29th week of pregnancy because of vaginal bleeding suggesting the placental abruption. The previous preclinical study by the same authors did not present any toxic influence of atosiban on rabbit's embryo development and human sperm motility (Pierzyński et al.,2007).

Moraloglu et al. (Moraloglu et al.,2010) presented the first prospective, randomized, placebo-controlled clinical trial involving the administration the oxytocin antagonists before embryo transfer. 180 women undergoing intracytoplasmic sperm injection who had top-quality embryos were randomly allocated into treatment and control groups. The studied patients received intravenous administration of atosiban before embryo transfer with a total administered dose of 3.75 mg. In the control group, the patients received placebo. The implantation rate per transfer in the atosiban patients was 20.4%, which was significantly higher than in the control group 12.6%. The miscarriage rates between studied group presented 16.7% in the atosiban patients group and 24.4% in the control group. These results indicated that atosiban increases the implantation rate after embryo transfer procedure. These results suggest that the treatment with the oxytocin antagonists before embryo transfer could be effective in priming of the uterus for implantation.

5. The role of endometrial structure

There are multiple studies that have supported or refuted the relationship between endometrial features such as thickness, length or pattern and the implantation rate (Bassil,2001; Kovacs et al.,2003; Richter et al.,2007; Zhang et al.,2005; Rinaldi et al.,1996). The data regarding the role of endometrial thickness as a predictor of implantation outcomes is still controversial. Most of the authors suggested that there is a trigger of endometrial thicknesses correlating with a significant reduction in the implantation rate (Bassil,2001; Weissman et al.,1999; Rinaldi et al.,1996). Some investigators tried to evaluate the endometrial pattern on the day of hCG administration, the day of oocyte retrieval or the day of embryo transfer and find some predicting markers of successful embryo implantation (Dickey et al.,1992; Rashidi et al.,2005), but the results did not show any statistically significant results. Fanchin et al. (Fanchin et al.,2000) proposed the assessment of the dynamics of endometrial growth to the triple layer together with endometrial thickness and endometrial echogenicity as prognostic markers in IVF treatment.

In IVF cycles, the prediction of the time of implantation window seems to be more difficult than in natural cycles. In stimulated cycles in comparison to natural, the excessive, non-physiological hormones serum concentrations can be responsible for the different biochemical and biophysical changes in endometrium and can have different influence on embryo implantation. The endometrial changes in the days preceding the oocyte retrieval are important to clarify the impact of endometrial features in the prediction of a successful embryo implantation. The progression of the histological transformation of the endometrial layer and its receptivity can also differ depending on the type of the COH protocol and the doses and kinds of gonadotropins. Hormone dependant endometrial cell proliferation and differentiation seem to have an important value in endometrial receptivity and successful implantation (Bourgain et al.,2002; Bourgain,2004). The changes to endometrial echogenicity and structure are caused by rising progesterone serum levels and determine the implantation window (Fanchin et al.,2000; Bourgain et al.,2002).

The differences between endometrial dating in stimulated and natural cycles were presented in Bourgain et al. study (Bourgain et al.,2002). The rapid onset of secretory changes in endometrium was observed in IVF cycles on the day of the oocyte retrieval, corresponding to at least the second day after ovulation in natural cycles. These endometrial changes in IVF cycles were no longer visible after the second day after the oocyte retrieval and could be connected with the rapid increase of serum progesterone concentration appearing between the day of hCG administration and the day of oocyte retrieval. The implantation rate in IVF cycles seems to be not associated with progesterone serum levels, but progesterone can correlate with endometrial printing. The study showed that IVF cycles presented a significantly advanced endometrial maturation on the day of the oocyte retrieval when compared to natural cycles on the day of ovulation. No pregnancies were observed when the endometrial maturation was advanced for more than three days on the day of hCG administration.

Some authors (Kovacs et al.,2003; Richter et al.,2007) reported a significant increase of implantation rate observed with increase of endometrial thickness, independent from the patients' age and embryo quality. The mean endometrial thickness was greater in the cycles resulting in pregnancy than in the cycles not resulting in pregnancy (11.9 mm, and 11.3 mm respectively), but these differences were are not large. Authors also found a significant trend presenting a decrease in spontaneous miscarriages with an increase of endometrial thickness. Dickey et al. (Dickey et al.,1992) did not find significant differences in the pregnancy rate between patients with endometrial thickness of 9-13 mm and 14 mm assessed on the day of hCG administration. Weissman et al. (Weissman et al.,1999) suggested that the threshold of an endometrial thickness of 14-15mm on the day of hCG administration a negative influence on implantation rates. Schild et al. (Schild et al.,2001) did not observed pregnancies in patients with an endometrial thickness of more than 15 mm on the day of embryo transfer, or more than 16 mm on the day of oocyte retrieval. Other investigators (Rinaldi et al.,1996) observed correlations between a minimal endometrial thickness of 9- 10 mm and higher implantation rates. Some authors (Kupesic et al.,2001; Schild et al.,2001) did not observe successful implantations when the endometrium was thinner than 7 mm.

In the study by Kuć et al. (Kuć et al.,2011), relatively higher implantation rates were achieved if the endometrium thickness ranged between 12 and13 mm and at least one good-quality blastocyst was transferred in a double embryo transfer. The study showed that the endometrial thickness on the day of the triple layer appearance in the long GnRH agonist protocol and GnRH antagonist protocol was connected with a higher implantation rate. This was a first study analysing the dynamism of endometrial growth to triple layer in three different controlled ovarian stimulation protocols. The pregnancy rate in the GnRH antagonist protocol was statistically dependent on the time of the appearance of the triple layer as well as on the endometrial thickness on the day of the triple layer appearance. In the long GnRH agonist protocol only the endometrial thickness on the day of the triple layer appearance exerted an influence on the implantation rate. If the time between the first day of the appearance of the triple layer and the day of the hCG administration was longer than six days, no implantations were observed. The appearance of the triple layer after the 13th day of stimulation was connected with the lack of implantations. The time of the appearance of the endometrial triple layer in COH cycles can be essential for endometrial dating and receptivity, as well as for the implantation window.

The monitoring of patients on the day of hCG administration together with the day of ET could results in some useful information regarding successful implantation, than on any other day of treatment. The assessment of endometrial echogenicity performed at the end of the late follicular phase in IVF cycles was tested in search of a prognostic factor for embryo implantation (Giannaris et al.,2008; Richter et al.,2007; Schild et al.,2001). Some studies presented the hypothesis that endometrial features in the late follicular phase can predict the IVF outcomes, especially assessment of endometrial pattern and thickness (Scioscia et al.,2009; Giannaris et al.,2008; Richter et al.,2007; Zhang et al.,2005; Kovacs et al.,2003; Dietterich et al.,2002).

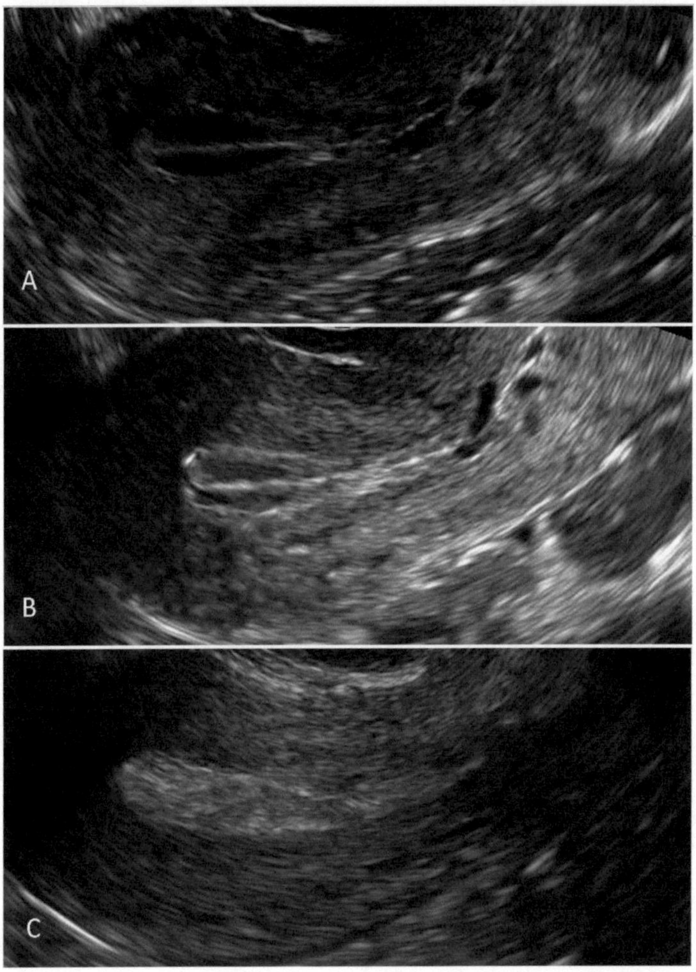

Fig. 10. Echogenicity of endometrial layer: A - hypoechogenic; B - isoechogenic; C - hyperechogenic.

Some studies showed that the endometrial echogenicity (Figure 10) on the day of hCG administration or embryo transfer can be a predictive marker of IVF outcomes (Basir et al.,2002; Fanchin et al.,2000). Fanchin et al. (Fanchin et al.,2000) confirmed the influence of endometrial echogenicity on the implantation rate. High endometrial echogenicity assessed in ultrasound examination on the day of hCG administration was connected with the lower implantation rate, but in this study the endometrial echogenic pattern was not evaluated on the day of embryo transfer. The intensity of hyperechogenic transformation observed on the day of hCG administration may denote an acceleration of secretory changes in endometrium. Premature exposure of the endometrium to progesterone during the follicular phase in stimulated cycles can also lead to a faster progression of the endometrial echogenicity during the early luteal phase and can be associated with the lower implantation rate (Fanchin et al.,2000). The relationship between endometrial echogenicity observed during ultrasound examination and implantation rate was presented also in Kuć et al. study (Kuć et al.,2011). The hyperechogenic endometrium on the day of hCG administration was associated with the low pregnancy rate, but only in patients undergoing the long GnRH agonist protocol.

Some investigators oppose the role of endometrial echogenicity in predicting the successful implantation, and they do not find a positive correlation between endometrial thickness and endometrial pattern with implantation rate. The authors claimed that endometrial growth and its pattern during the controlled ovarian hyperstimulation did not influence on the implantation rate (Bassil,2001; Kupesic et al.,2001; Rashidi et al.,2005).

Zhang et al. (Zhang et al.,2005) showed a significant correlation between the endometrial thickness, the length of gonadotropins administration and their influence on implantation rates. Controlled ovarian hyperstimulation last longer than 11 days corresponded with thinner endometrium and lower implantation rate. Authors also suggested that in some groups of patients, the implantation rate can depend on the endometrial thickness, and the implantation rate was statistically unaffected by endometrial thickness when good-quality embryos were transferred.

Endometrial parameters could be helpful predictors of the successful implantation, but they should be analyzed in a multivariate analysis rather than used alone. The most precise evaluation of the impact that endometrial features have on the implantation rate should be carried out on patients with a single, high quality blastocyst transfer.

6. Conclusions

In conclusions, successful embryo implantation requires a genetically and morphologically healthy embryo as well as developed receptive endometrium. The interactions between the embryo and endometrial layer during implantation have been not still completely understood. Nowadays, most of investigators recommend single blastocyst transfer on the 5th day after OR, if sufficient number of good quality embryos is cultured on the 3rd day. Uterine contractions at the time of embryo transfer negatively affect embryo implantation, but the methods for assessing uterine activity are not sensitive enough. The constant progress in biomedical sciences allows in the future finding the new markers dating endometrial receptivity, and implantation window, as well as better selection of the cultured embryos.

7. Acknowledgement

The author would like to acknowledge Professor Waldemar Kuczyński MD PhD (Centre for Reproductive Medicine KRIOBANK, Białystok, Poland) for chapter revision support as well as Piotr Sieczyński MSc PhD (Centre for Reproductive Medicine KRIOBANK, Białystok, Poland) for help in editing the embryological images.

8. References

Alikani, M., Calderon, G., Tomkin, G., Garrisi, J., Kokot, M., & Cohen, J. (2000). Cleavage anomalies in early human embryos and survival after prolonged culture in-vitro. *Hum Reprod* 15 (12):2634-43.

Ayoubi, J.M., Epiney, M., Brioschi, P.A., Fanchin, R., Chardonnens, D., & de Ziegler, D. (2003). Comparison of changes in uterine contraction frequency after ovulation in the menstrual cycle and in in vitro fertilization cycles. *Fertil Steril* 79 (5):1101-5.

Balaban, B., Yakin, K., & Urman, B. (2006). Randomized comparison of two different blastocyst grading systems. *Fertil Steril* 85 (3):559-63.

Basir, G.S., O, W.S., So, W.W., Ng, E.H., & Ho, P.C. (2002). Evaluation of cycle-to-cycle variation of endometrial responsiveness using transvaginal sonography in women undergoing assisted reproduction. *Ultrasound Obstet Gynecol* 19 (5):484-9.

Bassil, S. (2001). Changes in endometrial thickness, width, length and pattern in predicting pregnancy outcome during ovarian stimulation in in vitro fertilization. *Ultrasound Obstet Gynecol* 18 (3):258-63.

Bernabeu, R., Roca, M., Torres, A., & Ten, J. (2006). Indomethacin effect on implantation rates in oocyte recipients. *Hum Reprod* 21 (2):364-9.

Blake, D.A., Farquhar, C.M., Johnson, N., & Proctor, M. (2007). Cleavage stage versus blastocyst stage embryo transfer in assisted conception. *Cochrane Database Syst Rev* (4):CD002118.

Bourgain, C. (2004). [Endometrial biopsy in the evaluation of endometrial receptivity]. *J Gynecol Obstet Biol Reprod (Paris)* 33 (1 Pt 2):S13-7.

Bourgain, C., Ubaldi, F., Tavaniotou, A., Smitz, J., Van Steirteghem, A.C., & Devroey, P. (2002). Endometrial hormone receptors and proliferation index in the periovulatory phase of stimulated embryo transfer cycles in comparison with natural cycles and relation to clinical pregnancy outcome. *Fertil Steril* 78 (2):237-44.

Brezinova, J., Oborna, I., Svobodova, M., & Fingerova, H. (2009). Evaluation of day one embryo quality and IVF outcome--a comparison of two scoring systems. *Reprod Biol Endocrinol* 7:9.

Bulletti, C., & de Ziegler, D. (2005). Uterine contractility and embryo implantation. *Curr Opin Obstet Gynecol* 17 (3):265-76.

Bulletti, C., & de Ziegler, D. (2006). Uterine contractility and embryo implantation. *Curr Opin Obstet Gynecol* 18 (4):473-84.

Carrillo, A.J., Lane, B., Pridman, D.D., Risch, P.P., Pool, T.B., Silverman, I.H., & Cook, C.L. (1998). Improved clinical outcomes for in vitro fertilization with delay of embryo transfer from 48 to 72 hours after oocyte retrieval: use of glucose- and phosphate-free media. *Fertil Steril* 69 (2):329-34.

Charnock-Jones, D.S., Sharkey, A.M., Boocock, C.A., Ahmed, A., Plevin, R., Ferrara, N., & Smith, S.K. (1994). Vascular endothelial growth factor receptor localization and activation in human trophoblast and choriocarcinoma cells. *Biol Reprod* 51 (3):524-30.

Ciray, H.N., Ulug, U., & Bahceci, M. (2004). Transfer of early-cleaved embryos increases implantation rate in patients undergoing ovarian stimulation and ICSI-embryo transfer. *Reprod Biomed Online* 8 (2):219-23.

Ciray, N. (2007). Even early cleavage and day 2 embryo score. *Reprod Biomed Online* 14 (5):666; author reply 666.

Desai, N.N., Goldstein, J., Rowland, D.Y., & Goldfarb, J.M. (2000). Morphological evaluation of human embryos and derivation of an embryo quality scoring system specific for day 3 embryos: a preliminary study. *Hum Reprod* 15 (10):2190-6.

Dickey, R.P., Olar, T.T., Curole, D.N., Taylor, S.N., & Rye, P.H. (1992). Endometrial pattern and thickness associated with pregnancy outcome after assisted reproduction technologies. *Hum Reprod* 7 (3):418-21.

Dietterich, C., Check, J.H., Choe, J.K., Nazari, A., & Lurie, D. (2002). Increased endometrial thickness on the day of human chorionic gonadotropin injection does not adversely affect pregnancy or implantation rates following in vitro fertilization-embryo transfer. *Fertil Steril* 77 (4):781-6.

Dokras, A., Sargent, I.L., & Barlow, D.H. (1993). Human blastocyst grading: an indicator of developmental potential? *Hum Reprod* 8 (12):2119-27.

Fanchin, R., Ayoubi, J.M., Righini, C., Olivennes, F., Schonauer, L.M., & Frydman, R. (2001). Uterine contractility decreases at the time of blastocyst transfers. *Hum Reprod* 16 (6):1115-9.

Fanchin, R., Righini, C., Ayoubi, J.M., Olivennes, F., de Ziegler, D., & Frydman, R. (2000). New look at endometrial echogenicity: objective computer-assisted measurements predict endometrial receptivity in in vitro fertilization-embryo transfer. *Fertil Steril* 74 (2):274-81.

Fanchin, R., Righini, C., Olivennes, F., Taylor, S., de Ziegler, D., & Frydman, R. (1998). Uterine contractions at the time of embryo transfer alter pregnancy rates after in-vitro fertilization. *Hum Reprod* 13 (7):1968-74.

Fanchin, R., Righini, C., Schonauer, L.M., Olivennes, F., Cunha Filho, J.S., & Frydman, R. (2001). Vaginal versus oral E(2) administration: effects on endometrial thickness, uterine perfusion, and contractility. *Fertil Steril* 76 (5):994-8.

Fauque, P., Leandri, R., Merlet, F., Juillard, J.C., Epelboin, S., Guibert, J., Jouannet, P., & Patrat, C. (2007). Pregnancy outcome and live birth after IVF and ICSI according to embryo quality. *J Assist Reprod Genet* 24 (5):159-65.

Gardner, D.K., Lane, M., Stevens, J., Schlenker, T., & Schoolcraft, W.B. (2000). Blastocyst score affects implantation and pregnancy outcome: towards a single blastocyst transfer. *Fertil Steril* 73 (6):1155-8.

Giannaris, D., Zourla, A., Chrelias, C., Loghis, C., & Kassanos, D. (2008). Ultrasound assessment of endometrial thickness: correlation with ovarian stimulation and pregnancy rates in IVF cycles. *Clin Exp Obstet Gynecol* 35 (3):190-3.

Giorgetti, C., Hans, E., Terriou, P., Salzmann, J., Barry, B., Chabert-Orsini, V., Chinchole, J.M., Franquebalme, J.P., Glowaczower, E., Sitri, M.C., Thibault, M.C., & Roulier, R. (2007). Early cleavage: an additional predictor of high implantation rate following elective single embryo transfer. *Reprod Biomed Online* 14 (1):85-91.

Giudice, L. 2003. Implantation and endometrial function. In *Reproductive medicine: mollecular, cellular, and genetic fundaments.* , edited by B. F: Boca Roton: Parthenon Pub Group.

Kallen, B., Finnstrom, O., Lindam, A., Nilsson, E., Nygren, K.G., & Olausson, P.O. (2010). Blastocyst versus cleavage stage transfer in in vitro fertilization: differences in neonatal outcome? *Fertil Steril* 94 (5):1680-3.

Kawachiya, S., Bodri, D., Shimada, N., Kato, K., Takehara, Y., & Kato, O. (2011). Blastocyst culture is associated with an elevated incidence of monozygotic twinning after single embryo transfer. *Fertil Steril* 95 (6):2140-2.

Kissler, S., Siebzehnruebl, E., Kohl, J., Mueller, A., Hamscho, N., Gaetje, R., Ahr, A., Rody, A., & Kaufmann, M. (2004). Uterine contractility and directed sperm transport assessed by hysterosalpingoscintigraphy (HSSG) and intrauterine pressure (IUP) measurement. *Acta Obstet Gynecol Scand* 83 (4):369-74.

Kitlas, A., Oczeretko, E., Swiatecka, J., Borowska, M., & Laudanski, T. (2009). Uterine contraction signals--application of the linear synchronization measures. *Eur J Obstet Gynecol Reprod Biol* 144 Suppl 1:S61-4.

Kovacs, P., Matyas, S., Boda, K., & Kaali, S.G. (2003). The effect of endometrial thickness on IVF/ICSI outcome. *Hum Reprod* 18 (11):2337-41.

Kuć, P., Kuczyńska, A., Topczewska, M., Tadejko, P., & Kuczyński, W. (2011). The dynamics of endometrial growth and the triple layer appearance in three different controlled ovarian hyperstimulation protocols and their influence on IVF outcomes. *Gynecol Endocrinol* 27 (11): 867–873.

Kupesic, S., Bekavac, I., Bjelos, D., & Kurjak, A. (2001). Assessment of endometrial receptivity by transvaginal color Doppler and three-dimensional power Doppler ultrasonography in patients undergoing in vitro fertilization procedures. *J Ultrasound Med* 20 (2):125-34.

Ludwig, M., Schopper, B., Katalinic, A., Sturm, R., Al-Hasani, S., & Diedrich, K. (2000). Experience with the elective transfer of two embryos under the conditions of the german embryo protection law: results of a retrospective data analysis of 2573 transfer cycles. *Hum Reprod* 15 (2):319-24.

Moon, H.S., Park, S.H., Lee, J.O., Kim, K.S., & Joo, B.S. (2004). Treatment with piroxicam before embryo transfer increases the pregnancy rate after in vitro fertilization and embryo transfer. *Fertil Steril* 82 (4):816-20.

Moraloglu, O., Tonguc, E., Var, T., Zeyrek, T., & Batioglu, S. (2010). Treatment with oxytocin antagonists before embryo transfer may increase implantation rates after IVF. *Reprod Biomed Online* 21 (3):338-43.

Paiva, P., Salamonsen, L.A., Manuelpillai, U., Walker, C., Tapia, A., Wallace, E.M., & Dimitriadis, E. (2007). Interleukin-11 promotes migration, but not proliferation, of human trophoblast cells, implying a role in placentation. *Endocrinology* 148 (11):5566-72.

Papanikolaou, E.G., Camus, M., Kolibianakis, E.M., Van Landuyt, L., Van Steirteghem, A., & Devroey, P. (2006). In vitro fertilization with single blastocyst-stage versus single cleavage-stage embryos. *N Engl J Med* 354 (11):1139-46.

Papanikolaou, E.G., Fatemi, H., Venetis, C., Donoso, P., Kolibianakis, E., Tournaye, H., Tarlatzis, B., & Devroey, P. (2010). Monozygotic twinning is not increased after single blastocyst transfer compared with single cleavage-stage embryo transfer. *Fertil Steril* 93 (2):592-7.

Pierzyński, P., Gajda, B., Smorag, Z., Rasmussen, A.D., & Kuczyński, W. (2007). Effect of atosiban on rabbit embryo development and human sperm motility. *Fertil Steril* 87 (5):1147-52.

Pierzyński, P., Reinheimer, T.M., & Kuczyński, W. (2007). Oxytocin antagonists may improve infertility treatment. *Fertil Steril* 88 (1):213 e19-22.

Poindexter, A.N., 3rd, Thompson, D.J., Gibbons, W.E., Findley, W.E., Dodson, M.G., & Young, R.L. (1986). Residual embryos in failed embryo transfer. *Fertil Steril* 46 (2):262-7.

Rabotti, C., Mischi, M., van Laar, J.O., Oei, S.G., & Bergmans, J.W. (2009). Myometrium electromechanical modeling for internal uterine pressure estimation by electrohysterography. *Conf Proc IEEE Eng Med Biol Soc* 2009:6259-62.

Racowsky, C., Combelles, C.M., Nureddin, A., Pan, Y., Finn, A., Miles, L., Gale, S., O'Leary, T., & Jackson, K.V. (2003). Day 3 and day 5 morphological predictors of embryo viability. *Reprod Biomed Online* 6 (3):323-31.

Rashidi, B.H., Sadeghi, M., Jafarabadi, M., & Tehrani Nejad, E.S. (2005). Relationships between pregnancy rates following in vitro fertilization or intracytoplasmic sperm injection and endometrial thickness and pattern. *Eur J Obstet Gynecol Reprod Biol* 120 (2):179-84.

Rehman, K.S., Bukulmez, O., Langley, M., Carr, B.R., Nackley, A.C., Doody, K.M., & Doody, K.J. (2007). Late stages of embryo progression are a much better predictor of clinical pregnancy than early cleavage in intracytoplasmic sperm injection and in vitro fertilization cycles with blastocyst-stage transfer. *Fertil Steril* 87 (5):1041-52.

Richter, K.S., Bugge, K.R., Bromer, J.G., & Levy, M.J. (2007). Relationship between endometrial thickness and embryo implantation, based on 1,294 cycles of in vitro fertilization with transfer of two blastocyst-stage embryos. *Fertil Steril* 87 (1):53-9.

Rinaldi, L., Lisi, F., Floccari, A., Lisi, R., Pepe, G., & Fishel, S. (1996). Endometrial thickness as a predictor of pregnancy after in-vitro fertilization but not after intracytoplasmic sperm injection. *Hum Reprod* 11 (7):1538-41.

Saldeen, P., & Sundstrom, P. (2005). Nuclear status of four-cell preembryos predicts implantation potential in in vitro fertilization treatment cycles. *Fertil Steril* 84 (3):584-9.

Schild, R.L., Knobloch, C., Dorn, C., Fimmers, R., van der Ven, H., & Hansmann, M. (2001). Endometrial receptivity in an in vitro fertilization program as assessed by spiral artery blood flow, endometrial thickness, endometrial volume, and uterine artery blood flow. *Fertil Steril* 75 (2):361-6.

Scioscia, M., Lamanna, G., Lorusso, F., Serrati, G., Selvaggi, L.E., & Depalo, R. (2009). Characterization of endometrial growth in proliferative and early luteal phase in IVF cycles. *Reprod Biomed Online* 18 (1):73-8.

Scott, L. (2003). Pronuclear score as a predictor of embryo development. *Reprod Biomed Online* 6:201-214.

Scott, L., Alvero, R., Leondires, M., & Miller, B. (2000). The morphology of human pronuclear embryos is positively related to blastocyst development and implantation. *Hum Reprod* 15 (11):2394-403.

Scott, L.A., & Smith, S. (1998). The successful use of pronuclear embryo transfers the day following oocyte retrieval. *Hum Reprod* 13 (4):1003-13.

Simon, C., Gimeno, M.J., Mercader, A., Frances, A., Garcia Velasco, J., Remohi, J., Polan, M.L., & Pellicer, A. (1996). Cytokines-adhesion molecules-invasive proteinases. The missing paracrine/autocrine link in embryonic implantation? *Mol Hum Reprod* 2 (6):405-24.

Skiadas, C.C., Jackson, K.V., & Racowsky, C. (2006). Early compaction on day 3 may be associated with increased implantation potential. *Fertil Steril* 86 (5):1386-91.

Terriou, P., Giorgetti, C., Hans, E., Salzmann, J., Charles, O., Cignetti, L., Avon, C., & Roulier, R. (2007). Relationship between even early cleavage and day 2 embryo score and assessment of their predictive value for pregnancy. *Reprod Biomed Online* 14 (3):294-9.

Terriou, P., Sapin, C., Giorgetti, C., Hans, E., Spach, J.L., & Roulier, R. (2001). Embryo score is a better predictor of pregnancy than the number of transferred embryos or female age. *Fertil Steril* 75 (3):525-31.

Tesarik, J., & Greco, E. (1999). The probability of abnormal preimplantation development can be predicted by a single static observation on pronuclear stage morphology. *Hum Reprod* 14 (5):1318-23.

Weissman, A., Gotlieb, L., & Casper, R.F. (1999). The detrimental effect of increased endometrial thickness on implantation and pregnancy rates and outcome in an in vitro fertilization program. *Fertil Steril* 71 (1):147-9.

White, C.A., Dimitriadis, E., Sharkey, A.M., Stoikos, C.J., & Salamonsen, L.A. (2007). Interleukin 1 beta is induced by interleukin 11 during decidualization of human endometrial stromal cells, but is not released in a bioactive form. *J Reprod Immunol* 73 (1):28-38.

Zander-Fox, D.L., Tremellen, K., & Lane, M. (2011). Single blastocyst embryo transfer maintains comparable pregnancy rates to double cleavage-stage embryo transfer but results in healthier pregnancy outcomes. *Aust N Z J Obstet Gynaecol.*

Zhang, X., Chen, C.H., Confino, E., Barnes, R., Milad, M., & Kazer, R.R. (2005). Increased endometrial thickness is associated with improved treatment outcome for selected patients undergoing in vitro fertilization-embryo transfer. *Fertil Steril* 83 (2):336-40.

Zollner, U., Zollner, K.P., Hartl, G., Dietl, J., & Steck, T. (2002). The use of a detailed zygote score after IVF/ICSI to obtain good quality blastocysts: the German experience. *Hum Reprod* 17 (5):1327-33.

4

Immune Regulation of Human Embryo Implantation by Circulating Blood Cells

Hiroshi Fujiwara[1], Yukiyasu Sato[1], Atsushi Ideta[2], Yoshito Aoyagi[2], Yoshihiko Araki[3] and Kazuhiko Imakawa[4]

[1]Department of Gynecology and Obstetrics, Faculty of Medicine, Kyoto University, Kyoto,*
[2]Zen-noh Embryo Transfer Center, Kamishihoro, Katogun,
[3]Institute for Environmental & Gender-specific Medicine, Juntendo University Graduate School of Medicine, Urayasu-City,
[4]Laboratory of Animal Breeding, Graduate School of Agricultural and Life Sciences, The University of Tokyo, Tokyo,
Japan

1. Introduction

Mammalians have developed the part of the female genital tract, namely the uterus, to be a specific site that can receive embryo implantation. As a result, the mother must interact with the implanting embryo in the uterus, reconstruct maternal tissues during placentation and adapt maternal whole organs to accept embryo parasite. To induce the uterine environment to be favorable for embryo implantation, mammalian females in the reproductive stages periodically construct a unique endocrine organ, corpus luteum (CL), from the ovulated follicle. This newly constructed endocrine organ produces abundant amount of progesterone and induces the estrogen-primed endometrium to become a further differentiated stage that is suitable for embryo implantation (Yen, 1991). When the developing embryo enters the uterine cavity, a direct cross-talking of the embryo and the maternal endometrium is considered necessary to achieve a subsequent successful implantation of the embryo (Simón *et al.*, 2001). However, the precise mechanisms of the initial step of human embryo implantation remain unknown. Recently, accumulating evidence suggests that local immune cells at the implantation site actively contribute to embryo implantation (Lea and Sandra, 2007; Yoshinaga, 2008). In this chapter, we introduce new mechanisms by which circulating blood immune cells contribute to embryo implantation by inducing endometrial differentiation and promoting embryo-maternal cross-talk.

2. Regulation of ovarian function and differentiation by circulating immune cells

2.1 Endocrine regulation of human CL of pregnancy

In each menstrual cycle, human CL function continues only for 14 days. However, when becoming pregnant, the implanting embryo secretes human chorionic gonadotropin (HCG). This hormone is produced by the developing trophoblasts of the embryo and secreted into maternal blood circulation immediately after embryo invasion within the endometrium. HCG shares a receptor with luteinizing hormone (LH) and stimulates the function of CL of menstrual cycle in the ovary. This hormone also induces its transformation into CL of pregnancy to further produce progesterone, which in turn maintains embryo implantation in the uterus. Accordingly, there is a systemic crosstalk between the implantation embryo and mother through blood circulation system from the very early stages of human pregnancy. In this process, CL of pregnancy is an essential organ and it has been believed that HCG is a major regulator of human CL of pregnancy (Yen, 1991)(Fig. 1).

However, there are several lines of basic studies and clinical evidence to suggest that human CL of pregnancy is also regulated by different mechanisms (Rao *et al.*, 1977; Shima *et al.*, 1987). For example, in patients with ectopic pregnancy or natural abortion, despite a high HCG level in blood, progesterone production by the CL decreases and abortion proceeds (Alam *et al.*, 1999). Text books say that rapid and continuous increase in HCG concentration is necessary to maintain CL of pregnancy. However, LH/HCG receptor system does not need such a high concentration for its activation. On the other hand, chorionic gonadotropin is only detected in mare and primates (Murphy and Martinuk, 1991). Accordingly, regulatory mechanisms for CL of pregnancy are completely different among mammals. However, although many researchers have investigated additional essential hormones, no soluble factor other than HCG has been identified and the precise regulatory mechanisms remain unknown (Kratzer and Taylor, 1990).

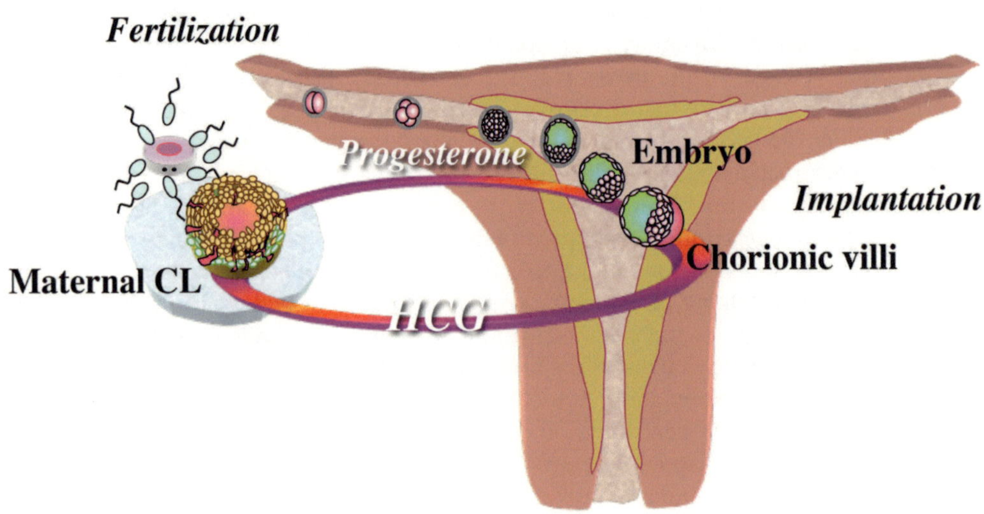

Fig. 1. Endocrine regulation of human early pregnancy

When being pregnant, human chorionic gonadotropin (HCG) that shares a receptor with LH, is secreted from the invading embryo and transmitted to the maternal ovary from the uterus by systemic blood circulation. Then, HCG stimulates corpus luteum to produce progesterone and this ovarian hormone is in turn transmitted to the uterus to maintain embryo implantation. Accordingly, there is a cross-talk between embryo and mother by endocrine system from the very early stage of human pregnancy.

2.2 Immune regulation of human CL of pregnancy

Based on the above background, we tried to identify the molecules that are expressed in human CL of pregnancy in order to clarify regulatory mechanism(s) that influence CL function and pregnancy. We found that several molecules that mediate interaction with T-lymphocytes were expressed on the luteal cell surface in the human CL of pregnancy (Fujiwara *et al.*, 1993; Hattori *et al.*, 1995). In general, immune cells are considered to enhance CL regression (Pate and Keyes, 2001). However, since these molecules such as HLA-DR and leukocyte functional antigen (LFA)-3/CD58 appear during CL formation, we speculated that interaction with immune cells plays some role in the functional and morphological transition from CL of menstrual cycle to CL of pregnancy.

After hatching, the human embryo takes an apposition, facing inner cell mass toward luminal epithelial layer, and then attaches to endometrial epithelial cells via trophectoderm layer. During this process, trophectoderm is activated to acquire invasive property and the attached embryo invades the endometrium as a mass through the epithelial layer, becoming buried within endometrial stromal tissue within 8-9 days after ovulation. Thereafter, trophoblast invasion transiently slows down and the lacunar spaces, which will become the intervillous spaces, are formed within the trophectoderm layer. Maternal blood gently flows in these spaces and then returns to the maternal systemic circulation (Boyd JD, Hamilton, 1970). At this stage, HCG is abundantly produced by the trophectoderm and the secreted HCG is transmitted to the ovary through the blood circulation, stimulating corpus luteum to produce progesterone via the LH/HCG receptor. During formation of the lacunar spaces, maternal blood cells including peripheral blood mononuclear cells (PBMC: lymphocytes and monocytes) are also considered to infiltrate here and these cells also return to the maternal systemic circulation including those in the ovary.

Taken together with the findings that the human CL expresses several molecules that can mediate direct interaction with T lymphocytes, we hypothesized that circulating immune cells contribute to the systemic crosstalk between embryo and mother (ovary) via blood circulation. It is theoretically sound to speculate that signals from the developing embryo in the genital tract are transmitted to the ovary by not only the endocrine system, but also the immune system, in other words, via not only soluble factors, but also circulating cells (Hattori *et al.*, 1995) (Fig. 2).

The maternal immune system recognizes the presence of the developing and implanting embryo in the Fallopian tube and the uterus by embryo- and species-specific signals such as degraded products of zona pellucida glycoprotein and/or HCG. Then, effector immune cells move to the ovary and the endometrium via blood circulation to regulate CL function and induce endometrial differentiation. The local immune cells at the implantation site also contribute to induction of embryo invasion, secreting chemoattractants by HCG stimulation.

To prove this hypothesis, we investigated the effects of PBMC derived from pregnant women in early pregnancy on progesterone production by human luteal cells in culture. We found that PBMC derived from women in early pregnancy promoted progesterone production as much as that by HCG stimulation, suggesting that circulating blood immune cells in early pregnancy enhance CL function (Hashii *et al.*, 1998). Based on these findings, we extended our hypothesis to the further concept that circulating immune cells transmit information about the presence of the developing embryo to various organs throughout the whole body and induce adequate functional change or differentiation in these organs to facilitate embryo implantation (Fujiwara, 2006).

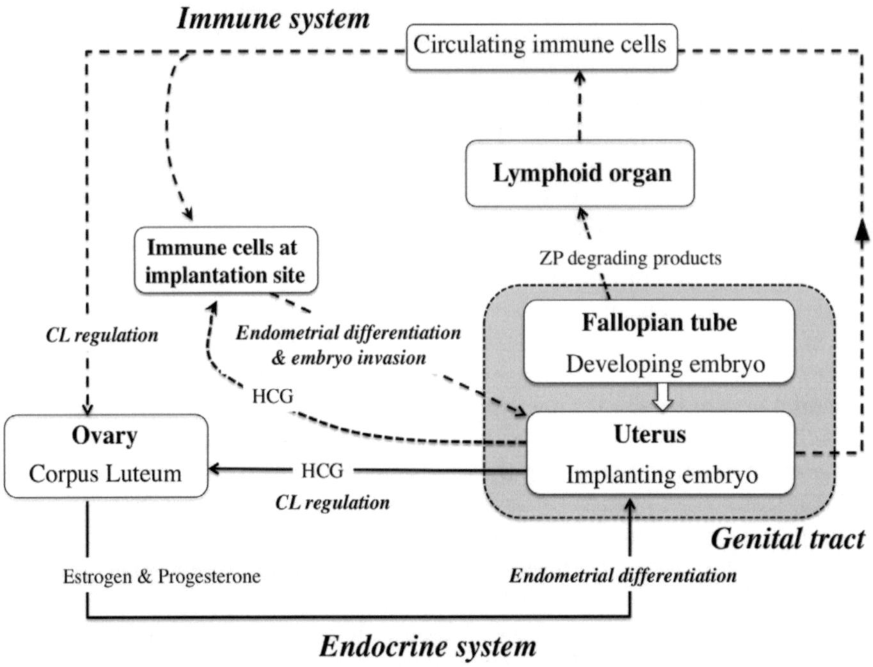

Fig. 2. Dual regulation of human embryo implantation by hormones and circulating immune cells

3. Regulation of endometrial differentiation by circulating immune cells

In human CL, LH/HCG receptor expression was already disappeared on 14th day after ovulation (Takao et al., 1997). When becoming pregnant, serum HCG arise around 11 days after ovulation. However, at this stage CL regression has already started. So, to achieve smooth transformation into CL of pregnancy, it is reasonable to expect that immune cells transmit information of the developing embryo to CL before embryo implantation. To support this speculation, HLA-DR and leukocyte functional antigen (LFA)-3/CD58 that can mediate direct interaction with T lymphocytes were expressed on human CL during corpus luteum formation.

3.1 Immune regulation of endometrial differentiation in mice

To investigate the above idea, we first examined the effects of circulating immune cells on endometrial differentiation and embryo implantation using mouse implantation experiments. When blastocysts were transferred into the uterine cavity of pseudopregnant recipient mice that had been mated with vasectomized male mice, successful implantation was only achieved during 3-5 days after ovulation when the endometrium was adequately differentiated. This period is called the "implantation window" (Psychoyos, 1993; Dey, 1996). However, when spleen cells, stocked circulating immune cells, were obtained from pregnant day 4 mice (before attachment stage) and were administered to pseudopregnant mice, embryo implantation was induced prior to the implantation window (1-2 days after ovulation) when embryos cannot normally be implanted (Takabatake et al., 1997a). Then we examined direct effect of spleen cells and observed that T-cell-rich population more effectively promoted embryo implantation (Takabatake et al., 1997b). In contrast to pregnant mice, spleen cells derived from diestrus or pseudopregnant mice had no effects. These findings indicated that before hatching stage, immune cells in early pregnancy have changed their functions to promote embryo implantation. This also suggests that developing embryo is necessary for functional change of immune cells.

In order to examine the direct effects of the splenocytes on endometrial differentiation, we used a delayed implantation model in which pseudopregnant mice were treated with daily progesterone supplementation following an oophorectomy on post-ovulatory day 3. In this model, in the absence of ovarian estrogen, blastocysts that are transferred into the uterine cavity remain floating in the luminal spaces, and the exogenous administration of estrogen induces expression of leukemia inhibitory factor (LIF) in the endometrium, restarting embryo implantation (Bhatt et al., 1991). Interestingly, instead of estrogen, intravenous administration of splenocytes derived from early pregnancy restarted embryo implantation along with induction of LIF expression (Takabatake et al., 1997b). These results indicated that circulating immune cells could encourage early endometrial differentiation that was necessary for subsequent embryo implantation. These findings suggest that endometrial differentiation just prior to embryo attachment can be achieved by dual control of the endocrine and immune systems (Fig. 2).

Notably, it was demonstrated that thymocytes from non-pregnant immature mice, especially CD8-negative population, could promote embryo implantation along with induction of LIF expression in the uterus. This indicates that there is a certain immune cell population that can induce endometrial differentiation and embryo implantation even in non-pregnant mice (Fujita et al., 1998).

3.2 Immune regulation of human endometrial receptivity

Implantation window is also supposed to exist in women. However, there has been no study to directly prove this window. Therefore, we then examined whether or not human endometrial receptivity really changes during menstrual cycle and immune cells can affect endometrial receptivity. To examine this issue, we first developed an attachment assay using a human choriocarcinoma-derived BeWo cell mass that mimics a human blastocyst and a human endometrial epithelial cell monolayer culture. In this assay, high attachment rates were observed in endometrial culture derived from women in the mid-luteal phase, supporting that there is an implantation window in human endometrium. Importantly, when these endometrial cells were co-cultured with autologous PBMC, attachment rates significantly increased in the culture derived from women in the late proliferative and early secretory phases, showing that autologous PBMC promote human endometrial cell receptivity *in vitro* (Kosaka *et al.*, 2003). These findings led us to think about the possible clinical application of autologous circulating immune cells to treatment for patients suffering with repeated implantation failures.

4. Maternal recognition of the human developing embryos by the immune system

4.1 HCG as a specific embryonal signal to the immune system

In order to receive information of the presence of the human developing embryo, the immune system must recognize the embryo-specific signals from the developing embryo in the female genital tract. First, we focused on the embryo-specific hormone, HCG, which is secreted from the developing and implanting human embryo. In invasion assays using murine embryo and BeWo cells, PBMC derived from women in early pregnancy promoted murine trophectoderm and BeWo cell invasion more than those obtained from non-pregnant women. It was also shown that this effect was exerted by soluble chemoattractive factors that were secreted by PBMC. Importantly, when PBMC derived from non-pregnant women were incubated with HCG, HCG-treated PBMC promoted invasion more than non-treated PBMC (Nakayama *et al.*, 2002; Egawa *et al.*, 2002). These findings suggest that HCG can change PBMC functions to facilitate embryo implantation.

Several decades ago, HCG crudely purified from urine was reported to suppress immune reactions (Adcock *et al.*, 1973). However, it was later shown that highly purified HCG had no effect on lymphocyte function (Muchmore and Blaese, 1997). Accordingly, the effects of HCG on immune cell function have been controversial for a long time. Ten years ago, we found that recombinant-HCG enhanced IL-8 production by human monocytes at relatively high concentrations via activation of NF-κB. HCG shares a receptor with LH to commonly access the LH/HCG receptor. However, the so-called LH/HCG receptor was not detected on the cell surface of monocytes. Therefore, it was speculated that there was a different pathway besides the LH/HCG-R system, which could respond to high HCG concentration. It should be noticed that HCG is an evolutionarily current hormone that is detected in primates (Cole, 2007). The most important difference between LH and HCG is the presence of abundant sugar chains at the C-terminal of the HCG β-subunit. Notably, binding of HCG on the cell surface of the monocytes and HCG-induced IL-8 production were inhibited by an exogenous excess of mannose, suggesting that HCG can regulate PBMC function through sugar chain receptors, which is a primitive regulatory mechanism in the immune system (Kosaka *et al.*, 2002). It should also be noted that the sugar chains of purified HCG are largely cleaved before urine production (Cole, 2009).

A high concentration of HCG is locally produced at the embryo implantation site. It is well known that the initial change around the implantation site is an increase in vascular permeability, leading to recruitment of certain immune cells to the area. Recently, it was reported that human trophoblasts invading the implantation site produce hyperglycosylated HCG, and that the hyperglycosylated HCG up-regulates trophoblast invasion in humans (Handschuh *et al.*, 2007). Therefore, it is reasonable to speculate that HCG stimulates endometrial immune cells to produce chemoattractants and vasodilators and that these cytokines in turn induce embryo invasion (Fujiwara, 2006).

To support our proposal, Kane et al. reported that HCG induced proliferation of uterine natural killer cells via the mannose receptor (Kane *et al.*, 2009). In addition, Schumacher et al., demonstrated that high HCG levels at very early pregnancy stages ensure regulatory T cells to migrate to the site of contact between paternal antigens and maternal immune cells and to orchestrate immune tolerance toward the fetus (Schumacher *et al.* 2009). Furthermore,

Wan et al. proposed that HCG contributed to the maternal-fetal tolerance during pregnancy by inducing dendritic cells toward a tolerogenic phenotype (Wan *et al.*, 2008).

4.2 Maternal recognition of the developing embryo in the Fallopian tube by the immune system

The findings from mouse implantation experiments suggest that functional changes in the immune system have already occurred in the early stage of pregnancy when the developing embryo passes through the Fallopian tube. In support of this speculation, it was also reported that intraepithelial lymphocytes of human oviduct, which were identified as CD8-positive T lymphocytes, expressed both estrogen receptor-β and membrane progesterone receptor. The number of Ki-67- and estrogen receptor-positive intraepithelial lymphocytes fluctuated during menstrual cycle in the normal oviducts and significantly increased in tubal pregnancy oviducts, suggesting their involvement in immune reactions during early pregnancy (Ulziibat et al, 2006).

In order to accurately identify the embryo, the maternal immune system must distinguish non-self tissues belonging to the same species from those of other organisms. The immune system must also discriminate between developing embryos and unfertilized eggs. However, since the embryo is surrounded by the zona pellucida, immune cells cannot directly interact with the embryo in the Fallopian tube. Therefore, it is speculated that the developing embryo actively releases species-specific and embryo-specific factors into the Fallopian tube. However, it appears difficult for the embryo to produce a sufficient amount of such soluble factors to successfully activate the maternal immune system at such an early stage in its development.

Since it was shown that the sugar chains of the HCG effectively activate immune cells, we then paid attention to the zona pellucida that contains abundant glycoproteins. It is well known that the zona pellucida is composed of glycoproteins that mediate species-specific interaction between spermatozoa and oocytes (Florman and Ducibella, 2006). Accordingly, the zona pellucida can be considered an abundant store of species- and oocyte-specific glycoproteins. In addition, in contrast to unfertilized oocytes, the developing embryo actively degrades the zona pellucida. During fertilization, the zona pellucida of fertilized oocytes can be a target for acrosomal enzymes of sperm and cortical granules of oocytes (Oura and Toshimori, 1990; Tanii *et al.*, 2001) and developing embryos further degrade the zona pellucida in order to achieve hatching. Thus, degradation products of zona pellucida glycoproteins may be released from fertilized oocytes/developing embryos into the Fallopian tube. Accordingly, we hypothesized that degradation products of zona pellucida glycoproteins can be an embryonal signal that transmits information about the presence of the developing embryo to the immune system in the female genital tract (Fujiwara *et al.*, 2009).

Taken together, we propose that degraded products of zona pellucida glycoprotein and HCG are important candidates for embryo- and species-specific signals for maternal recognition by the immune system (Fig. 1).

5. Clinical application

As a growing clinical problem in reproductive medicine, increasing attention has been paid to repeated implantation failure in infertile patients who had undergone in vitro fertilization

(IVF) therapy. Unfortunately, no effective therapy had been developed. Based on our original findings, we developed a novel therapy using autologous PBMC. In this treatment, autologous PBMC are pre-incubated with HCG and then administrated into the uterine cavity prior to blastocyst transfer in order to induce endometrial differentiation that facilitates subsequent embryo implantation. We applied this therapy to patients who had experienced implantation failure in IVF therapy and found that PBMC treatment effectively improved pregnancy and implantation rates (Yoshioka *et al.*, 2006). Several possible mechanisms relevant to this procedure can be demonstrated as follows. 1) PBMC may induce endometrial differentiation that facilitates embryo attachment. 2) Although PBMC are autologous cells from the patient, the induction of PBMC by themselves is expected to evoke favorable inflammatory reactions in the uterine cavity *in vivo*. 3) PBMC can secrete proteases that may effectively change the function or structure of surface molecules expressed on endometrial luminal epithelial cells. 4) PBMC can move from the uterine cavity toward the endometrial stromal tissue, creating a leading pathway for subsequent embryo attachment and invasion (Yoshioka *et al.*, 2006; Fujiwara *et al.*, 2009b).

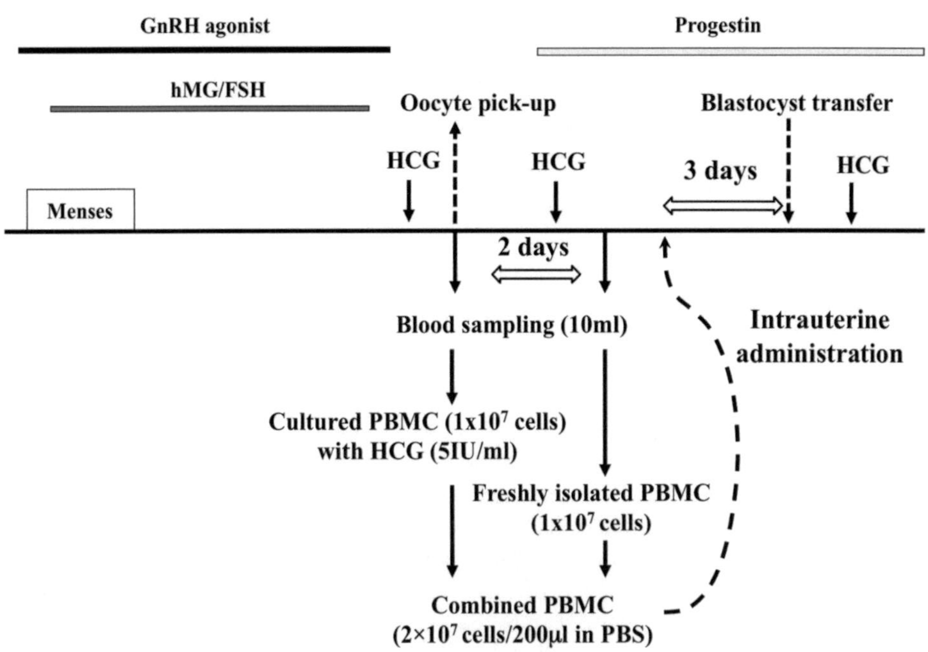

Fig. 3. Clinical protocol of PBMC treatment in IVF therapy

In our clinical protocol, PBMC are isolated at the time of oocyte pick-up, and activated with HCG. After 2-day incubation, PBMC are isolated again and the freshly collected PBMC are combined with the cultured PBMC and they are administrated into uterine cavity 3 days before blastocyst transfer.

In accordance with these clinical findings, Ideta et al. reported that administration of autologous PBMC in the uterine cavity increases pregnancy rates in bovine embryo transfer (Ideta et al., 2009). In addition, it was also observed that HCG-non-treated autologous PBMC were effective for patient with repeated implantation failures in IVF therapy

(Okitsu et al., 2011). These findings suggest that the application of autologous PBMC is an effective therapy for infertile patients suffering from repeated implantation failures.

6. Conclusion

In conclusion, we described a novel concept that immune cells receive information about the presence of a developing embryo and transmit this information through blood circulation to the whole body, inducing functional changes or differentiation in various organs, which facilitate human embryo implantation in cooperation with the endocrine system. Importantly, when the endocrine mechanism does not adequately operate, alternative mechanisms involving the immune system can be applied to infertility therapy. In the future, further clarification of the precise mechanisms for maternal recognition of the developing embryo by the immune system will contribute to our understanding the physiology of human embryo implantation and to developing more effective therapies using autologous immune cells along with further improvement in the breeding of domestic animals.

7. References

Adcock Ew 3d, Teasdale T, August CS, Cox S, Meschia G, Ballaglia TC, Naughton MA. Human chorionic gonadotropin: its possible role in maternal lymphocyte suppression. *Science* 1973; 181: 845-847.

Alam V, Altieri E, Zegers-Hochschild F. Preliminary results on the role of embryonic human chorionic gonadotrophin in corpus luteum rescue during early pregnancy and the relationship to abortion and ectopic pregnancy. *Hum Reprod* 1999; 14:2375-2378.

Bhatt H, Brunet LJ, Stewart CL. Uterine expression of leukemia inhibitory factor coincides with the onset of blastocyst implantation. *Proc Natl Acad Sci USA* 1991; 88: 11408–11412.

Boyd JD, Hamilton WJ. *The Human Placenta*. W. Cambridge, Heffer & Sons Ltd. 1970

Cole LA. Hyperglycosylated hCG. *Placenta* 2007; 28: 977-986.

Cole LA. New discoveries on the biology and detection of human chorionic gonadotropin. *Reprod Biol Endocrinol* 2009; 26:7:8.

Dey SK. Implantation. In: Adashi, E.Y.et al. eds. Reproductive Endocrinology, Surgery, and Technology. Philadelphia, Lippincott–Raven 1996: 421–434.

Egawa H, Fujiwara H, Hirano T, Nakayama T, Higuchi T, Tatsumi K, Mori T, Fujii S. Peripheral blood mononuclear cells in early pregnancy promote invasion of human choriocarcinoma cell line, BeWo cells. *Hum Reprod* 2002; 17: 473-480.

Florman HM, Ducibella T. Fertilization in Mammals. In: Neill, J.D. eds. Knobil and Neill's Physiology of Reproduction. St Louis, Elsevier Academic Press 2006; 55-112.

Fujita K, Nakayama T, Takabatake K, Higuchi T, Fujita J, Maeda M, Fujiwara H, Mori T. Administration of thymocytes derived from non-pregnant mice induces an endometrial receptive stage and leukaemia inhibitory factor expression in the uterus. *Hum Reprod* 1998; 13: 2888-2894.

Fujiwara H, Ueda M, Imai K, et al. Human leukocyte antigen-DR is a differentiation antigen for human granulosa cells. *Biol Reprod* 1993; 49: 705-715.

Fujiwara H. Hypothesis: Immune cells contribute to systemic cross-talk between the embryo and mother during early pregnancy in cooperation with the endocrine system. *Reprod Med Biol* 2006; 5: 19-29.

Fujiwara H, Araki Y, Toshimori K. Is the zona pellucida an intrinsic source of signals activating maternal recognition of the developing mammalian embryo? *J Reprod Immunol* 2009a; 81: 1-8.

Fujiwara H, Ideta A, Araki Y, Takao Y, Sato Y, Tsunoda N, Aoyagi Y, Konishi I. Immune system cooperatively supports endocrine system-primed embryo implantation. *J Mammal Ova Res* 2009b; 26: 122-128.

Handschuh K, Guibourdenche J, Tsatsaris V, Guesnon M, Laurendeau I, Evain-Brion D, Fournier T. Human chorionic gonadotropin produced by the invasive trophoblast but not the villous trophoblast promotes cell invasion and is down-regulated by peroxisome proliferator-activated receptor-γ. *Endocrinology* 2007; 148: 5011-5019.

Hashii K, Fujiwara H, Yoshioka S, et al. Peripheral blood mononuclear cells stimulate progesterone production by luteal cells derived from pregnant and non-pregnant women: possible involvement of interleukin-4 and interleukin-10 in corpus luteum function and differentiation. *Hum Reprod* 1998; 13: 2738-2744.

Hattori N, Ueda M, Fujiwara H, Fukuoka M, Maeda M, Mori T. Human luteal cells express leukocyte functional antigen (LFA)-3. *J Clin Endocrinol Metab* 1995; 80: 78-84.

Ideta A, Sakai S, Nakamura Y, Urakawa M, Hayama K, Tsuchiya K, Fujiwara H, Aoyagi Y. Administration of peripheral blood mononuclear cells into the uterine horn to improve pregnancy rate following bovine embryo transfer. *Anim Reprod Sci.* 2010 117:18-23.

Kane N, Kelly R, Saunders PT, Critchley HO. Proliferation of uterine natural killer cells is induced by human chorionic gonadotropin and mediated via the mannose receptor. *Endocrinology*. 2009 150: 2882-2888.

Kosaka K, Fujiwara H, Tatsumi K, et al. Human chorionic gonadotropin (HCG) activates monocytes to produce interleukin-8 via a different pathway from luteinizing hormone/HCG receptor system. *J Clin Endocrinol Metab* 2002; 87: 5199-5208.

Kosaka K, Fujiwara H, Tatsumi K, et al. Human peripheral blood mononuclear cells enhance cell-cell interaction between human endometrial epithelial cells and BeWo-cell spheroids. *Hum Reprod* 2003; 18: 19-25.

Kratzer PG, Taylor RN. Corpus luteum function in early pregnancies is primarily determined by the rate of change of human chorionic gonadotropin levels. *Am J Obstet Gynecol* 1990; 163: 1497-1502.

Lea RG, Sandra O. Immunoendocrine aspects of endometrial function and implantation. *Reproduction* 2007; 134: 389-404.

Muchmore AV, Blaese RM. Immunoregulatory properties of fractions from human pregnancy urine: evidence that human chorionic gonadotropin is not responsible. *J Immunol* 1977; 118: 881-886.

Murphy BD, Martinuk SD. Equine chorionic gonadotropin. *Endocr Rev* 1991; 12: 27-44.

Nakayama T, Fujiwara H, Maeda M, Inoue T, Yoshioka S, Mori T, Fujii S. Human peripheral blood mononuclear cells (PBMC) in early pregnancy promote embryo invasion in vitro: HCG enhances the effects of PBMC. *Hum Reprod* 2002; 17: 207-212.

Oura C, Toshimori K. Ultrastructural studies on the fertilization of mammalian gametes. In: Jeon KW, Friedlander M. eds. Int Rev Cytol. Academic Press Inc. 1990; 105-151.

Okitsu O, Kiyokawa M, Oda T, Miyake K, Sato Y, Fujiwara H. Intrauterine administration of autologous peripheral blood mononuclear cells increased clinical pregnancy rates in frozen/thawed embryo transfer cycle of patients with repeated implantation failure. *J Reprod Immunol.* 2011, in press.

Pate JL, Keyes PL. Immune cells in the corpus luteum: friends or foes? *Reproduction* 2001; 122: 665-676.

Psychoyos A. The implantation window: basic and clinical aspects. In: Mori, T. et al. eds. Perspectives in Assisted Reproduction. Ares Serono Symposia, Rome 1993 57–62.

Rao CV, Griffin LP, Carman FRJr. Gonadotropin receptors in human corpora lutea of the menstrual cycle and pregnancy. *Am J Obstet Gynecol* 1977; 128: 146-153.

Simón C, Dominguez F, Remohí J, Pellicer A. Embryo effects in human implantation: embryonic regulation of endometrial molecules in human implantation. *Ann N Y Acad Sci* 2001; 943: 1-16.

Schumacher A, Brachwitz N, Sohr S, Engeland K, Langwisch S, Dolaptchieva M, Alexander T, Taran A, Malfertheiner SF, Costa SD, Zimmermann G, Nitschke C, Volk HD, Alexander H, Gunzer M, Zenclussen AC. Human chorionic gonadotropin attracts regulatory T cells into the fetal-maternal interface during early human pregnancy. *J Immunol.* 2009 182:5488-97.

Shima K, Kitayama S, Nakano R. Gonadotropin binding sites in human ovarian follicles and corpora lutea during the menstrual cycle. *Obstet Gynecol* 1987; 69: 800-806.

Takabatake K, Fujiwara H, Goto Y, et al. Intravenous administration of splenocytes in early pregnancy changes the implantation window in mice. *Hum Reprod* 1997a; 12: 583-585.

Takabatake K, Fujiwara H, Goto Y, et al. Splenocytes in early pregnancy promote embryo implantation by regulating endometrial differentiation in mice. *Hum Reprod* 1997b; 12: 2102-2107.

Tanii I, Oh-oka T, Yoshinaga K, Toshimori K. A mouse acrosomal cortical matrix protein, MC41, has ZP2-binding activity and forms a complex with a 75-kDa serine protease. *Dev Biol* 2001; 238. 332-341.

Ulziibat, S., Ejima, K., Shibata, Y., Hishikawa, Y., Kitajima, M., Fujishita, A., Ishimaru, T., Koji, T. 2006. Identification of estrogen receptor beta-positive intraepithelial lymphocytes and their possible roles in normal and tubal pregnancy oviducts. *Hum. Reprod.* 21, 2281-2289.

Wan H, Versnel MA, Leijten LM, van Helden-Meeuwsen CG, Fekkes D, Leenen PJ, Khan NA, Benner R, Kiekens RC. Chorionic gonadotropin induces dendritic cells to express a tolerogenic phenotype. *J Leukoc Biol.* 2008 83:894-901.

Yen SSC. Endocrine-metabolic adaptations in pregnancy. In: Yen SSC and Jaffe RB eds. Reproductive Endocrinology. 3rd ed. Philadelphia, Saunders 1991; 936-981.

Yoshinaga K. Review of factors essential for blastocyst implantation for their modulating effects on the maternal immune system. *Semin Cell Dev Biol* 2008; 19: 161-169.

Yoshioka S, Fujiwara H, Nakayama T, Kosaka K, Mori T, Fujii S. Intrauterine administration of autologous peripheral blood mononuclear cells promotes implantation rates in patients with repeated failure of IVF-embryo transfer. *Hum Reprod* 2006; 21: 3290-3294.

5

The Future of Human Embryo Culture Media – Or Have We Reached the Ceiling?

Deirdre Zander-Fox[1] and Michelle Lane[2]
[1]Repromed, Adelaide, SA,
[2]University of Adelaide, Department of Obstetrics and Gynaecology, Adelaide, SA,
Australia

1. Introduction

Within the embryology laboratory one of the central components is embryo culture media. The fundamental goal/role of the laboratory and therefore the culture media has been to maintain the inherent viability of the gametes/embryos before replacement to the mother. Over the last 10-15 years there have been major advancements in this area, with culture media developing from simple salt solutions into highly complex defined media, specifically designed to reduce stress to the embryo and maintain high pregnancy rates. As a direct result of these advancements in culture media formulation and increased awareness of the contribution of QA/QC, single embryo transfer is now a realistic outcome for a majority of patients. Although the role of culture media in stress reduction and viability maintenance may have reached its ceiling, with likely only incremental increases in pregnancy rates to be made in the future, there may be a new role for culture media as a therapeutic device evolving from the goal of maintaining the inherent viability to improving the viability of the gametes and embryos.

This chapter will discuss the development of the pre-implantation embryo, the evolution of embryo culture media up until the present day and hypothesize on the future of this technology.

2. Pre-implantation embryo physiology

The development of embryo culture media has undergone dramatic transition since the 1950's where originally embryos were cultured in media designed to support somatic cell development (reviewed by:(Biggers 1987). Research into mammalian preimplantation embryo development has highlighted that somatic cells and the mammalian embryo are completely different in their metabolic requirements, biosynthetic pathways and also likely in their epigenome. As a result it was established several decades ago that somatic cell culture media is ill-equipped to support optimal development of the pre-implantation embryo (Bavister 1995; Brinster 1965a). This has ultimately resulted in present day culture media being designed around the stage specific nutrient requirements of the embryo as well as factoring in what is present in the natural in vivo reproductive tract environment (Gardner and Leese 1990; Leese 1988).

However, before one can understand the progression of culture media development it is imperative to understand the complex changes that the embryo undergoes as it divides from the zygote to the blastocyst stage. Animal models are frequently utilised to study the nutrient requirements of the mammalian pre-implantation embryo and murine preimplantation development is often used as model for the human as the nutrient requirements and developmental milestones are similar.

The preimplantation embryo, defined as development from the 2 pro-nuclear (2PN) stage to the blastocyst, is highly complex. It is therefore easiest to consider development in two distinct stages, pre-compaction and post-compaction, although this in reality may be a significant over simplification.

2.1 Pre-compaction stage embryo

Initially the oocyte and early embryo are relatively quiescent cells reflecting the fact that the egg has sat dormant in the ovary for many years. Each cell undergoes a series of reductive mitotic divisions called 'cleavage', during which time the total size of the embryo does not change. Thus with each division the size of the cells, or blastomeres, is reduced, which assists in restoring the exaggerated cytoplasmic:nuclear ratio back to levels more traditionally observed in somatic cells (Johnson 1988).

At these early stages the embryo is completely reliant on its mitochondria to produce energy via oxidative phosphorylation of pyruvate (or lactate and carboxylic acids from the 2-cell stage) and cannot metabolise glucose possibly due to a block to the regulatory glycolytic enzyme phosphofruktokinase (Barbehenn *et al.* 1974). The early embryo is also considered to be metabolically quiescent, in that it has a low metabolic rate and has low biosynthetic activity which results in a high ATP:ADP ratio. In fact its respiratory quotient is similar to that of bone (Leese 1991; Leese and Barton 1984). The mitochondria themselves at these early stages are also quite immature with an ovoid shape and small area of inner mitochondrial membrane for energy transport. The cleavage stage embryo also appears to be more susceptible to stress exposure, as it has a limited ability to regulate against alterations in pH, osmotic stress and reactive oxygen species due to a lack of many key homeostatic mechanisms that are routinely found in most all somatic cells (Baltz *et al.* 1991; Harvey *et al.* 1995; Lane 2001) (Figure 1).

During these early stages of development, the in vivo embryo resides in the protective environment of the oviduct which mirrors its requirements with supply of high levels of pyruvate and lower levels of glucose and protective substrates such as non- essential amino acids (Gardner *et al.* 1996; Leese 1988). There are also pH gradients as well as lower levels of oxygen that are conducive to an oxidative based metabolism (Fischer and Bavister 1993; Maas *et al.* 1977).

2.2 Post-compaction embryo

Following the cleavage stages, the pre-implantation embryo undergoes a change in morphology by compacting and forming a morula, at which stage the human embryo has reached the cornua of the uterus. Compaction typically occurs between the 8 and 12 cell stage in the human and involves the blastomeres flattening into one another to maximise cell-cell contact, resulting in the polarisation of the cells (Gallicano 2001; Ziomek and Johnson 1980). Complete activation of the embryonic genome also occurs at this time (although genomic transcription increases progressively over time with transcription as early as the 4- to 8-cell stage in the human) and there is the development of increasing transcription such that by the blastocyst stage the embryo has highly developed homeostatic systems. Once compaction has occurred the embryo now begins the process of cavitation, which results in the formation of the blastocyst. Initially the outer cells of the embryo begin to elaborate their junctional complexes, in particular ion transport systems and tight junctions in preparation for cavity formation (Watson *et al.* 2004). At this stage the Na+/K+-ATPase establishes and maintains an ionic gradient across the trophectoderm, which promotes water accumulation across the epithelium due to movement of water through aquaporins (Watson *et al.* 2004). This, combined with the tight junctions, maintains this water in the centre of the embryo, resulting in a fluid-filled cavity. During this time the embryo undergoes cellular differentiation into two distinct cell types: inner cell mass (ICM) and trophectoderm (TE). The TE forms the outer rim of the embryo, surrounding the blastocoelic cavity, which contains blastocoelic fluid, and the ICM is located eccentrically within the blastocoelic cavity against the TE. The major difference between these two cell types is that the TE cells are now committed to certain differentiative pathways where they will eventually form extra-embryonic tissue (placenta and yolk sac) (Gardner 1975), whereas the ICM is still totipotent and will eventually form the fetus as well as contributing to the yolk sac and allantois (Gardner 1975; Gardner and Rossant 1979).

Due to the high energy requirements at these later stages, the embryo now readily consumes glucose in a balance with cytoplasmic and mitochondrial metabolism and the metabolic quotient in the blastocyst reflects that commonly seen in highly proliferating tissues. The embryo resides in the uterus at this stage and the difference in the embryo itself is mirrored by the vastly different environment that the uterus provides in comparison to the oviduct with high levels of glucose and both non-essential essential amino acids and lower levels of lactate and pyruvate (Gardner *et al.* 1996; Gardner and Leese 1990; Leese 1988) (Figure 1).

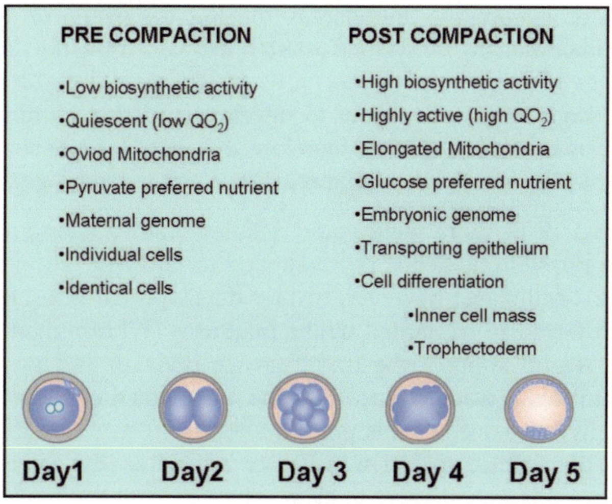

Fig. 1. Dynamics of preimplantation embryo physiology.

3. Embryo culture

3.1 Preimplantation embryo culture: the past

The ability to culture tissue samples was pioneered in the early 1900s, and during this time the importance of using a biologically defined media was acknowledged. A biologically defined medium was beneficial in that it could be reproduced at different times and in different laboratories. It can also be varied in a controlled manner and is free of enzyme activities that may interfere with the responses being studied (Biggers 1971). The design of chemically defined media accelerated in the 1940s, as media was designed to support the growth of plant and animal cells. Following this the culture of mammalian pre-implantation embryos began in the late 1940s. At this time ill-defined culture media were used for embryo culture that primarily occurred using the rabbit as a model (Biggers 1987).

The possibility of experimentally studying the mammalian pre-implantation embryo in vitro was first realised by Whitten, who reported that 8-cell mouse embryos could develop to the blastocyst stage when cultured in a simple chemically defined media based on Krebs-Ringer bicarbonate, supplemented with glucose bovine plasma albumin, antibiotics and utilising a CO_2-bicarbonate buffering system (Whitten 1956). At this point embryo stages prior to the 8-cell would not grow; however, the crucial observation was made the following year that lactate was needed to support early embryo development, and, for the first time, 2-cell embryos were able to be grown to the blastocyst stage in culture (Brinster 1963; Whitten 1957). Subsequently, it was also shown that pyruvate, oxaloacetate and phosphoenolpyruvate could substitute lactate and that when used in combination, pyruvate and lactate in the media resulted in increased blastocyst yield from 2-cells, compared to when they are used alone (Brinster 1965b). These studies were of fundamental importance, as they demonstrated that the early embryo was unlike a somatic cell in that it cannot utilise glucose for development and, instead, requires a more simple sugar in the form of lactate and pyruvate. The following year the transfer of these blastocysts into surrogate mothers produced offspring that appeared outwardly normal, demonstrating that the culture environment produced viable blastocysts (McLaren and Biggers 1958).

These pioneering studies lay the foundation for the discovery of the exact substrate requirements of the mammalian embryo and assisted in overcoming the developmental blocks seen in varying stages of embryo development. It was discovered that mouse embryos from the 1-cell to 2-cell stage require pyruvate to develop, and this requirement seems to be universal among all mammalian species: therefore it is now an essential component of all media for pre-implantation embryo development (Whittingham and Biggers 1967).

During the 1960s and 1970s there were many detailed studies trying to understand more about basic embryo physiology. When pyruvate and lactate were supplied, mouse zygotes would cleave to the 2-cell stage; however, further development was blocked unless the 2-cells were then transferred to explanted oviduct cultures (Whittingham and Biggers 1967) and only pyruvate would support the first cleavage division and nuclear maturation of mouse oocytes. From this it was deduced that the metabolism of the oocyte and the 1-cell embryo were virtually the same. At this point it was also discovered that the ability of the embryo to survive the culture period was highly reliant on the mouse strain. Using F1 hybrids of inbred strains it was possible to grow embryos from the 1-cell to the blastocyst in simple media of a modified salt and protein composition (Whitten and Biggers 1968).

However, 1-cell embryos from random-bred strains would not develop and it took another 20 years of research before this problem was overcome. This research led to the discovery of the 'substrate triad' of pyruvate, lactate and glucose, as together they could support the development of some inbred mouse strain embryos from the 1-cell to the blastocyst (Bavister 1995). These substrates are still the cornerstone of most all culture media for mammalian preimplantation embryos including the human.

The seminal discovery that the human oocyte could be successfully fertilized in vitro (Edwards et al. 1969), shifted the focus to the human embryo. During this period a variety of media was used involving both simple and complex media formulations containing bovine serum albumin (BSA) or serum. As early as 1970 it was reported that the human embryo could be cultured up to the 16-cell stage in vitro (Edwards *et al.* 1970). Following this progress many studies were undertaken to try and support the in vitro development of species, other than the mouse and rabbit, using semi-defined serum-free media; however, this was met with limited success due to the poor knowledge of substrate requirements for each species. Most studies from this period appeared to assume that substrate requirements for all species were similar to that of the mouse and rabbit. But it has now become apparent that although some aspects are the same, each species needs to be assessed independently and the media modified depending on substrate requirements (Bavister 1995).

Although some success was found in growing embryos from a variety of species, such as monkey and cattle, these were mainly grown in complex media containing blood serum. They resulted in low blastocyst yield and did not increase the knowledge on the varying requirements of embryos from different species (Bavister 1995). It was also noted, that the majority of useful laboratory animals displayed 'blocks in development' that precluded complete pre-implantation development in culture. A variety of methods were trialled to try and overcome these blocks, such as transferring cytoplasm from non-blocking embryos into those displaying developmental blocking; however, the reason for these blocks remained unknown (Muggleton-Harris *et al.* 1982).

The need to overcome these developmental blocks was the focus of research during the late 1980s onwards. This was mainly due to the need to obtain complete pre-implantation development in vitro for the livestock industry, in particular using oocytes from abattoir cattle ovaries. Unlike in the human and primate, early cleavage stage embryos of most species will not survive if transferred into the uterus. Thus it is necessary to maintain in vitro development up to stages (morula and blastocyst) that are attuned with uterine transfer. Complete embryo development was also required to obtain comparative data between species, other than inbred mice and rabbits, for research purposes and also for other livestock industries.

The developmental blocks were attributed to artefacts of the culture environment, and the stage of the block appeared to be species-specific (Bavister 1995). It was also noted that the blocks were perhaps genetically derived as inbred mouse strains were able to develop from the 1-cell stage to the blastocyst; however, random-bred strains displayed the 2-cell block. Interestingly, it was discovered that these blocks in development coincided with the activation of the embryonic genome, which occurs at different stages depending on the species (Telford *et al.* 1990). These developmental blocks were able to be overcome by co-culture; the growth of embryos alongside the growth of somatic tissue such as endothelial, fibroblast or ovarian cells (Allen and Wright 1984; Gandolfi and Moor 1987). Although this culturing system was able to facilitate the development of blastocysts that formed offspring after transfer, further investigations into the requirements of the embryo has resulted in the development of media systems that can facilitate blastocyst development without co-culture which eliminates the risks associated with co-culturing human embryos alongside animal somatic cells such as the transfer of bovine spongiform encephslopathy (Bavister 1995).

Many studies have shown that the environmental requirements of the pre-implantation embryo change as the embryo progresses along the female reproductive tract. Changes in morphology and ultrastructures accompany alterations in energy transport mechanisms and responsiveness to growth factors as the embryo develops and moves from the oviduct to the uterine environment (Bavister 1995). It has also been shown that changes in mitochondrial morphology accompany embryo development and that these changes may be particularly significant in relationship to the perturbed metabolism that is seen in cultured embryos (Hillman and Tasca 1969). From this it was hypothesised that perhaps the developmental blocks seen were due to inadequate energy production, as many studies have demonstrated that the addition of certain nutrients or energy substrates can overcome developmental blocks in embryo development (Brinster 1963; Whitten 1957).

Continual research into the requirements of the developing embryo led to the generation of more defined culture media, which could support the growth of a mammalian embryo from the zygote to the blastocyst stage; however, this growth was associated with decreased development and viability along with altered gene expression and perturbed mitochondrial homeostasis (Gardner and Lane 1993; Lane and Gardner 1994).

3.2 Human embryo culture: the present

The first 20-25 years of human IVF treatments were almost exclusively resulting from the culture of embryos to day 2 or in some cases day 3 before transfer to the uterus. The human and primate are the only 2 species where the embryo has the plasticity required for this asynchronous transfer however; this early transfer to the uterus was necessitated by an inability to grow the human embryo in culture beyond these stages at high rates.

This was a result of the lack of understanding regarding the physiology or nutrient requirements of the preimplantation human embryo. Therefore, the culture media used for the early years of human IVF were those designed for tissue culture and were either simple salt solutions or complex tissue culture media. 'Simple' media such as Tryode's or Earle's T6 medium consisted of balanced salt solutions with added carbohydrates glucose, pyruvate and lactate and were commonly supplemented with patient's serum. These media lacked many components that we now know are important for maintaining embryo physiology and health such as amino acids. Alternatively, embryos were grown in tissue culture media that were designed to support immortal cell lines in culture and were more complex containing salts supplemented with carbohydrates, amino acids, vitamins, nucleic acids and metal ions and include media such as Ham's F-10, MEM or TCM-199 (Lane 2001; Menezo *et al.* 1984). None of these media were designed to support embryo development and they contained many components that have subsequently been shown to be detrimental to embryo development in vitro such as high levels of glucose, metal ions and hormones (Bowden *et al.* 1993; Brown and Whittingham 1991; Pinsino *et al.* 2010; Quinn 1995;

Takahashi and First 1992; Van Winkle and Campione 1982; Vidal and Hidalgo 1993). In fact early attempts to culture the human embryo for prolonged periods in these media resulted in low blastocyst development rates and implantation rates between 5-10%. This contrasted with the rates of >60% implantation following uterine lavage (Buster 1985; Buster *et al.* 1985).

As the human embryo shows enormous plasticity and the pregnancy rates after IVF in a variety of media formulations from the very simple to the highly complex were very similar; little research was invested into human embryo culture media formulations in the early years. However, in the early 1990's studies on animal model data began to indicate that the embryo had different nutrient requirements compared to somatic cells and that culture media for embryo development needed to be specifically designed for this purpose.

Initially a media named B2 was produced that utilised a complex array of amino acids and serum albumin followed by media designed by Quinn called HTF (human tubal fluid) that, although based on a simple base media construct, contained the same potassium concentrations seen in the human reproductive tract and resulted in improved embryo development (Menezo *et al.* 1984; Quinn *et al.* 1985). This media is still used in some laboratories to this day for human embryo culture to day2 or day3 of development before transfer back into the uterus.

During this period, further scientific research emerged that demonstrated that the nutrient requirements of the mammalian preimplantation embryo were not only different from somatic cells but also that the requirements for the embryo change through the developmental period so that what is beneficial at one time point may cause developmental delay if given at another. One vital discovery was the switch from pyruvate-lactate metabolism in the early stages of development to glucose metabolism after activation of the embryonic genome. This, along with the issues surrounding the presence of inorganic phosphate, resulted in further modifications to culture media via the removal of phosphate and glucose, further improving embryo culture conditions (Quinn 1995). Although during this period, cleavage stage embryos were successfully grown and transferred resulting in pregnancies; these media designs still did not permit efficient development of the late stage embryo.

To try and facilitate the growth of the human blastocyst, research was conducted into the components found in oviduct and uterine fluid. These studies demonstrated that there are significant changes in the concentrations of metabolites and nutrients such as lactate, pyruvate and glucose within the tract, and that changes in these concentrations not only occur because of location but also during the stage of the menstrual cycle (Gardner and Leese 1990; Leese 1988) (Figure 2).

Furthermore, it was also discovered that amino acids play a crucial role in embryo development, and their concentrations also vary at different regions in the tract, such that a specific group of amino acids are required for early embryo development; however, late stage embryo development requires a different subset of amino acids (Bavister and Arlotto 1990; Gardner and Lane 1996; Gardner *et al.* 1996; Gwatkin 1969).

These studies eventually led to the design and implementation of sequential culture media, which was tailored to meet the metabolic and nutritional needs of specific stages of embryo development (Gardner 1998). This culture media design was an improvement on the current human culture media designs, which were single phase, and, although they were able to support limited blastocyst development, did not take into account the different nutritional needs of different stages of embryo development (Menezo *et al.* 1984; Quinn 1995; Quinn *et al.* 1985). The widespread use of sequential media has resulted in a change in clinical IVF to later stage embryos being transferred. Meta-analysis of outcomes following IVF determined that the highest rates of implantation and pregnancy resulted in the transfer of the later stage embryo to the tract compared to the earlier embryo. However, interestingly, this increase in implantation rate was dependent on the use of sequential media formulations rather than single media formulations in agreement with the studies on animal models.

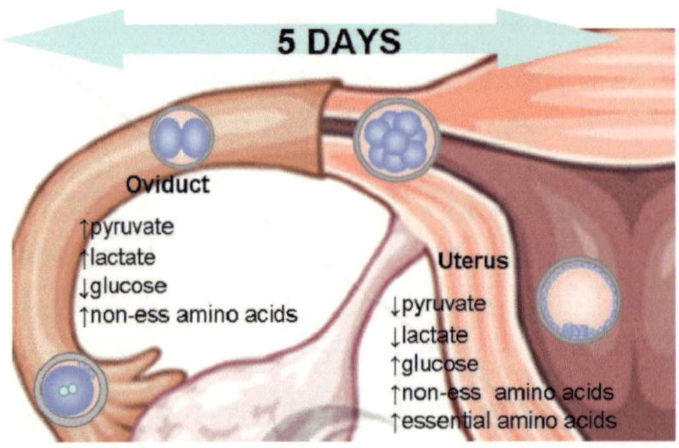

Fig. 2. Nutrient contents of the female reproductive tract and preimplantation embryo development.

4. Culture media components

In order to understand the different culture media available for use on the human embryo it is essential to understand the literature behind each of the key components in the formulation. The significance of this is becoming more apparent with the recent publication that different culture media may program the human embryo such that birthweight parameters are altered. Therefore, there is an increasing imperative to understand the components of the culture media and how they interact with the developing embryo.

4.1 Nutrients

Carbohydrates

The pre-implantation embryo relies on different energy sources at different stages of development to generate ATP. As highlighted earlier, the early stages of development appear reliant on pyruvate as an energy source (Biggers and Stern 1973; Leese and Barton 1984). Pyruvate is oxidised directly by mitochondria via oxidative phosphorylation to yield ATP, and the early embryo can utilise this mechanism only, to derive the majority of its energy.

Lactate can also be an important energy source; however, lactate cannot support the first cleavage division in the mouse embryo and causes abnormal changes in the pronuclei (Whittingham 1969). Despite this, lactate can support development from the 2-cell stage and is a regulator of pyruvate uptake. Previous studies have shown that a greater proportion of 2-cell embryos develop when both pyruvate and lactate are in the media compared to when either energy source is present by itself (Brinster 1965b). This is because pyruvate facilitates the conversion of lactate to pyruvate, and, conversely, lactate regulates the uptake and metabolism of pyruvate and that the regulation is based on the stage of embryo development (Biggers and Stern 1973; Lane and Gardner 2000). Studies have demonstrated that pyruvate uptake at the human pre-compaction stage is high and glucose uptake is very low; however, after compaction, a switch occurs and glucose uptake is high and pyruvate uptake decreases (Gardner and Leese 1986; Leese and Barton 1984). Together with the increased levels of these nutrients present in the oviduct, pyruvate and lactate are present in the first phase of sequential culture media in an increased amount compared to glucose (Table 1).

Glucose metabolism is also used to generate energy; however, this occurs in the later stage embryo only. Glucose is used by almost all mammalian cells as the primary energy source and so the early embryo is unique in that it lacks the ability to metabolise glucose. Experiments have demonstrated that the zygote and 2-cell mouse embryo cannot develop in the presence of glucose alone (Biggers *et al.* 1967; Brinster 1965a; Whitten 1957). In contrast the 8-cell mouse embryo will develop in the presence of glucose alone, and in other species, such as the rabbit, only the blastocyst stage will develop in the presence of glucose alone (Brinster and Thomson 1966; Daniel and Krishnan 1967; Whitten 1956). Glucose is taken up by the cells and converted to pyruvate by a series of reactions of the Embden-Meyerhof pathway in the cytosol. Further studies on the mouse have demonstrated that glucose is essential for the development of the blastocyst and in particular the ICM is entirely dependent on glycolysis for energy. As a result of these collective findings along with the the increased levels of glucose present in the uterus, glucose is present in the second phase of sequential culture media in an amount similar to that measured in the uterus and higher than that for the cleavage stage embryo (Table 1).

	Pyruvate (mM)	Lactate (mM)	Glucose (mM)
Oviduct	0.32	10.5	0.5
G-1 (cleavage stage)	0.32	10.5	0.5
Uterus	0.1	5.87	3.15
G-2 (blastocyst stage)	0.1	5.87	3.15

Table 1. Concentration of carbohydrates in human oviduct and uterine fluid and concentration of carbohydrates in G-1 and G-2 sequential media (Gardner and Lane 1998; Gardner *et al.* 1996).

Amino acids

The reproductive tract also contains significant concentrations of amino acids (Fahning *et al.* 1967; Lane and Gardner 1997b; Miller and Schultz 1987). Furthermore, the oocyte and embryo itself maintain an endogenous pool of amino acids as well as possessing specific amino acid transporters (Van Winkle 1988). The beneficial effect of amino acids is believed to be due to their use as a metabolic substrate and also their ability to act as osmolyte and a regulator of intracellular pH (Edwards *et al.* 1998; Van Winkle *et al.* 1990). Amino acids also play an essential role as chelators and anti-oxidants and can regulate metabolism and cell differentiation (Gardner 1998; Lane and Gardner 1997a; Lane and Gardner 2005; Lindenbaum 1973; Liu and Foote 1995; Martin and Sutherland 2001).

Several studies have investigated the utilisation and importance of amino acids to the embryo and, in turn, their importance in embryo culture media (Bavister and Arlotto 1990; Brinster 1971; Carney and Bavister 1987; Gardner and Lane 1996; Gardner *et al.* 1994; Gwatkin 1969; Kane and Bavister 1988; Kane *et al.* 1986; Kaye *et al.* 1982; Lane and Gardner 1997a; Lane and Gardner 1997b; McKiernan *et al.* 1995; Pinyopummintr and Bavister 1996; Schultz *et al.* 1981). Multiple studies have shown that amino acid transport is critical for early embryo development, even a brief exposure to media without added amino acids can be detrimental to the developing embryo by reducing development to the blastocyst stage and decreasing blastocyst cell numbers (Gardner and Lane 1996).

In particular, it has been shown that the addition of Eagle's non-essential amino acids and glutamine significantly increases development of the zygote to blastocyst stage, alleviate 2-cell blocking, increases the rate of compaction and increase fetal development after transfer (Devreker *et al.* 1998; Gardner and Lane 1993; Gardner and Lane 1996; Lane and Gardner 1997b; McKiernan *et al.* 1995). In contrast zygotes cultured to the blastocyst stage in the presence of essential amino acids show a significant reduction in blastocyst cell number (Gardner and Lane 1993). Together these studies demonstrate that while non-essential amino acids and glutamine support growth from the zygote to the blastocyst stage throughout development, the presence of essential amino acids for the first 48 hours of culture have a negative impact on cellular division. Interestingly, in contrast to their lack of effect in earlier stages, essential amino acids from the 8-cell to blastocyst stage increase cleavage rates, increase development of the ICM and increase fetal development after transfer (Lane and Gardner 1997a). Therefore, non-essential amino acids are usually added to both phases of sequential media for their roles as chealtors and osmolytes and essential amino acids are added in the second phase as the metabolism of the embryo becomes more complex and more similar to that of a somatic cell.

4.2 Ammonium

Traditionally embryos are cultured in media at 37 °C. However, at 37 °C components of the media such as amino acids begin to break down spontaneously forming by-products such as ammonium.

Initial studies that assessed the effect of amino acids on embryo development discovered that if embryos were cultured in the absence of amino acids, culture media renewal at 48 hours did not alter blastocyst development. In comparison, if amino acids were present in the culture media, blastocyst development was significantly increased if the culture media was renewed after both 48 and 72 hours when compared to 96 hours in the same media.

Embryo quality was also improved after media renewal, with an increase being seen in blastocyst cell number (Gardner and Lane 1993). A subsequent study demonstrated that media renewal also resulted in increased implantation and fetal weights after transfer and reduced fetal defects when comparing to embryo cultured in the same media continuously (Lane and Gardner 1994). These studies determined that spontaneous breakdown of amino acids and de-amination of amino acids by the embryos themselves resulted in a toxic build-up of ammonium. In particular, glutamine is considered to be the most volatile amino acid and is responsible for the majority of ammonium produced (Gardner and Lane 1993; Lane and Gardner 1995). However, there are now stable di-peptide forms of glutamine available such as alanyl-L-glutamine or glycyl-L-glutamine, which result in significantly lower levels of ammonium production (Gardner and Lane 1993; Lane and Gardner 2003).

As a result of these studies it is essential that any media containing glutamine is handled carefully. Most all media for clinical IVF have avoided this issue by including the stable di-peptide forms of glutamine.

4.3 Macromolecules

Serum has been used for many years to supplement somatic cell tissue culture media as it provides multiple beneficial factors including amino acids and vitamins (Bavister 1995). Initially as embryos were cultured in media developed for somatic cell culture; it is understandable that serum was also added to embryo culture. The preimplantation embryo is exposed to a variety of macromolecules such as albumin and hyaluronan in the reproductive tract, which are beneficial for embryo development, however in vivo the embryo is never exposed to serum (Leese 1988). Despite this, initial culture media designs were supplemented with whole serum which contains a large amount of unknown factors and due to its nature is highly variable in its composition. Serum has been demonstrated to be detrimental to embryo development as it causes metabolic, genetic and morphological changes in the blastocyst cultured in the presence of serum from the 1-cell stage and also results in abnormal increases in lamb offspring weight due to its presence during culture of sheep embryos (Gardner *et al.* 1994; Thompson *et al.* 1995). Aside from the significant impact serum has on embryo development, serum can be embryo toxic and each batch of serum contains differing levels of metabolites, growth factors, hormones and protein making it impossible to standardise culture conditions within a laboratory (Maurer 1992). Serum is now no longer added to human embryo culture media and instead media is often supplemented by serum albumin. Albumin is the most abundant macromolecule present in the female reproductive tract and has multiple benefits as it not only can negate the toxic effects associated with colloidal osmotic pressure but also assists in gamete and embryo manipulation by altering surface tension and preventing gametes and embryos from sticking to the culture vessel (Gardner 2008). Although serum albumin is determined to be free from biological contamination, such as HIV, before it is added to human culture media, the ability to screen for other contaminants such as prions is currently not available. This therefore makes recombinant serum albumin a more appealing choice and also allows for the elimination of small impurities such as fatty acids which often contaminate serum albumin fractions (Hanson and Ballard 1968).

Glycosaminoglycans are present at high levels in the reproductive tract fluid It has also been shown that hyaluronan levels increase in the uterus around the time of implantation, embryos express the receptor for hyaluronan (CD44) throughout development and CD44 is also expressed in the stroma of the endometrium (Behzad *et al.* 1994; Campbell *et al.* 1995; Zorn *et al.* 1995). Hyaluronan can also be synthesised in a pure form eliminating the issues of contamination by viral particles and prions. Studies have demonstrated that the presence of hyaluronan instead of serum albumin in mouse embryo culture media can result in increased rates of implantation and that exposure of blastocysts to hyaluronan prior to transfer also increases implantation rates (Gardner *et al.* 1999). Hyaluronan also increases cryotolerance in multiple species and assists in the maintenance of embryo ultrastructure (Lane *et al.* 2003; Palasz *et al.* 2006). Further, transfer of embryos in a medium with hyaluronan has been demonstrated to increase implantation rates in the human (Bontekoe *et al.* 2009).

4.4 Growth factors

During preimplantation development, the embryo is exposed to a variety of growth factors and cytokines present within the female reproductive tract (Hardy and Spanos 2002). These factors mediate cross-talk between the embryo and maternal tissue to facilitate development and implantation and are produced by both the embryo and also the maternal environment therefore posing the question of: should embryo culture media be supplemented with growth factors and cytokines?

Insulin and insulin like growth factor (IGF) ligands have received considerable research attention as they are involved in cell proliferation and glucose transport. Insulin and IGF are present at the 8-cell stage murine embryo and have also been detected in the reproductive tract (Henemyre and Markoff 1999; Heyner *et al.* 1989). Insulin and IGF improve in vitro maturation outcomes in a variety of species and the addition of insulin and IGF ligands to culture media increases cell proliferation, blastocyst development rates and increases ICM cell numbers in the mouse (Gardner and Kaye 1991; Guler *et al.* 2000; Harvey and Kaye 1992; Kaye and Gardner 1999; Makarevich and Markkula 2002). In addition the presence of IGF can also protect against the negative effects of oxidative stress (Kurzawa *et al.* 2002). Due to this insulin is now a component of some culture media available for human IVF.

Two growth factors that have received considerable attention are TGF-β (transforming growth factor beta) and GM-CSF (granulocyte-macrophage colony stimulating factor); however there are many more possible candidates which are being investigated such as EGF (epidermal growth factor), LIF (leukaemia inhibitory factor) and IGF (insulin-like growth factor).

TGF-β belongs to a large gene family and has multiple roles within the cell including enhancing cell growth, differentiation and formation of extracellular matrix (Paria and Dey 1990). TGF-β has been demonstrated to be produced by preimplantation mouse embryos suggesting a possible role via autocrine and paracrine mechanisms (Rappolee *et al.* 1988; Slager *et al.* 1991). Another study has demonstrated that the late stage embryo (8-cell to blastocyst) has the ability to bind radiolabeled TGF-β demonstrating that the embryo has the potential to react to TGF-β signalling and the addition of TGF-β to embryo culture media increases development to the blastocyst stage (Paria and Dey 1990; Paria *et al.* 1992).

GM-CSF is involved in cellular proliferation and differentiation and is produced by epithelial cells of the oviduct and uterus (Robertson *et al.* 1992; Zhao and Chegini 1994). The GM-CSF receptor is expressed by both cell lineages of the blastocyst and embryos exposed to GM-CSF in culture have increased blastocyst development and increases glucose transport and hatching rates (Robertson *et al.* 2001; Sjoblom *et al.* 1999). Exposure of mouse embryos to GM-CSF in culture also resulted in the suppression of stress response genes such as *Hspa5* and *Bax* (Chin *et al.* 2009). Together these results suggest that both TGF-β and GM-CSF may play an important role in embryo development and differentiation, and the addition of these growth factors to human embryo culture media may improve blastocyst development and ultimately implantation rates.

That being said, studies have also demonstrated the possible inhibitory effects of growth factors on embryo development where the addition of multiple growth factors to embryo culture media from the 2-cell stage, including both mouse and human recombinant-CSF, significantly inhibited blastocyst development (Hill *et al.* 1987). Therefore great care must be taken when adding growth factors as what is beneficial at one stage may be inhibitory at another.

5. The future of human culture media: from maintenance to rescue

To date the philosophy of the laboratory and therefore function of the culture medium has been in maintaining the inherent viability of the gamete/embryo until they are returned to the female reproductive tract. This philosophy has worked well such that results from around the world indicate that more than 85% of women under the age of 35 should expect to conceive with a single embryo transfer within 12-18 months of IVF treatment. It is therefore likely that, in these patient groups where there are healthy gametes with a high inherent viability, the culture media that we currently use functions at a level that is suitable, providing maximal outcomes for these patients.

However, what about the increasing patient groups where the inherent viability of the gametes that we receive maybe reduced or low? For example in western society there has been a shift toward delaying childbearing for a variety of social reasons. Concomitantly there has been an increase in the number of women of advanced maternal age seeking assisted reproductive technologies to artificially compensate for this loss of fecundity. Previous research has demonstrated that significant perturbations occur in oocytes as maternal age increases. For example, increases in reactive oxygen species (ROS) in oocytes has been linked to increasing maternal age and it has been hypothesised that oocytes may be particularly susceptible to ROS damage while dormant in the ovary, potentially damaging lipids, proteins and DNA(Eichenlaub-Ritter *et al.* 2010; Miquel and Fleming 1984; Tarin *et al.* 1998a; Tarin 1996). This increase in ROS is proposed to be due to 'leaky mitochondria' as high energy electrons are transported along the electron transport chain and are leaked into the cytoplasm resulting the the formation of ROS such as superoxide anion (O^{2-}), hydrogen peroxide (H_2O_2) and hydroxyl free radical (OH·) which can then damage the oocyte (Tarin *et al.* 1998a; Tarin *et al.* 1998b).

It is these older patients that become repeat cyclers and where the current technology is frequently unable to provide the 'holy grail' of a viable embryo for transfer. This presents a large knowledge gap in our treatment strategies and it is therefore not unreasonable to suggest that this will become the focus of advancements in the future.

5.1 Repair of mitochondrial function: quenching ROS

Perturbations to mitochondrial function and increased ROS levels are associated with the onset of many diseases including Parkinson's, Huntington's and Alzheimer's and is also linked to the aging process. Due to this fact, mitochondrial therapeutics are being investigated to try and improve mitochondrial function and possibly repair the damage associated with aging and disease (Chen ; Hoekstra *et al.* ; Pashkow 2011). Similarly in the oocyte and embryo one of the common observations after either in vivo (e.g. aging) or in vitro stress is a reduction in mitochondrial function that is often observed before any changes in developmental measures can be seen. These perturbations in mitochondrial activity and the balance of cytoplasmic and mitochondrial metabolism are associated with reduced rates of development and also reduced implantation and fetal development in animal models. One of the main causes of this decline in mitochondrial function is likely the production of ROS.

ROS can be produced by a variety of metabolic pathways however in the embryo is primarily produced by oxidative phosphorylation (OXPHOS) as a by-product of metabolism. Oxidative stress is responsible for damage to lipids by inducing peroxidation (Nasr-Esfahani *et al.* 1990), protein inactivation via inducing the formation of disulphide bonds (Gutteridge and Halliwell 1989) and DNA strand breaks (Lopes *et al.* 1998). In particular mitochondrial DNA (mDNA) is particularly susceptible to ROS damage due to its lack of histones and, due to the fact that mDNA encodes vital subunits for the OXPHOS pathway, this can result in metabolic dysfunction (Guerin *et al.* 2001). As the oocyte and embryo relies so heavily on mitochondrial metabolism, damage to mitochondrial DNA may result in decreased generation of ATP, damaging the oocyte and resultant embryo (Eichenlaub-Ritter *et al.* 2004). ATP levels in oocytes and embryos are positively correlated with the proportion of embryos that reach the blastocyst stage and has been linked to their implantation potential (Quinn and Wales 1973; Van Blerkom *et al.* 1995).

Aging in many tissue types has been linked to increased levels of oxidative stress, in particular increased maternal age has been associated with decreased mitochondrial membrane potential and activity, increased prevelance of mDNA deletions and a decline in antioxidant levels within the oocyte. Therefore it has been hypothesised that the decline in oocyte viability seen with advanced maternal age may be due to oxidative stress (Keefe *et al.* 1995; Tarin 1996; Wilding *et al.* 2001; Wilding *et al.* 2003). In addition advanced maternal age has also been associated with increased rates of aneuploidy, in particular trisomy, which may increase in frequency due to decreased energy generation which results in impaired chromosome alignment and spindle activity (Wilding *et al.* 2005). Decreased mitochondrial membrane potential has also been linked to increased rates of chaotic mosaicism, further supporting this hypothesis (Wilding *et al.* 2003). Together this information demonstrates that increased ROS coupled with decreasing levels of antioxidant can result in large amount of cellular damage, cumulatively resulting in decreased oocyte and embryo viability (Figure 3).

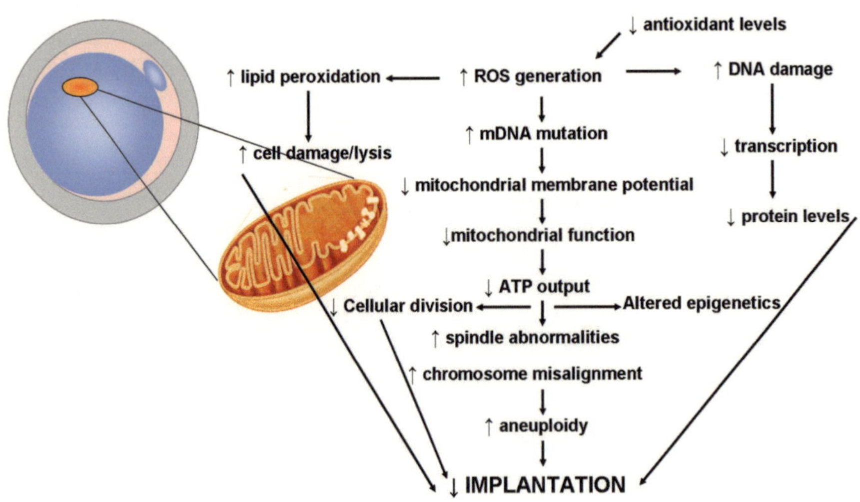

Fig. 3. Proposed model of cellular damage and the link to decreased implantation the in the aged oocyte.

In vivo the oocyte and embryo are protected from ROS by oxygen scavangers or metal-binding proteins, such as albumin or transferrin, present in oviduct and uterine fluid (Guerin *et al.* 2001). The oocyte and embryo also contain numerous compounds which have antioxidant function including pyruvate, cysteamine, taurine and hypotaurine, glutathione (GSH) and Co-enzyme Q10 as well as enzymatic mechanisms such as superoxide dismutase (SOD) and catalase (Bentinger *et al.* 2007; El Mouatassim *et al.* 1999; Gardiner and Reed 1994; Guerin and Menezo 1995; Guyader-Joly *et al.* 1998; Lapointe *et al.* 1998).

Animal studies have demonstrated that supplementing culture media with SOD or catalase increases blastocyst development rates and assists in overcoming the 2-cell block often seen in the mouse however the addition of these enzymes is very expensive and not always effective (Li *et al.* 1993; Noda *et al.* 1991; Payne *et al.* 1992).

Vitamins are another important source of antioxidants and have been demonstrated to decrease hydrogen peroxide (H_2O_2) levels in sperm when semen preparation media is supplemented with Vitamin C and E (Donnelly *et al.* 1999). Vitamin supplementation has also been demonstrated to be of benefit when administered orally as in the aged mouse model, oral supplementation with vitamins C and E reduces age associated perturbations in segregation of chromosomes and spindle arrangement (Tarin *et al.* 1998b).

Similarly some amino acids can also act as antioxidants for example hypotaurine has been demonstrated to neutralise hydroxyl radicals therefore preventing sperm lipid peroxidation (Alvarez and Storey 1983). During this process hypotaurine is converted to taurine which then has further antioxidant effects by neutralising cytotoxic aldehydes. Hypotaurine has been added to culture media demonstrating beneficial effects on blastocyst development in a variety of species including the human (Barnett and Bavister 1992; Devreker and Hardy 1997; Dumoulin *et al.* 1992) and is frequently seen in bovine embryo culture media.

However despite their obvious benefit, antioxidants must be used with care as often they can have a negative impact on development; in particular thiols such as CSH have been shown to decrease blastocyst development at concentrations greater than 250μm/l and that a delicate balance in redox state must be maintained as significant alterations may lead to cell cycle arrest and embryo death (Guyader-Joly *et al.* 1998; Liu *et al.* 1999).

As oxidative stress may be in part responsible for the aging of the oocyte, the addition of antioxidants to culture media may be the next step in trying to rescue mitochondrial function and therefore ATP production. Today's culture media formulations do contain some antioxidants, in particular pyruvate, and low levels of amino acids, however the current concentrations of these components has most often been established based on their function as a nutrient and not as an antioxidant.

One factor, Coenzyme Q10 (CoQ10) is not only an antioxidant, but is also part of the respiratory chain complex. CoQ10 is primarily found in its reduced form of ubiquinol, thereby having the ability to oxidise free radicals, and levels have been shown to be decreased in the aged cell (Bentinger *et al.* 2007; Sohal and Forster 2007). The oral supplementation of CoQ10 has been used successfully in the treatment of hypertension, congenative heart failure and Parkinson's, all of which are associated with mitochondrial dysfunction (Langsjoen and Langsjoen 2008; Rosenfeldt *et al.* 2003; Winkler-Stuck *et al.* 2004). In addition oral supplementation of CoQ10 to rats decreases the incidence of mitochondrial complex I deletion often associated with aging and increases mitochondrial activity in the oocyte up to the level seen in young control mice (Bentov *et al.* 2009; Ochoa *et al.* 2011).

Due to being water insoluble, CoQ10 is difficult to use in culture media, however CoQ10 has been added to bovine in vitro culture (via nano-particle technology) and subsequently improved cleavage rates, blastocyst development and cell numbers as well as ATP production (Stojkovic *et al.* 1999). In addition synthetic analogues such as Co-enzyme Q2 (CoQ2) and idebnenone have been developed for use in vitro and have been shown to reduce rates of lipid peroxidation as well as stimulating mitochondrial electron flow and increasing oxidation of Complex II (Briere *et al.* 2004; Imada *et al.* 2008). It is therefore possible that the addition of components, such as CoQ10, CoQ2 and idebenone to culture media, may not only assist in quenching ROS, but also may stimulate OXPHOS resulting in increased mitochondrial function and ultimately improved oocyte viability.

5.2 Future gazing: customised culture media

Evidence of the metabolic changes that occurs with age have demonstrated that the aged oocyte is very different to an oocyte obtained from a young woman, however increased maternal age is not the only condition that alters the oocyte. The increasing rates of obesity within the Western population and the negative effect obesity has on fecundity has lead to increasing rates of obese women accessing assisted reproductive treatment. Obesity is associated with decreased conception rates (even in those women with regular ovulation) and increased rates of miscarriage possibly indicative of an effect of obesity on peri-conception events such oocyte and embryo quality and viability (Robker 2008; van der Steeg *et al.* 2008). The follicular environment of obese women is different to women with normal BMI as follicular fluid from obese women contains increased levels of insulin, lactate, triglycerides and C-reactive protein, all of which may contribute to the decreased fecundity seen in obese women (Robker *et al.* 2009). In animal models, mice fed a high fat diet exhibit increased levels of intracellular lipid within the oocyte and reduced mitochondrial membrane potential as well as decreased blastocyst development and decreased blastocyst cell number compared to control fed mice (Igosheva *et al.* 2010; Minge *et al.* 2008; Wu *et al.* 2010). This therefore demonstrates that, as with advanced maternal age, the oocytes from obese women are different to oocytes from women of normal weight. This example can also be applied to altered maternal diet (such as high/low protein intake or under-nutrition), diabetes and smoking as well as pathologies such as polycystic ovarian syndrome, all of which have been linked to altered oocyte and embryo physiology and or molecular make up (Depa-Martynow *et al.* 2006; Kwong *et al.* 2000; Ludwig *et al.* 1999; McEvoy *et al.* 1997; Qiao and Feng 2011; Shiloh *et al.* 2004; Wynn and Wynn 1988).

This therefore poses the question: If not all oocytes/embryos are created equal, then why do we treat them as such?

The environment in which the oocyte is grown can have a significant impact on the genetic, epigenetic and molecular and metabolic makeup of the embryo, therefore should customised culture media be designed to factor in these differences and try and rescue the inherent viability of the oocyte and embryo by reversing the perturbations induced by sub-optimal environmental conditions. In addition, although this chapter has not covered the topic of sperm, it would be remiss to neglect the contribution of sperm health to embryo viability. The impact of paternal age, weight and health can also impact greatly on the ability of the embryo to implant and develop into healthy offspring and as IVF culture media possibly moves from maintenance to repair, sperm health should also be considered and factored into gamete culture media design. It is these concepts that are likely to drive changes in culture media formulations in the future.

6. Conclusion

Since embryo culture was first introduced in the 1940's, research has demonstrated that the mammalian embryo is unique in its development, as unlike a somatic cell, it requires specific nutrients at differing stages as it develops from a relatively quiescent single cell into the highly active blastocyst. As a result, embryo culture media formulations have also developed in the hope of providing the necessary nutrient requirements when they are needed by the embryo. However since the development of sequential culture media systems, innovation into culture media design has remained somewhat static. This begs the question of: have we reached the ceiling of culture media design?

Present day media formulation are primarily focused on maintenance of oocyte viability however with the decreased oocyte viability associated with advanced maternal age, obesity as well as a range of other in vivo stresses such as under-nutrition, smoking and pathologies such as endometriosis, it is possible that current culture conditions need to move to being therapeutic in design to try and reverse the damage induced by these conditions.

However before this can be achieved we must first understand what 'goes wrong' in the oocyte and the embryo before we can implement a strategy to restore function and improve viability. Increasing our knowledge as to how the molecular function of the egg contributes to the viability of the embryo is essential for IVF culture media design to move into the next phase of oocyte and embryo repair.

7. References

Allen RL, Wright RW, Jr. (1984) In vitro development of porcine embryos in coculture with endometrial cell monolayers or culture supernatants. *J Anim Sci* 59, 1657-61.

Alvarez JG, Storey BT (1983) Taurine, hypotaurine, epinephrine and albumin inhibit lipid peroxidation in rabbit spermatozoa and protect against loss of motility. *Biol Reprod* 29, 548-55.

Baltz JM, Biggers JD, Lechene C (1991) Two-cell stage mouse embryos appear to lack mechanisms for alleviating intracellular acid loads. *J Biol Chem* 266, 6052-7.

Barbehenn EK, Wales RG, Lowry OH (1974) The explanation for the blockade of glycolysis in early mouse embryos. *Proc Natl Acad Sci U S A* 71, 1056-60.

Barnett DK, Bavister BD (1992) Hypotaurine requirement for in vitro development of golden hamster one-cell embryos into morulae and blastocysts, and production of term offspring from in vitro-fertilized ova. *Biol Reprod* 47, 297-304.

Bavister BD (1995) Culture of preimplantation mammalian embryos: Facts and Artifacts. *Hum Reprod Update* 1, 91-148.

Bavister BD, Arlotto T (1990) Influence of single amino acids on the development of hamster one-cell embryos in vitro. *Mol Reprod Dev* 25, 45-51.

Behzad F, Seif MW, Campbell S, Aplin JD (1994) Expression of two isoforms of CD44 in human endometrium. *Biol Reprod* 51, 739-47.

Bentinger M, Brismar K, Dallner G (2007) The antioxidant role of coenzyme Q. *Mitochondrion* 7 Suppl, S41-50.

Bentov Y, Esfandiari N, Burstein E, Casper RF (2009) The use of mitochondrial nutrients to improve the outcome of infertility treatment in older patients. *Fertil Steril* 93, 272-5.

Biggers J (1987) Pioneering mammalian embryo culture. In 'The Mammalian Preimplantation Embryo'. (Ed. BD Bavister) pp. 1-22. (Plenum Publishing: New York)

Biggers JD, Stern S (1973) Metabolism of the preimplantation mammalian embryo. *Adv Reprod Physiol* 6, 1-59.

Biggers JD, Whitten, W.K. and Whittingham, D.G (1971) The culture of mouse embryos in vitro. In 'Methods in Mammalian Embryology'. (Ed. JC Daniel). (W.H.Freeman: San Francisco)

Biggers JD, Whittingham DG, Donahue RP (1967) The pattern of energy metabolism in the mouse oocyte and zygote. *Proc Natl Acad Sci U S A* 58, 560-7.

Bontekoe S, Blake D, Heineman MJ, Williams EC, Johnson N (2009) Adherence compounds in embryo transfer media for assisted reproductive technologies. *Cochrane Database Syst Rev*, CD007421.

Bowden HC, Tesh JM, Ross FW (1993) Effects of female sex hormones in whole embryo culture. *Toxicol In Vitro* 7, 799-802.

Briere JJ, Schlemmer D, Chretien D, Rustin P (2004) Quinone analogues regulate mitochondrial substrate competitive oxidation. *Biochem Biophys Res Commun* 316, 1138-42.

Brinster RL (1963) A Method for in Vitro Cultivation of Mouse Ova from Two-Cell to Blastocyst. *Exp Cell Res* 32, 205-8.

Brinster RL (1965a) Studies on the Development of Mouse Embryos in Vitro. Ii. The Effect of Energy Source. *J Exp Zool* 158, 59-68.

Brinster RL (1965b) Studies on the development of mouse embryos in vitro. IV. Interaction of energy sources. *J Reprod Fertil* 10, 227-40.

Brinster RL (1971) Uptake and incorporation of amino acids by the preimplantation mouse embryo. *J Reprod Fertil* 27, 329-38.

Brinster RL, Thomson JL (1966) Development of eight-cell mouse embryos in vitro. *Exp Cell Res* 42, 308-15.

Brown JJ, Whittingham DG (1991) The roles of pyruvate, lactate and glucose during preimplantation development of embryos from F1 hybrid mice in vitro. *Development* 112, 99-105.

Buster JE (1985) Embryo donation by uterine flushing and embryo transfer. *Clin Obstet Gynaecol* 12, 815-24.

Buster JE, Bustillo M, Rodi IA, Cohen SW, Hamilton M, Simon JA, Thorneycroft IH, Marshall JR (1985) Biologic and morphologic development of donated human ova recovered by nonsurgical uterine lavage. 153, 211-7.

Campbell S, Swann HR, Aplin JD, Seif MW, Kimber SJ, Elstein M (1995) CD44 is expressed throughout pre-implantation human embryo development. *Hum Reprod* 10, 425-30.

Carney EW, Bavister BD (1987) Stimulatory and inhibitory effects of amino acids on the development of hamster eight-cell embryos in vitro. *J In Vitro Fert Embryo Transf* 4, 162-7.

Chen CM Mitochondrial dysfunction, metabolic deficits, and increased oxidative stress in Huntington's disease. *Chang Gung Med J* 34, 135-52.

Chin PY, Macpherson AM, Thompson JG, Lane M, Robertson SA (2009) Stress response genes are suppressed in mouse preimplantation embryos by granulocyte-macrophage colony-stimulating factor (GM-CSF). *Hum Reprod* 24, 2997-3009.

Daniel JC, Jr., Krishnan RS (1967) Amino acid requirements for growth of the rabbit blastocyst in vitro. *J Cell Physiol* 70, 155-60.

Depa-Martynow M, Jedrzejczak P, Taszarek-Hauke G, Josiak M, Pawelczyk L (2006) [The impact of cigarette smoking on oocytes and embryos quality during in vitro fertilization program]. *Przegl Lek* 63, 838-40.

Devreker F, Hardy K (1997) Effects of glutamine and taurine on preimplantation development and cleavage of mouse embryos in vitro. *Biol Reprod* 57, 921-8.

Devreker F, Winston RM, Hardy K (1998) Glutamine improves human preimplantation development in vitro. *Fertil Steril* 69, 293-9.

Donnelly ET, McClure N, Lewis SE (1999) The effect of ascorbate and alpha-tocopherol supplementation in vitro on DNA integrity and hydrogen peroxide-induced DNA damage in human spermatozoa. *Mutagenesis* 14, 505-12.

Dumoulin JC, Evers JL, Bras M, Pieters MH, Geraedts JP (1992) Positive effect of taurine on preimplantation development of mouse embryos in vitro. *J Reprod Fertil* 94, 373-80.

Edwards LJ, Williams DA, Gardner DK (1998) Intracellular pH of the mouse preimplantation embryo: amino acids act as buffers of intracellular pH. *Hum Reprod* 13, 3441-8.

Edwards RG, Bavister BD, Steptoe PC (1969) Early stages of fertilization in vitro of human oocytes matured in vitro. *Nature* 221, 632-5.

Edwards RG, Steptoe PC, Purdy JM (1970) Fertilization and cleavage in vitro of preovulator human oocytes. *Nature* 227, 1307-9.

Eichenlaub-Ritter U, Vogt E, Yin H, Gosden R (2004) Spindles, mitochondria and redox potential in ageing oocytes. *Reprod Biomed Online* 8, 45-58.

Eichenlaub-Ritter U, Wieczorek M, Luke S, Seidel T (2010) Age related changes in mitochondrial function and new approaches to study redox regulation in mammalian oocytes in response to age or maturation conditions. *Mitochondrion* 11, 783-96.

El Mouatassim S, Guerin P, Menezo Y (1999) Expression of genes encoding antioxidant enzymes in human and mouse oocytes during the final stages of maturation. *Mol Hum Reprod* 5, 720-5.

Fahning ML, Schultz RH, Graham EF (1967) The free amino acid content of uterine fluids and blood serum in the cow. *J Reprod Fertil* 13, 229-36.

Fischer B, Bavister BD (1993) Oxygen tension in the oviduct and uterus of rhesus monkeys, hamsters and rabbits. *J Reprod Fertil* 99, 673-9.

Gallicano GI (2001) Composition, regulation, and function of the cytoskeleton in mammalian eggs and embryos. *Front Biosci* 6, D1089-108.

Gandolfi F, Moor RM (1987) Stimulation of early embryonic development in the sheep by co-culture with oviduct epithelial cells. *J Reprod Fertil* 81, 23-8.

Gardiner CS, Reed DJ (1994) Status of glutathione during oxidant-induced oxidative stress in the preimplantation mouse embryo. *Biol Reprod* 51, 1307-14.

Gardner DK (1998) Changes in requirements and utilization of nutrients during mammalian preimplantation embryo development and their significance in embryo culture. *Theriogenology* 49, 83-102.

Gardner DK (2008) Dissection of culture media for embryos: the most important and less important components and characteristics. *Reprod Fertil Dev* 20, 9-18.

Gardner DK, Lane M (1993) Amino acids and ammonium regulate mouse embryo development in culture. *Biol Reprod* 48, 377-85.

Gardner DK, Lane M (1996) Alleviation of the '2-cell block' and development to the blastocyst of CF1 mouse embryos: role of amino acids, EDTA and physical parameters. *Hum Reprod* 11, 2703-12.

Gardner DK, Lane M (1998) Culture of viable human blastocysts in defined sequential serum-free media. *Hum Reprod* 13 Suppl 3, 148-59; discussion 160.

Gardner DK, Lane M, Calderon I, Leeton J (1996) Environment of the preimplantation human embryo in vivo: metabolite analysis of oviduct and uterine fluids and metabolism of cumulus cells. *Fertil Steril* 65, 349-53.

Gardner DK, Lane M, Spitzer A, Batt PA (1994) Enhanced rates of cleavage and development for sheep zygotes cultured to the blastocyst stage in vitro in the absence of serum and somatic cells: amino acids, vitamins, and culturing embryos in groups stimulate development. *Biol Reprod* 50, 390-400.

Gardner DK, Leese HJ (1986) Non-invasive measurement of nutrient uptake by single cultured pre-implantation mouse embryos. *Hum Reprod* 1, 25-7.

Gardner DK, Leese HJ (1990) Concentrations of nutrients in mouse oviduct fluid and their effects on embryo development and metabolism in vitro. *J Reprod Fertil* 88, 361-8.

Gardner DK, Rodriegez-Martinez H, Lane M (1999) Fetal development after transfer is increased by replacing protein with the glycosaminoglycan hyaluronan for mouse embryo culture and transfer. *Hum Reprod* 14, 2575-80.

Gardner HG, Kaye PL (1991) Insulin increases cell numbers and morphological development in mouse pre-implantation embryos in vitro. *Reprod Fertil Dev* 3, 79-91.

Gardner RL, Papaioannou, V.E (1975) Differentiation in the trophectoderm and inner cell mass. In 'The early development of mammals'. (Ed. ME Balls, Wild, A.E) pp. 107-132. (Cambridge Uni Press: London)

Gardner RL, Rossant J (1979) Investigation of the fate of 4-5 day post-coitum mouse inner cell mass cells by blastocyst injection. *J Embryol Exp Morphol* 52, 141-52.

Guerin P, El Mouatassim S, Menezo Y (2001) Oxidative stress and protection against reactive oxygen species in the pre-implantation embryo and its surroundings. *Hum Reprod Update* 7, 175-89.

Guerin P, Menezo Y (1995) Hypotaurine and taurine in gamete and embryo environments: de novo synthesis via the cysteine sulfinic acid pathway in oviduct cells. *Zygote* 3, 333-43.

Guler A, Poulin N, Mermillod P, Terqui M, Cognie Y (2000) Effect of growth factors, EGF and IGF-I, and estradiol on in vitro maturation of sheep oocytes. *Theriogenology* 54, 209-18.

Gutteridge JM, Halliwell B (1989) Iron toxicity and oxygen radicals. *Baillieres Clin Haematol* 2, 195-256.

Guyader-Joly C, Guerin P, Renard JP, Guillaud J, Ponchon S, Menezo Y (1998) Precursors of taurine in female genital tract: effects on developmental capacity of bovine embryo produced in vitro. *Amino Acids* 15, 27-42.

Gwatkin RB (1969) Nutritional requirements for post-blastocyst development in the mouse. Amino acids and protein in the uterus during implantation. *Int J Fertil* 14, 101-5.

Hanson RW, Ballard FJ (1968) Citrate, pyruvate, and lactate contaminants of commercial serum albumin. *J Lipid Res* 9, 667-8.

Hardy K, Spanos S (2002) Growth factor expression and function in the human and mouse preimplantation embryo. *J Endocrinol* 172, 221-36.

Harvey MB, Arcellana-Panlilio MY, Zhang X, Schultz GA, Watson AJ (1995) Expression of genes encoding antioxidant enzymes in preimplantation mouse and cow embryos and primary bovine oviduct cultures employed for embryo coculture. *Biol Reprod* 53, 532-40.

Harvey MB, Kaye PL (1992) Insulin-like growth factor-1 stimulates growth of mouse preimplantation embryos in vitro. *Mol Reprod Dev* 31, 195-9.

Henemyre C, Markoff E (1999) Expression of insulin-like growth factor binding protein-4, insulin-like growth factor-I receptor, and insulin-like growth factor-I in the mouse uterus throughout the estrous cycle. *Mol Reprod Dev* 52, 350-9.

Heyner S, Smith RM, Schultz GA (1989) Temporally regulated expression of insulin and insulin-like growth factors and their receptors in early mammalian development. *Bioessays* 11, 171-6.

Hill JA, Haimovici F, Anderson DJ (1987) Products of activated lymphocytes and macrophages inhibit mouse embryo development in vitro. *J Immunol* 139, 2250-4.

Hillman N, Tasca RJ (1969) Ultrastructural and autoradiographic studies of mouse cleavage stages. *Am J Anat* 126, 151-173.

Hoekstra JG, Montine KS, Zhang J, Montine TJ Mitochondrial therapeutics in Alzheimer's disease and Parkinson's disease. *Alzheimers Res Ther* 3, 21.

Igosheva N, Abramov AY, Poston L, Eckert JJ, Fleming TP, Duchen MR, McConnell J (2010) Maternal diet-induced obesity alters mitochondrial activity and redox status in mouse oocytes and zygotes. *PLoS One* 5, e10074.

Imada I, Sato EF, Kira Y, Inoue M (2008) Effect of CoQ homologues on reactive oxygen generation by mitochondria. *Biofactors* 32, 41-8.

Johnson M, Everitt, B. (1988) 'Essential Reproduction.' (Blackwell Scientific Publications: Oxford)

Kane MT, Bavister BD (1988) Protein-free culture medium containing polyvinylalcohol, vitamins, and amino acids supports development of eight-cell hamster embryos to hatching blastocysts. *J Exp Zool* 247, 183-7.

Kane MT, Carney EW, Bavister BD (1986) Vitamins and amino acids stimulate hamster blastocysts to hatch in vitro. *J Exp Zool* 239, 429-32.

Kaye PL, Gardner HG (1999) Preimplantation access to maternal insulin and albumin increases fetal growth rate in mice. *Hum Reprod* 14, 3052-9.

Kaye PL, Schultz GA, Johnson MH, Pratt HP, Church RB (1982) Amino acid transport and exchange in preimplantation mouse embryos. *J Reprod Fertil* 65, 367-80.

Keefe DL, Niven-Fairchild T, Powell S, Buradagunta S (1995) Mitochondrial deoxyribonucleic acid deletions in oocytes and reproductive aging in women. *Fertil Steril* 64, 577-83.

Kurzawa R, Glabowski W, Baczkowski T, Brelik P (2002) Evaluation of mouse preimplantation embryos exposed to oxidative stress cultured with insulin-like growth factor I and II, epidermal growth factor, insulin, transferrin and selenium. *Reprod Biol* 2, 143-62.

Kwong WY, Wild AE, Roberts P, Willis AC, Fleming TP (2000) Maternal undernutrition during the preimplantation period of rat development causes blastocyst abnormalities and programming of postnatal hypertension. *Development* 127, 4195-202.

Lane M (2001) Mechanisms for managing cellular and homeostatic stress in vitro. *Theriogenology* 55, 225-36.

Lane M, Gardner DK (1994) Increase in postimplantation development of cultured mouse embryos by amino acids and induction of fetal retardation and exencephaly by ammonium ions. *J Reprod Fertil* 102, 305-12.

Lane M, Gardner DK (1995) Removal of embryo-toxic ammonium from the culture medium by in situ enzymatic conversion to glutamate. *J Exp Zool* 271, 356-63.

Lane M, Gardner DK (1997a) Differential regulation of mouse embryo development and viability by amino acids. *J Reprod Fertil* 109, 153-64.

Lane M, Gardner DK (1997b) Nonessential amino acids and glutamine decrease the time of the first three cleavage divisions and increase compaction of mouse zygotes in vitro. *J Assist Reprod Genet* 14, 398-403.

Lane M, Gardner DK (2000) Lactate regulates pyruvate uptake and metabolism in the preimplantation mouse embryo. *Biol Reprod* 62, 16-22.

Lane M, Gardner DK (2003) Ammonium induces aberrant blastocyst differentiation, metabolism, pH regulation, gene expression and subsequently alters fetal development in the mouse. *Biol Reprod* 69, 1109-17.

Lane M, Gardner DK (2005) Mitochondrial malate-aspartate shuttle regulates mouse embryo nutrient consumption. *J Biol Chem* 280, 18361-7.

Lane M, Maybach JM, Hooper K, Hasler JF, Gardner DK (2003) Cryo-survival and development of bovine blastocysts are enhanced by culture with recombinant albumin and hyaluronan. *Mol Reprod Dev* 64, 70-8.

Langsjoen PH, Langsjoen AM (2008) Supplemental ubiquinol in patients with advanced congestive heart failure. *Biofactors* 32, 119-28.

Lapointe S, Sullivan R, Sirard MA (1998) Binding of a bovine oviductal fluid catalase to mammalian spermatozoa. *Biol Reprod* 58, 747-53.

Leese HJ (1988) The formation and function of oviduct fluid. *J Reprod Fertil* 82, 843-56.

Leese HJ (1991) Metabolism of the preimplantation mammalian embryo. *Oxf Rev Reprod Biol* 13, 35-72.

Leese HJ, Barton AM (1984) Pyruvate and glucose uptake by mouse ova and preimplantation embryos. *J Reprod Fertil* 72, 9-13.

Li J, Foote RH, Simkin M (1993) Development of rabbit zygotes cultured in protein-free medium with catalase, taurine, or superoxide dismutase. *Biol Reprod* 49, 33-7.

Lindenbaum A (1973) A survey of naturally occurring chelating ligands. *Adv Exp Med Biol* 40, 67-77.

Liu L, Trimarchi JR, Keefe DL (1999) Thiol oxidation-induced embryonic cell death in mice is prevented by the antioxidant dithiothreitol. *Biol Reprod* 61, 1162-9.

Liu Z, Foote RH (1995) Effects of amino acids on the development of in-vitro matured/in-vitro fertilization bovine embryos in a simple protein-free medium. *Hum Reprod* 10, 2985-91.

Lopes S, Jurisicova A, Sun JG, Casper RF (1998) Reactive oxygen species: potential cause for DNA fragmentation in human spermatozoa. *Hum Reprod* 13, 896-900.

Ludwig M, Finas DF, al-Hasani S, Diedrich K, Ortmann O (1999) Oocyte quality and treatment outcome in intracytoplasmic sperm injection cycles of polycystic ovarian syndrome patients. *Hum Reprod* 14, 354-8.

Maas DH, Storey BT, Mastroianni L, Jr. (1977) Hydrogen ion and carbon dioxide content of the oviductal fluid of the rhesus monkey (Macaca mulatta). *Fertil Steril* 28, 981-5.

Makarevich AV, Markkula M (2002) Apoptosis and cell proliferation potential of bovine embryos stimulated with insulin-like growth factor I during in vitro maturation and culture. *Biol Reprod* 66, 386-92.

Martin PM, Sutherland AE (2001) Exogenous amino acids regulate trophectoderm differentiation in the mouse blastocyst through an mTOR-dependent pathway. *Dev Biol* 240, 182-93.

Maurer HR (1992) Towards serum-free, chemically defined media for mammalian cell culture. In 'Animal Cell Culture: A Practical Approach'. (Ed. RI Freshney) pp. 15-46. (Oxford University Press: Oxford)

McEvoy TG, Robinson JJ, Aitken RP, Findlay PA, Robertson IS (1997) Dietary excesses of urea influence the viability and metabolism of preimplantation sheep embryos and may affect fetal growth among survivors. *Anim Reprod Sci* 47, 71-90.

McKiernan SH, Clayton MK, Bavister BD (1995) Analysis of stimulatory and inhibitory amino acids for development of hamster one-cell embryos in vitro. *Mol Reprod Dev* 42, 188-99.

McLaren, Biggers JD (1958) Successful development and birth of mice cultivated in vitro as early as early embryos. *Nature* 182, 877-8.

Menezo Y, Testart J, Perrone D (1984) Serum is not necessary in human in vitro fertilization, early embryo culture, and transfer. *Fertil Steril* 42, 750-5.

Miller JG, Schultz GA (1987) Amino acid content of preimplantation rabbit embryos and fluids of the reproductive tract. *Biol Reprod* 36, 125-9.

Minge CE, Bennett BD, Norman RJ, Robker RL (2008) Peroxisome proliferator-activated receptor-gamma agonist rosiglitazone reverses the adverse effects of diet-induced obesity on oocyte quality. *Endocrinology* 149, 2646-56.

Miquel J, Fleming JE (1984) A two-step hypothesis on the mechanisms of in vitro cell aging: cell differentiation followed by intrinsic mitochondrial mutagenesis. *Exp Gerontol* 19, 31-6.

Muggleton-Harris A, Whittingham DG, Wilson L (1982) Cytoplasmic control of preimplantation development in vitro in the mouse. *Nature* 299, 460-2.

Nasr-Esfahani MH, Aitken JR, Johnson MH (1990) Hydrogen peroxide levels in mouse oocytes and early cleavage stage embryos developed in vitro or in vivo. *Development* 109, 501-7.

Noda Y, Matsumoto H, Umaoka Y, Tatsumi K, Kishi J, Mori T (1991) Involvement of superoxide radicals in the mouse two-cell block. *Mol Reprod Dev* 28, 356-60.

Ochoa JJ, Pamplona R, *et al.* (2011) Age-related changes in brain mitochondrial DNA deletion and oxidative stress are differentially modulated by dietary fat type and coenzyme Q. *Free Radic Biol Med* 50, 1053-64.

Palasz AT, Rodriguez-Martinez H, Beltran-Brena P, Perez-Garnelo S, Martinez MF, Gutierrez-Adan A, De la Fuente J (2006) Effects of hyaluronan, BSA, and serum on bovine embryo in vitro development, ultrastructure, and gene expression patterns. *Mol Reprod Dev* 73, 1503-11.

Paria BC, Dey SK (1990) Preimplantation embryo development in vitro: cooperative interactions among embryos and role of growth factors. *Proc Natl Acad Sci U S A* 87, 4756-60.

Paria BC, Jones KL, Flanders KC, Dey SK (1992) Localization and binding of transforming growth factor-beta isoforms in mouse preimplantation embryos and in delayed and activated blastocysts. *Dev Biol* 151, 91-104.

Pashkow FJ (2011) Oxidative Stress and Inflammation in Heart Disease: Do Antioxidants Have a Role in Treatment and/or Prevention? *Int J Inflam* 2011, 514623.

Payne SR, Munday R, Thompson JG (1992) Addition of superoxide dismutase and catalase does not necessarily overcome developmental retardation of one-cell mouse embryos during in-vitro culture. *Reprod Fertil Dev* 4, 167-74.

Pinsino A, Turturici G, Sconzo G, Geraci F (2010) Rapid changes in heat-shock cognate 70 levels, heat-shock cognate phosphorylation state, heat-shock transcription factor, and metal transcription factor activity levels in response to heavy metal exposure during sea urchin embryonic development. *Ecotoxicology* 20, 246-54.

Pinyopummintr T, Bavister BD (1996) Effects of amino acids on development in vitro of cleavage-stage bovine embryos into blastocysts. *Reprod Fertil Dev* 8, 835-41.

Qiao J, Feng HL (2011) Extra- and intra-ovarian factors in polycystic ovary syndrome: impact on oocyte maturation and embryo developmental competence. *Hum Reprod Update* 17, 17-33.

Quinn P (1995) Enhanced results in mouse and human embryo culture using a modified human tubal fluid medium lacking glucose and phosphate. *J Assist Reprod Genet* 12, 97-105.

Quinn P, Kerin JF, Warnes GM (1985) Improved pregnancy rate in human in vitro fertilization with the use of a medium based on the composition of human tubal fluid. *Fertil Steril* 44, 493-8.

Quinn P, Wales RG (1973) The relationships between the ATP content of preimplantation mouse embryos and their development in vitro during culture. *J Reprod Fertil* 35, 301-9.

Rappolee DA, Brenner CA, Schultz R, Mark D, Werb Z (1988) Developmental expression of PDGF, TGF-alpha, and TGF-beta genes in preimplantation mouse embryos. *Science* 241, 1823-5.

Robertson SA, Mayrhofer G, Seamark RF (1992) Uterine epithelial cells synthesize granulocyte-macrophage colony-stimulating factor and interleukin-6 in pregnant and nonpregnant mice. *Biol Reprod* 46, 1069-79.

Robertson SA, Sjoblom C, Jasper MJ, Norman RJ, Seamark RF (2001) Granulocyte-macrophage colony-stimulating factor promotes glucose transport and blastomere viability in murine preimplantation embryos. *Biol Reprod* 64, 1206-15.

Robker RL (2008) Evidence that obesity alters the quality of oocytes and embryos. *Pathophysiology* 15, 115-21.

Robker RL, Akison LK, Bennett BD, Thrupp PN, Chura LR, Russell DL, Lane M, Norman RJ (2009) Obese women exhibit differences in ovarian metabolites, hormones, and gene expression compared with moderate-weight women. *J Clin Endocrinol Metab* 94, 1533-40.

Rosenfeldt F, Hilton D, Pepe S, Krum H (2003) Systematic review of effect of coenzyme Q10 in physical exercise, hypertension and heart failure. *Biofactors* 18, 91-100.

Schultz GA, Kaye PL, McKay DJ, Johnson MH (1981) Endogenous amino acid pool sizes in mouse eggs and preimplantation embryos. *J Reprod Fertil* 61, 387-93.

Shiloh H, Lahav-Baratz S, Koifman M, Ishai D, Bidder D, Weiner-Meganzi Z, Dirnfeld M (2004) The impact of cigarette smoking on zona pellucida thickness of oocytes and embryos prior to transfer into the uterine cavity. *Hum Reprod* 19, 157-9.

Sjoblom C, Wikland M, Robertson SA (1999) Granulocyte-macrophage colony-stimulating factor promotes human blastocyst development in vitro. *Hum Reprod* 14, 3069-76.

Slager HG, Lawson KA, van den Eijnden-van Raaij AJ, de Laat SW, Mummery CL (1991) Differential localization of TGF-beta 2 in mouse preimplantation and early postimplantation development. *Dev Biol* 145, 205-18.

Sohal RS, Forster MJ (2007) Coenzyme Q, oxidative stress and aging. *Mitochondrion* 7 Suppl, S103-11.

Stojkovic M, Westesen K, Zakhartchenko V, Stojkovic P, Boxhammer K, Wolf E (1999) Coenzyme Q(10) in submicron-sized dispersion improves development, hatching, cell proliferation, and adenosine triphosphate content of in vitro-produced bovine embryos. *Biol Reprod* 61, 541-7.

Takahashi Y, First NL (1992) In vitro development of bovine one-cell embryos: Influence of glucose, lactate, pyruvate, amino acids and vitamins. *Theriogenology* 37, 963-78.

Tarin J, Ten J, Vendrell FJ, de Oliveira MN, Cano A (1998a) Effects of maternal ageing and dietary antioxidant supplementation on ovulation, fertilisation and embryo development in vitro in the mouse. *Reprod Nutr Dev* 38, 499-508.

Tarin JJ (1996) Potential effects of age-associated oxidative stress on mammalian oocytes/embryos. *Mol Hum Reprod* 2, 717-24.

Tarin JJ, Vendrell FJ, Ten J, Cano A (1998b) Antioxidant therapy counteracts the disturbing effects of diamide and maternal ageing on meiotic division and chromosomal segregation in mouse oocytes. *Mol Hum Reprod* 4, 281-8.

Telford NA, Watson AJ, Schultz GA (1990) Transition from maternal to embryonic control in early mammalian development: a comparison of several species. *Mol Reprod Dev* 26, 90-100.

Thompson JG, Gardner DK, Pugh PA, McMillan WH, Tervit HR (1995) Lamb birth weight is affected by culture system utilized during in vitro pre-elongation development of ovine embryos. *Biol Reprod* 53, 1385-91.

Van Blerkom J, Davis PW, Lee J (1995) ATP content of human oocytes and developmental potential and outcome after in-vitro fertilization and embryo transfer. *Hum Reprod* 10, 415-24.

van der Steeg JW, Steures P, *et al.* (2008) Obesity affects spontaneous pregnancy chances in subfertile, ovulatory women. *Hum Reprod* 23, 324-8.

Van Winkle LJ (1988) Amino acid transport in developing animal oocytes and early conceptuses. *Biochim Biophys Acta* 947, 173-208.

Van Winkle LJ, Campione AL (1982) Toxic effects of Zn++ and Cu++ on mouse blastocysts in vitro. *Experientia* 38, 354-6.

Van Winkle LJ, Haghighat N, Campione AL (1990) Glycine protects preimplantation mouse conceptuses from a detrimental effect on development of the inorganic ions in oviductal fluid. *J Exp Zool* 253, 215-9.

Vidal F, Hidalgo J (1993) Effect of zinc and copper on preimplantation mouse embryo development in vitro and metallothionein levels. *Zygote* 1, 225-9.

Watson AJ, Natale DR, Barcroft LC (2004) Molecular regulation of blastocyst formation. *Anim Reprod Sci* 82-83, 583-92.

Whitten WK (1956) Culture of tubal mouse ova. *Nature* 177, 96.

Whitten WK (1957) Culture of tubal ova. *Nature* 179, 1081-2.

Whitten WK, Biggers JD (1968) Complete development in vitro of the pre-implantation stages of the mouse in a simple chemically defined medium. *J Reprod Fertil* 17, 399-401.

Whittingham DG (1969) The failure of lactate and phosphoenolpyruvate to support development of the mouse zygote in vitro. *Biol Reprod* 1, 381-6.

Whittingham DG, Biggers JD (1967) Fallopian tube and early cleavage in the mouse. *Nature* 213, 942-3.

Wilding M, Dale B, Marino M, di Matteo L, Alviggi C, Pisaturo ML, Lombardi L, De Placido G (2001) Mitochondrial aggregation patterns and activity in human oocytes and preimplantation embryos. *Hum Reprod* 16, 909-17.

Wilding M, De Placido G, De Matteo L, Marino M, Alviggi C, Dale B (2003) Chaotic mosaicism in human preimplantation embryos is correlated with a low mitochondrial membrane potential. *Fertil Steril* 79, 340-6.

Wilding M, Di Matteo L, Dale B (2005) The maternal age effect: a hypothesis based on oxidative phosphorylation. *Zygote* 13, 317-23.

Winkler-Stuck K, Wiedemann FR, Wallesch CW, Kunz WS (2004) Effect of coenzyme Q10 on the mitochondrial function of skin fibroblasts from Parkinson patients. *J Neurol Sci* 220, 41-8.

Wu LL, Dunning KR, Yang X, Russell DL, Lane M, Norman RJ, Robker RL (2010) High-fat diet causes lipotoxicity responses in cumulus-oocyte complexes and decreased fertilization rates. *Endocrinology* 151, 5438-45.

Wynn M, Wynn A (1988) Nutrition around conception and the prevention of low birthweight. *Nutr Health* 6, 37-52.

Zhao Y, Chegini N (1994) Human fallopian tube expresses granulocyte-macrophage colony stimulating factor (GM-CSF) and GM-CSF alpha and beta receptors and contain immunoreactive GM-CSF protein. *J Clin Endocrinol Metab* 79, 662-5.

Ziomek CA, Johnson MH (1980) Cell surface interaction induces polarization of mouse 8-cell blastomeres at compaction. *Cell* 21, 935-42.

Zorn TM, Pinhal MA, Nader HB, Carvalho JJ, Abrahamsohn PA, Dietrich CP (1995) Biosynthesis of glycosaminoglycans in the endometrium during the initial stages of pregnancy of the mouse. *Cell Mol Biol (Noisy-le-grand)* 41, 97-106.

6

Benzo[a]pyrene and Human Embryo

Shi Jiao[1], Bingci Liu[2] and Meng Ye[2]
[1]*The Key Laboratory of Nutrition and Metabolism, Institute for Nutritional Sciences, Shanghai Institute for Biological Sciences, Chinese Academy of Sciences, Shanghai,*
[2]*Institute of Occupational Health and Poison Control, Chinese Center for Disease Control and Prevention, Beijing, P.R. China*

1. Introduction

Benzo[a]pyrene (B[a]P) is a typical compound of the polycyclic aromatic hydrocarbons (PAHs), compounds that are usually generated through the combustion of fossil fuels, wood, and other organic materials and are found in significant amounts in diesel exhaust, cigarette smoke, charcoal-broiled foods, and industrial waste-by-products (Boström et al, 2000). B[a]P is readily absorbed following inhalation, oral, and dermal routes of administration (Knafla et al, 2006). B[a]P absorption activates the aryl hydrocarbon receptor (AhR), which forms an active transcription factor heterodimer with the AhR nuclear translocator (ARNT), and induces the expression of a group of genes called the Ah gene battery, including the cytochrome P450 1A1 (CYP1A1), CYP1A2, and CYP1B1 genes (Shimizu et al, 2000; Nebert et al, 2000).

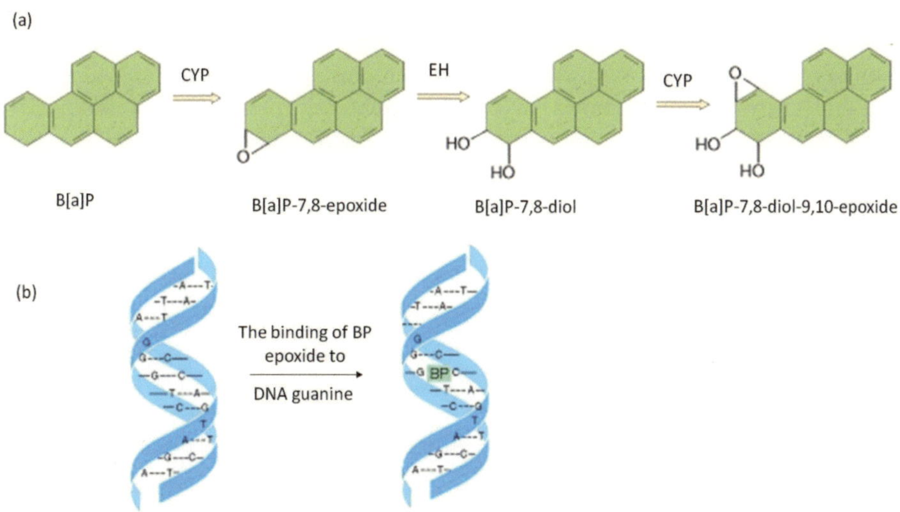

Fig. 1. The metabolic conversion of benzo[a]pyrene into a mutagen. (a) Benzo[a]pyrene goes through several steps as it is made more water soluble prior to excretion. (b) One of the intermediates in this process, B[a]P-7,8-diol-9,10-epoxide, is capable of reacting with guanine in DNA. This reaction leads to a distortion of the DNA molecule and mutations.

Several P450 enzymes are involved in key steps in the oxidation of B[a]P, and CYP1A1 has been demonstrated to be the most active in this oxidation in mammals (Chung et al, 2007). CYP1A1 activates B[a]P to B[a]P-7,8-epoxide, which through hydration by epoxide hydrolase (EH) is metabolized to (+/-)-B[a]P-trans-7,8-dihydrodiol (DHD). B[a]P-7,8-DHD may then serve as a substrate for a second CYP-dependent oxidation reaction, generating the ultimate carcinogenic metabolite r-7,t-8- dihydrodiol-t-9,10-oxy-7,8,9,10-tetrahydrobenzo[a]pyrene (BPDE-I) (Fig 1a). In the nucleus, the diol- epoxides may covalently bind to DNA, mainly forming deoxyguanoside-DNA adducts, which may result in misreplication and mutagenesis (Kaina, 2003) (Fig 1b).

2. Effects of benzo[a]pyrene on reproduction

Adverse reproductive effects were observed in several studies with B[a]P. Exposure of male and female zebrafish to B[a]P impaired reproduction in zebrafish (Hoffmann and Oris, 2006). Intraperitoneal administration of B[a]P to rat embryos has resulted in stillbirths, resorptions, and malformations; decreases in follicular growth and corpora lutea; and in testicular changes (Luijten et al, 2008). Subcutaneous injections of B[a]P produced increased resorptions in rats and direct embryonal injection led to decreased fetal survival in mice (Pereraa et al, 2005). In utero exposure to B[a]P has produced adverse reproductive effects in mice (Legraverend, et al, 1984). Dietary administration of doses as low as 10 mg/kg during gestation caused reduced fertility and reproductive capacity in offspring (Mackenzie and Angevine, 1981) and treatment by gavage with 120 mg/kg/day during gestation caused stillbirths and malformations (Legraverend et al, 1984).

2.1 Benzo[a]pyrene and male fertility

Spermatogenesis is carefully controlled to produce mature spermatozoa from spermatogonial stem cells in three major stages – the mitotic stage, the meiotic stage and the maturation stage (Verhofstad et al, 2010). Germ cells are susceptible for the induction of mutations during mitotic and meiotic divisions, because cell turnover is a prerequisite for fixation of DNA damage into mutations (Somers et al, 2002). Changes in the DNA sequence can be induced by exposure to chemicals during life, but may also be inherited via mutations in the spermatogonial stem cells, in that way increasing the risk of developing abnormalities or diseases in the offspring (Vilarino-Guell et al, 2003). B[a]P related DNA damages were observed at all stages of spermatogenesis (Zenzes et al, 1999), which were associated with significantly decreased sperm counts (Verhofstad et al, 2009).

Although B[a]P has been studied with respect to sperm DNA adducts (Kao et al, 1998) and apoptosis (Whitfield et al, 2002), few studies have evaluated its possible effect on sperm motion characteristics. Because the motion characteristics, hyperactivation status, and acrosomal reaction of spermatozoa indicate functional status and fertilizing potential (Cheo et al, 1997), it is worthwhile to note whether B[a]P has any effect on these parameters (Fig 2). A study of adult male F-344 rats showed that subchronic exposure to inhaled B[a]P contributed to reduced testicular and epididymal function (NTP, 2000). Moreover, some studies have proved that escalating hypermotility of spermatozoa occurs with increasing concentrations of B[a]P as a result of premature capacitation (Zenzes, 2000). B[a]P treatment can significantly decrease the percentage of halo formation, and the hyperactivation status attained due to B[a]P treatment induces false acrosomal reactions in the spermatozoa (Yauk et al, 2008).

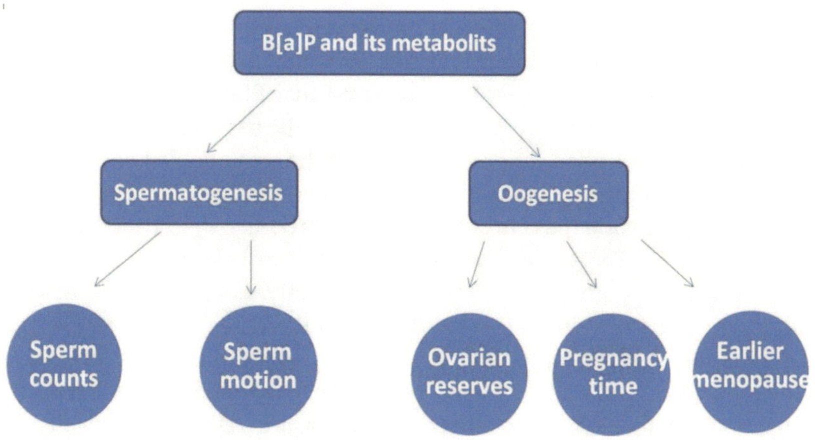

Fig. 2. Influence of benzo[a]pyrene on male and female fertility.

2.2 Benzo[a]pyrene and female fertility

Ovarian function can be compromised by exposure to toxic chemicals (Younglai et al, 2007). In addition, the ovary itself can be affected resulting in disturbances in oocyte maturation and/or destruction of the oocyte. The mechanism of B[a]P-mediated ovotoxicity may be indirect (Fig 2), since oocytes at all stages of development are surrounded by follicular cells (Hombach-Klonisch et al, 2005). A loss in integrity of this follicular wall by B[a]P may compromise its ability to maintain oocyte viability (El Nemr et al, 1998). Extensive damages of ovarian follicles would also impair steroid hormone production which, in turn, affects the endocrine balance and results in ovarian failure (Shiverick and Salafa, 1999). The carcinogenic metabolite (BPDE-I) is a diol epoxide derivative of B[a]P which binds predominantly to the 2-amino group of DNA guanosine and forms adducts. In ovarian tissue, BPDE-DNA adducts were detected in oocytes and luteal cells in ovaries of adult women who were exposed to cigarette smoke from smoking themselves or from second-hand smoke (Wright et al, 2006).

B[a]P was reported to cross the placenta in mice, rats, and guinea pigs following maternal injection, dermal, or inhalation exposure to B[a]P (Karttunena et al, 2010). Evidence from human studies indicates that BPDE-DNA adducts have been found in the placentas of smoking mothers (Motejlek et al, 2006). In addition, prolonged time to pregnancy, earlier mean age of menopause, altered ovarian steroidogenesis, and depleted ovarian reserves, have all been observed in women who smoke compared to non-smokers (Younglai et al, 2005). Inhalation exposure of pregnant rats or mice to B[a]P resulted in decreased numbers of live pups at birth (Archibong et al, 2002; Wu et al, 2003). Injection of B[a]P to pregnant rats resulted in decreased fetal weight and increased fetal death (Bui et al, 2003). Administration of B[a]P by ingestion to pregnant rats resulted in an increased number of stillborn pups (Perera et al, 2004). Injection of pregnant mice with B[a]P also resulted in measurable changes in some enzymes in lungs (pyruvate kinase and lactic acid dehydrogenase) of exposed fetuses (Parman and Wells, 2002).

3. Mechanisms of benzo[a]pyrene on reproductive toxicity

3.1 Oxidative stress and damage

B[a]P has been proved to be able to enhance the generation of reactive oxygen species (ROS) by inducing cytochrome P450 enzymes and free radiocals produced by B (a) P metabolism (Ji and Shen, 2009). Numerous studies demonstrated that B[a]P can induce oxidative DNA damage and the formation of teratogenic ROS, and B[a]P have been postulated, at least in part, to be involved in the underlying mechanisms in the teratogenicity of B[a]P (Wells et al, 2009). Most ROS are too unstable to travel beyond the cell, which are capable of damaging every molecule present inside the cell: carbohydrates, proteins, lipids and the DNA (Kovacic and Somanathan, 2006). Teratogenicity likely depends to a large extent upon a balance between the pathogenic pathways of xenobiotic bioactivation, oxidative macromolecular damage and signal transduction on one hand, and on the other, the protective pathways of maternal elimination, embryonic detoxification of xenobiotic reactive intermediates and reactive oxygen species, and embryonic pathways for the detection and repair of oxidative DNA damage (Jeng et al, 2005). Accordingly, embryopathic risk is theoretically determined by the balance between the pathogenic and embryoprotective pathways. The risk of ROS-mediated teratogenesis can be enhanced by either genetic or environmental determinants that increase embryonic xenobiotic bioactivation or decrease one or more of the antioxidants, so the teratologically relevant processes of embryopathic xenobiotic bioactivation and reactive intermediate detoxification, ROS formation and their associated protective pathways involving antioxidants and antioxidative enzymes, and pathways for the repair of oxidative DNA damage, all lie exclusively within the embryo.

3.2 Apoptosis and cell cycle

B[a]P has been shown to induce apoptosis and necrosis in various cell types (Ko et al, 2004; Patil et al, 2009). There are two major mitochondria-dependent pathways involved in apoptosis. One is mediated by Bax, a proapoptotic member of the Bcl-2 family. After receiving death signals, Bax is activated and inserts into the mitochondrial membrane, causing cytochrome c release, which triggers downstream apoptotic pathway, including apoptosome formation, caspase cascade activation, and nuclear degradation (Teijido and Dejean, 2010). B[a]P has been shown to activate apoptotic pathways in a number of studies using mammalian cell lines (Jiang et al, 2011). Other study with B[a]P in JEG-3 (human trophoblastic) cells found no evidence of apoptosis based on analysis of cell cycle phase distribution, DNA fragmentation, or Bax or Bcl-2 levels, which may due to concentration or cell type specific (Drukteinis et al, 2005).

Cell cycle regulation has been increasingly recognized as one of the important mechanisms required for the teratogenicity of B[a]P during the past several years. As reported, B[a]P induces cell cycle arrest in MCF-7 (human breast carcinoma) and HELF (human embryo lung fibroblasts) cells, and altered expression of genes that affect cell cycle regulation (Khan and Dipple, 2000; Gao et al, 2005). Moreover, cell cycle phases showed an accumulation of cells in the G1 and G2 phase after B[a]P exposure (Vaziri et al, 1997; Zhu et al, 2005). It has also been shown that BPDE, the metabolite of B[a]P, can induce a G2/M accumulation (Wang et al, 2003). In line with these findings, G1-S arrest was observed in testis of B[a]P exposed male mice(Verhofstad et al, 2010). B[a]P produces growth inhibition involving

G2/M arrest in JEG-3 trophoblastic cells (Drukteinis et al, 2005). Expression of G2/M phase genes showed a trend towards a higher induction of these genes in testis of mice after B[a]P exposure.

We and other have demonstrated that B[a]P could stimulate cell proliferation through certain signaling pathways (Jiao et al, 2008; Gao et al, 2007; Tannheimer et al, 1998). In addition, B[a]P-induced cell proliferation is accompanied by increased G1/S transition (Gao et al, 2006; Jia et al, 2006). Cyclin D1 serves as a key sensor and integrator of extracellular signals of cells in early to mid-G1 phase, involved in regulation of cell proliferation and differentiation (Neumeister et al, 2003). Cyclin D1 in complex with its partner, cyclin-dependent kinase 4 (CDK4), phosphorylates the product of the retinoblastoma gene, the retinoblastoma protein (pRb), a well known tumor suppressor. The phosphorylated pRb releases the E2F family that plays an integral role in cell cycle progression by inducing the expression of gene required for S phase entry (Wang et al, 2004). In a previous study, we found that B[a]P exposure also induces cyclin D1 overexpression in HELFs (Du et al, 2006; Ye et al, 2008). Exposure of HELF cells to B[a]P obviously induced cyclin D1 transcription in a dose- and time-dependent manners (Jiao et al, 2008). Cyclin D1/CDK4-E2F-1/4 pathways are also involved in the cell cycle changes in B[a]P-treated HELFs, but these pathways have different patterns in response to low dose and high dose B[a]P treatment: in cells treated with 2 μmol/L B[a]P, cyclin D1 positively regulates the expression of E2F-1, whereas CDK4 negatively regulates the expression of E2F-4; in cells treated with 100 μmol/L B[a]P, both cyclin D1 and CDK4 negatively regulate the expression of E2F-4 (Ye et al, 2008). All the above studies have demonstrated that cell cycle changes are involved in the teratogenicity of B[a]P.

3.3 Aberrant signaling pathways

Oxidative and genotoxic stress induced by B[a]P, activate checkpoint mechanisms for cell cycle control and apoptosis involving the p53 pathway and $p21^{CIP1}$ in mammalian cells (Pääjärvi et al, 2008). The importance of DNA damage detection is supported by the enhanced teratogenicity of B[a]P in p53 knockout mice (Nicol et al, 1995). We noted that primary sensors of DNA damage and stress appear to be the phosphotidyl-inostitol-3-(PI-3) kinases such as DNA-dependent protein kinase (DNA-PK), ATM (ataxia-telangiectasiamutated), and/or ATR(ATM related), with activation of p53 involving phosphorylation on serine 15 (Laposa et al, 2004; Bhuller and Wells, 2006).We previously found that PI-3K pathway was implicated in activator factor 1 (AP-1) transactivation induced by B[a]P (Gao, et al., 2007). C-Jun, a primary member components of AP-1 families, have been proved to be required for B[a]P-induced cell cycle alternation (Jiao et al, 2008). The conventional position of the c-Jun protein in the signaling transduction cascades is close to mitogen activated protein kinase (MAPK) family (Kennedy and Davis, 2003). Two subgroups of the MAPK family, extracellular signaling regulated kinase (ERK) and c-Jun NH2-terminal kinase (JNK), have been demonstrated to be able to activate c-Jun activation in B[a]P-treated HELF (Jiao et al, 2007). Other evidence shows that NF-κB signaling pathway might be involved during in the teratogenicity of B[a]P (Li et al, 2004).

4. Future work

Evidence from molecular studies in vitro combined with results from complementary studies in embryo culture and in vivo suggest that B[a]P in animal models contribute to both constitutive origins of teratogenesis as well as a broad spectrum of B[a]P and its metabolites-initiated adverse developmental outcomes, including structural birth defects, traditionally referred to as teratogenesis, as well as developmental deficits and cancer in later postnatal life.

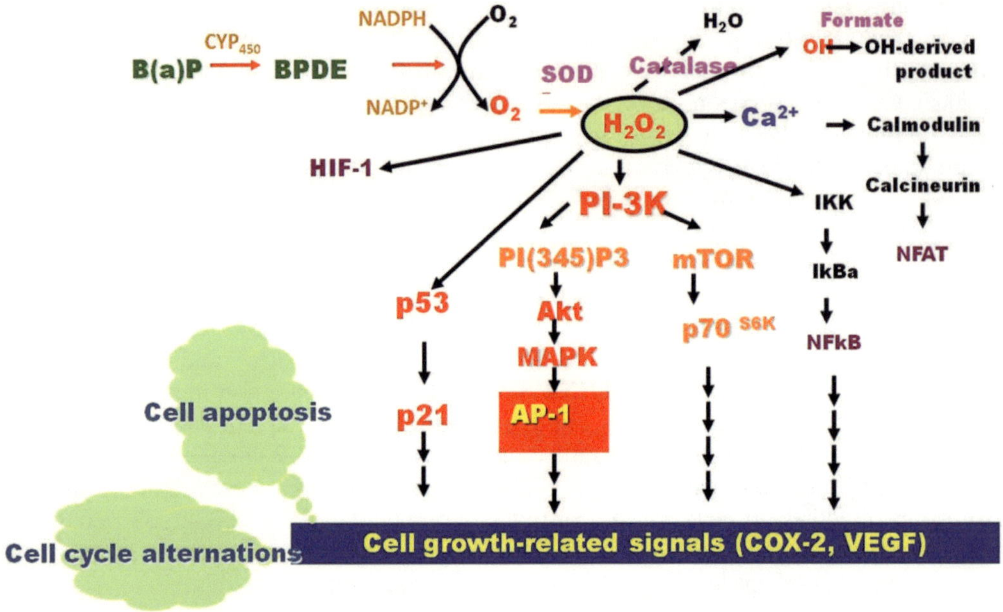

Fig. 3. Mechanism of benzo(a)pyrene-related reproduction toxicity.

At least some of probably mechanisms such as oxidative macromolecular damage, cell cycle alternation and signaling pathway aberrant activation, are involved in the the risk of teratogenesis of B[a]P (Fig 3). However, we still know relatively little about the full nature of B[a]P teratogenicity, particularly with regard to its signal transduction. It is likely that other important contributing signaling pathways remain to be discovered, and that more than one mechanism may contribute to the same adverse reproductive outcome. The results from animal studies provide a basis for similar evaluations in humans, for whom little information is available.

5. Acknowledgment

This work was supported by grants of National Natural Science Foundation of China (30972449, 30671747).

6. References

Archibong AE, Inyang F, Ramesh A, et al. (2002) Alteration of pregnancy related hormones and fetal survival in F-344 rats exposed by inhalation to benzo(a)pyrene. Reprod Toxicol 16: 801-808.

Bhuller Y & Wells PG. (2006) A developmental role for ataxia-telangiectasia mutated in protecting the embryo from spontaneous and phenytoin enhanced embryopathies in culture. Toxicol Sci. 93: 156-163.

Boström CE, Gerde P, Hanberg A, et al, (2002) Cancer risk assessment, indicators, and guidelines for polycyclic aromatic hydrocarbons in the ambient air. Environ Health Perspect 110: 451-488.

Bui QQ, Tran MB & West WL. (1986) A comparative study of the reproductive effects of methadone and benzo[a]pyrene in the pregnant and pseudopregnant rat. Toxicology 42: 195-204.

Cheo DL, Ruven HJ, Meira LB, et al. (1997) Characterization of defective nucleotide excision repair in XPC mutant mice. Mutat Res. 374: 1-9.

Chung JY, Kim JY, Kim YJ, et al. (2007) Cellular defense mechanisms against benzo[a]pyrene in testicular Leydig cells: implications of p53, aryl-hydrocarbon receptor, and cytochrome P450 1A1 status. Endocrinology. 148: 6134-6144.

Drukteinis JS, Medrano T, Ablordeppey E A, et al. (2005) Benzo[a]pyrene, but not 2,3,7,8-TCDD, Induces G2/M cell cycle arrest, p21CIP1 and p53 phosphorylation in human choriocarcinoma JEG-3 cells: a distinct signaling Pathway. Placenta, 26 Suppl A:S87-95.

Du H, Tang N, Liu B, et al. (2006) Benzo(a)pyrene-induced cell cycle progression is through ERKs/cyclin D1 pathway and requires the activation of JNKs and p38 mapk in human diploid lung fibroblasts. Mol Cell Biochem. 287: 78-89.

El Nemr A, Al Shawaf T, Sabatini L, et al. (1998) Effect of smoking on ovarian reserve and ovarian stimulation in in-vitro fertilization and embryo transfer. Hum Reprod . 13: 2192-2198.

Gao A, Liu B, Shi X, et al. (2006) Vitamin C inhibits benzo(a)pyrene-induced cell cycle changes partly via cyclin D1/E2F pathway in human embryo lung fibroblasts. Biomed. Environ. Science. 19: 239-244.

Gao A, Liu B, Shi X, et al. (2007) Phosphatidylinositol-3 kinase/Akt/p70S6K/AP-1 signaling pathway mediated benzo(a)pyrene-induced cell cycle alternation via cell cycle regulatory proteins in human embryo lung fibroblasts. Toxicol. Lett. 170: 30-41.

Guo N, Faller D V & Vaziri C. (2002) Carcinogen-induced S-phase arrest is Chk1 mediated and caffeine sensitive. Cell Growth Differ. 13: 77-86.

Hoffmann JL & Oris JT. (2006) Altered gene expression: A mechanism for reproductive toxicity in zebrafish exposed to benzo[a]pyrene. Aquat Toxicol. 78: 332-40.

Hombach-Klonisch S, Pocar P, Kietz S, et al. (2005) Molecular actions of polyhalogenated arylhydrocarbons (PAHs) in female reproduction. Current Medicinal Chemistry. 12: 599-616.

Jeng W, Wong AW, Ting-A-Kee R, et al. (2005). Methamphetamine- enhanced embryonic oxidative DNA damage and neurodevelopmental de?cits. Free Radic Biol Med 39: 317-326.

Ji HF & Shen L. (2009) Mechanisms of reactive oxygen species photogeneration by benzo[a]pyrene: A DFT study. J Mol Structure: THEOCHEM. 893: 6-8.

Jia X, Liu B, Shi X, et al. (2006) Inhibition of Benzo(a)pyrene-induced cell cycle progression by all-trans retinoic acid partly through cyclin D1/E2F-1 pathway in human embryo lung fibroblasts. Cell Biology International. 30: 183-189.

Jiang Y, Zhou X, Chen X, et al. (2011) Benzo(a)pyrene-induced mitochondrial dysfunction and cell death in p53-null Hep3B cells. Mutat Res. [Epub ahead of print]

Jiao S, Liu B, Gao A,et al. (2008) Benzo(a)pyrene-caused increased G1-S transition requires the activation of c-Jun through p53-dependent PI-3K/Akt/ERK pathway in human embryo lung fibroblasts.Toxicol Lett. 178: 167-175.

Jiao S, Liu B, Shi X, et al. (2006) JNK and ERK signaling pathways regulate Benzo(a)pyrene-induced c-Jun activation in human embryo lung fibroblasts. Zhonghua Lao Dong Wei Sheng Zhi Ye Bing Za Zhi. 25: 385-388.

Kaina B. (2003) DNA damage-triggered apoptosis: critical role of DNA repair, double-strand breaks, cell proliferation and signaling. Biochem Pharmacol 66: 1547-1554.

Kao SH, Chao HT & Wei YH. (1998) Multiple deletions of mitochondrial DNA are associated with the decline of motility and fertility of human spermatozoa. Mol Hum Reprod. 4: 657-666.

Karttunena V, Myllynenb P, Prochazkac G, et al. (2010) Placental transfer and DNA binding of benzo(a)pyrene in human placental perfusion. Toxicol Lett. 197: 75-81.

Kennedy Nj and Davis RJ. (2003) Role of JNK in tumor development. Cell Cycle 2:199-201.

Khan Q A & Dipple A (2000). Diverse chemical carcinogens fail to induce G1 arrest in MCF-7 cells. Carcinogenesis. 21:1611-1618.

Knafla A, Phillipps KA, Brecher RW, et al. (2006) Development of a dermal cancer slope factor for benzo[a]pyrene. Regul Toxico. Pharmaco. 45: 159-168.

Ko CB, Kim SJ, Park C, et al. (2004) Benzo(a)pyrene-induced apoptotic death of mouse hepatoma Hepa1c1c7 cells via activation of intrinsic caspase and mito- chondrial dysfunction. Toxicology. 199: 35-46.

Kovacic P & Somanathan R. (2006). Mechanisms of teratogenesis: electron transfer, reactive oxygen species and antioxidants. Birth Defects Research Part C: Embryo Today Reviews. 78: 308-325.

Laposa RR, Henderson JT, Xu E, et al. (2004) Atm-null mice exhibit enhanced radiation-induced birth defects and a hybrid form of embryonic programmed cell death indicating a teratological suppressor function for ATM. FASEB J 18: 896-898.

Legraverend C, Guenthner TM and Nebert DW. (1984) Importance of the route of administration for genetic differences in benzo[a]pyrene-induced in utero toxicity and teratogenicity. Teratology. 29: 35-47.

Li J, Chen H, Ke Q, et al. (2004) Differential effects of polycyclic aromatic hydrocarbons on transactivation of AP-1 and NF-kappaB in mouse epidermal cl41 cells. Mol Carcinog 40: 104-115.

Luijten M, Verhoef A, Westerman A, et al. (2008) Application of a metabolizing system as an adjunct to the rat whole embryo culture. Toxicology in Vitro. 22: 1332-1336.

MacKenzie, KM & Angevine DM. (1981) Infertility in mice exposed in uteroto benzo[a]pyrene. Biol. Reprod. 24: 183-191.

Motejlek K, Palluch F, Neulen J, et al. (2006) Smoking impairs angiogenesis during maturation of human oocytes. Fertil Steril. 86:186-191.

National Toxicology Program (NTP, 2000). Toxicology and Carcinogenesis Studies of Naphthalene (CAS No. 91-20-3) in F344/N Rats (Inhalation Studies). TR-500.

Nebert DW, Roe AL, Dieter MZ, et al.2000. Role of the aromatic hydrocarbon receptor and [Ah] gene battery in the oxidative stress response, cell cycle control, and apoptosis. Biochem Pharmacol, 59: 65-85.

Neumeister P, Pixley FJ, Xiong Y, et al. (2003) Cyclin D1 governs adhesion and motility of macrophages. Mol Biol Cell 14: 2005-2015.

Nicol CJ, Harrison ML, Laposa RR, et al. (1995) A teratologic suppressor role for p53 in benzo[a]pyrene-treated transgenic p53-deficient mice. Nat Genet 10:181-187.

Pääjärvi G, Jernström B, Seidel A, et al. (2008) Anti-diol epoxide of benzo[a]pyrene induces transient Mdm2 and p53 Ser15 phosphorylation, while anti-diol epoxide of dibenzo[a,l]pyrene induces a nontransient p53 Ser15 phosphorylation. Mol Carcinog. 47: 301-309.

Parman, T & Wells, PG. (2002) Embryonic prostaglandin H synthase-2 (PHS-2) expression and benzo[a]pyrene teratogenicity in PHS-2 knock-out mice. FASEB J. 16: 1001-1009.

Patil AJ, Gramajo AL, Sharma A, et al. (2009) Effects of benzo(e)pyrene on the retinal neurosensory cells and human microvascular endothelial cells in vitro. Curr. Eye Res. 34: 672-682.

Perera FP, Rauh V, Whyatt RM, et al. (2004) Molecular evidence of an interaction between prenatal environmental exposures and birth outcomes in a multiethnic population. Environ.Health Perspect. 112: 626-630.

Pereraa FP, Rauha V, Whyatt RM, et al. (2005) A summary of recent findings on birth outcomes and developmental effects of renatal ETS, PAH, and pesticide exposures. NeuroToxicology. 26: 573-587.

Pickford D & Morris LD. (1999) Effects of endocrine-disrupting contaminants on amphibian oogenesis: methoxychlor inhibits progesterone-induced maturation of xenopus laevis oocytes in vitro. Environ Health Perspect. 107: 285-292.

Research article

Shimizu, Y, Nakatsuru, Y, Ichinose, M, et al. (2000) Benz[a]pyrene carcinogenicity is lost in mice lacking the arylhydrocarbon receptor. Proc Natl Acad Sci USA 97: 779-782.

Shiverick KT & Salafa C. (1999) Cigarette smoking and pregnancy I: ovarian, uterine and placental effects. Placenta. 20: 265-272.

Somers CM, Yauk CL, White PA, et al. (2002) Air pollution induces heritable DNA mutations. Proc Natl Acad Sci USA. 99:15904-15907.

Tannheimer SL. Ethier SP, Caldwell KK, et al. (1998) Polycyclic aromatic hydrocarbon-induced alterations in tyrosine phosphorylation and insulin-like growth factor signaling pathways in the MCF-10A human mammary epithelial cell line. Carcinogenesis. 19: 1291-1297.

Teijido O & Dejean L. (2010) Upregulation of Bcl2 inhibits apoptosis-driven BAX insertion but favors BAX relocalization in mitochondria, FEBS Lett. 584: 3305-3310.

Vaziri C & Faller DV. (1997) A benzo[a]pyrene-induced cell cycle checkpoint resulting in p53-independent G1 arrest in 3T3 fibroblasts. J Biol Chem. 272: 2762-2769.

Verhofstad N, Pennings J L, van Oostrom CT, et al. (2010) Benzo(a)pyrene induces similar gene expression changes in testis of DNA repair proficient and deficient mice. BMC Genomics. 11:333-344.

Verhofstad N, van Oostrom CT, van Benthem J, et al. (2009) DNA adduct kinetics in reproductive tissues of DNA repair proficient and deficient male mice after oral exposure to benzo(a)pyrene. Environ Mol Mutagen. 51: 123-129.

Vilarino-Guell C, Smith AG and Dubrova YE. (2003) Germline mutation induction at mouse repeat DNA loci by chemical mutagens. Mutat Res. 526: 63-73.

Wang A, Gu J, Kremer K J, et al. (2003) Response of human mammary epithelial cells to DNA damage induced by BPDE: involvement of novel regulatory pathways. Carcinogenesis 24:225-234.

Wang C, Li Z, Fu M, et al. (2004) Signal transduction mediated by cyclin D1: from mitogens to cell proliferation: a molecular target with therapeutic potential. Cancer Treat Res. 119: 217-237.

Wells PG, McCallum GP, Chen CS, et al. (2009) Oxidative stress in developmental origins of disease: teratogenesis, neurodevelopmental de?cits, and cancer. Toxicol Sci. 108: 4-18.

Whitfield ML, Sherlock G, Saldanha AJ, et al. (2002) Identification of genes periodically expressed in the human cell cycle and their expression in tumors. Mol Biol Cell. 13: 1977-2000.

Wright KP, Trimarchi JR, Allsworth J, et al. (2006) The effect of female tobacco smoking on IVF outcomes. Hum Reprod. 21: 1930-1934.

Wu J, Ramesh A, Nayyar T, et al. (2003) Assessment of metabolites and AhR and CYP1A1 mRNA expression subsequent to prenatal exposure to inhaled benzo(a)pyrene. Int J Dev Neurosci. 21: 333-346.

Yauk C, Polyzos A, Rowan-Carroll A, et al. (2008) Germ-line mutations, DNA damage, and global hypermethylation in mice exposed to particulate air pollution in an urban/industrial location. Proc Natl Acad Sci USA. 105: 605-610.

Ye M, Liu B, Shi X, et al. (2008) Different patterns of Cyclin D1/CDK4-E2F-1/4 pathways in human embryo lung fibroblasts treated by benzo[a]pyrene at different doses. Biomed Environ Sci. 21: 30-36.

Younglai EV, Holloway AC & Foster WG. (2005) Environmental and occupational factors affecting fertility and IVF success. Hum Reprod Update. 11: 43-57.

Younglai EV, Wu YJ & Foster WG. (2007) Reproductive Toxicology of Environmental Toxicants: Emerging Issues and Concerns. Current Pharmaceutical Design. 13:, 3005-3019.

Zenzes MT, Bielecki R & Reed TE. (1999) Detection of benzo(a)pyrene diol epoxide-DNA adducts in sperm of men exposed to cigarette smoke. Fertil Steri. 72:330-335.

Zenzes MT. (2000) Smoking and reproduction: Gene damage to human gametes and embryos. Hum Reprod Update. 6: 122-131.

Zhu H, Smith C, Ansah C, et al. (2005) Responses of genes involved in cell cycle control to diverse DNA damaging chemicals in human lung adenocarcinoma A549 cells. Cancer Cell Int 5: 28.

Part 3

Organogenesis and Genetics

7

Developmental Anatomy of the Human Embryo – 3D-Imaging and Analytical Techniques

Shigehito Yamada[1], Takashi Nakashima[2], Ayumi Hirose[2], Akio Yoneyama[3], Tohoru Takeda[4] and Tetsuya Takakuwa[2]
[1]*Congenital Anomaly Research Center, Kyoto University,*
[2]*Human Health Science, Kyoto University,*
[3]*Central Research Laboratory, Hitachi Ltd.,*
[4]*Allied Health Sciences, Kitasato University,*
Japan

1. Introduction

Prenatal or antenatal development is a process during which the human embryo undergoes complex morphogenetic changes. To understand and characterize the dynamic events underlying human ontogenesis, it is useful to visualize embryonic structures in three-dimensions (3D). Classically, solid reconstruction and fine drawing have been the primary approaches used to model the architecture of the embryonic body. The most impressive wax models of staged human embryos are housed at the Carnegie Institution of Washington DC in the Human Developmental Anatomy Center (see Fig. 1 in Chapter 1). The wax plate technique of reconstruction was first introduced to human embryology by Gustav Born (1883), and later modified in the Carnegie Laboratory in Baltimore by Osborne O. Heard and his colleagues (Heard, 1951, Heard, 1953, Heard, 1957). The procedure involves embedding of human embryos in paraffin wax, followed by serial sectioning and histological staining. Wax plates were cut faithfully as the enlarged image of each section, and the wax plates were piled up for making the 3D embryonic structures. These reconstructed models allowed for the production of accurate drawings of human embryos, some of the most notable being those of James F. Didusch, a medical artist who added valuable information to the understanding of human prenatal development (O'Rahilly, 1988). However, both solid reconstruction and fine drawings used in classical embryology are time-consuming and require specific and rare skills.

In the past decades, the visualization of biological structures has been significantly facilitated by computer-assisted techniques, allowing for the three-dimensional reconstruction of human embryos from section images and offering the unique ability to manipulate reconstructed images. The difficulties that have hindered efforts in 3D reconstruction using two-dimensional image stacks revolve around the issues of section registration and distortion. A solution has come about with the advent of Episcopic Fluorescence Image Capture (EFIC), a novel imaging modality for the generation of high-resolution 3D reconstruction (Weninger and Mohun, 2002; see 2.2.1). With EFIC imaging, tissue autofluorescence is used to image the block face prior to cutting each section. Although the samples have been sliced and lost during the procedure, the optical resolution of EFIC was reported to reach approximately 5-6 μm (Yamada et al., 2010) and EFIC enables us to obtain 3D images with high-resolution comparable to the images of histological serial sections. On the other hand, remarkable progress has been made in nondestructive imaging technologies such as magnetic resonance (MR) imaging. MR imaging was originally developed as a non-invasive diagnostic tool in clinical medicine, but recent technological advances has promoted its application to detailed imaging and 3D reconstruction of tiny biological structures such as embryos (Smith, 1999, 2000, 2001, Smith et al., 1994, 1996, 1999; see 2.2.2), reaching a resolution close to 30 μm/pixel. X-ray technology is also widely used for non-destructive imaging of inner structures. Using the characteristics of X-rays as electromagnetic waves, phase-contrast X-ray imaging visualizes the phase-shift of X-ray passing through the samples and reconstructs 2D or 3D images of the samples in combination with computed tomography (Momose et al., 1996, Yoneyama et al., 2011). EFIC, MR microscopy, and phase-contrast X-ray computed tomography (CT) have all been applied to embryology. The imaging modalities are selected on the basis of their destructive vs. non-destructive features, the size of the samples and the desired resolution (Fig. 1).

Morphometrics refers to the quantitative analysis of forms, a concept that encompasses size and shape (Rohlf and Bookstein, 1990). While the qualitative morphological data obtained by classical modalities such as serial sections are not suitable for numerical conversion, the data obtained by 3D-imaging techniques (see 2.2) are easily converted for quantitative analyses. Three-dimensional morphometric analyses of human embryos from the Kyoto Collection are actively underway.

In this chapter, we will describe in detail modern modalities currently used for human embryo imaging and their applications to developmental anatomy.

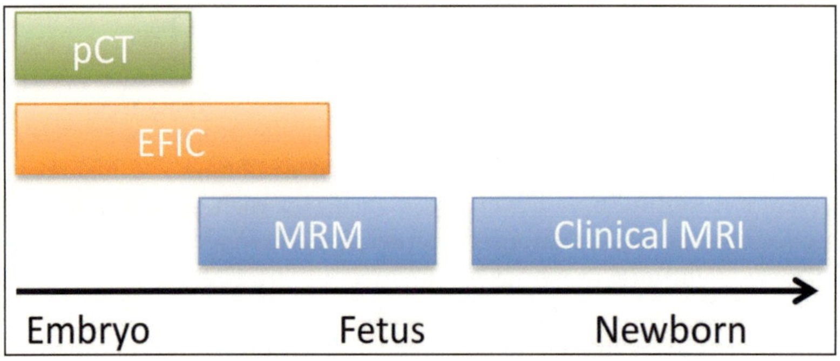

Fig. 1. Relationship between sample size and imaging techniques. pCT: phase-contrast X-ray computed tomography, EFIC: episcopic fluorescence image capture, MRM: magnetic resonance microscopy, Clinical MRI: magnetic resonance imaging for routine clinical use.

2. Imaging modalities for three-dimensional analyses

2.1 Digital reconstruction from serial sections

Classical reconstruction methods based on wax models have been described earlier. In "modern" computer-assisted reconstruction, stained histological sections are digitized using a digital camera equipped with a normal bright-field illumination. The color images of the serial sections (Fig. 2A) are then saved as TIFF files and a 3D reconstruction can be obtained using DeltaViewer (see 5. Appendix), a software designed to perform automated alignment and 3D reconstruction from serial sections. Once aligned, the images are then segmented using painting softwares (Fig. 2B) and 3D images are obtained (Fig. 2C). Further details on reconstruction procedures from serial sections can be found in previous publications (Yamada et al., 2007).

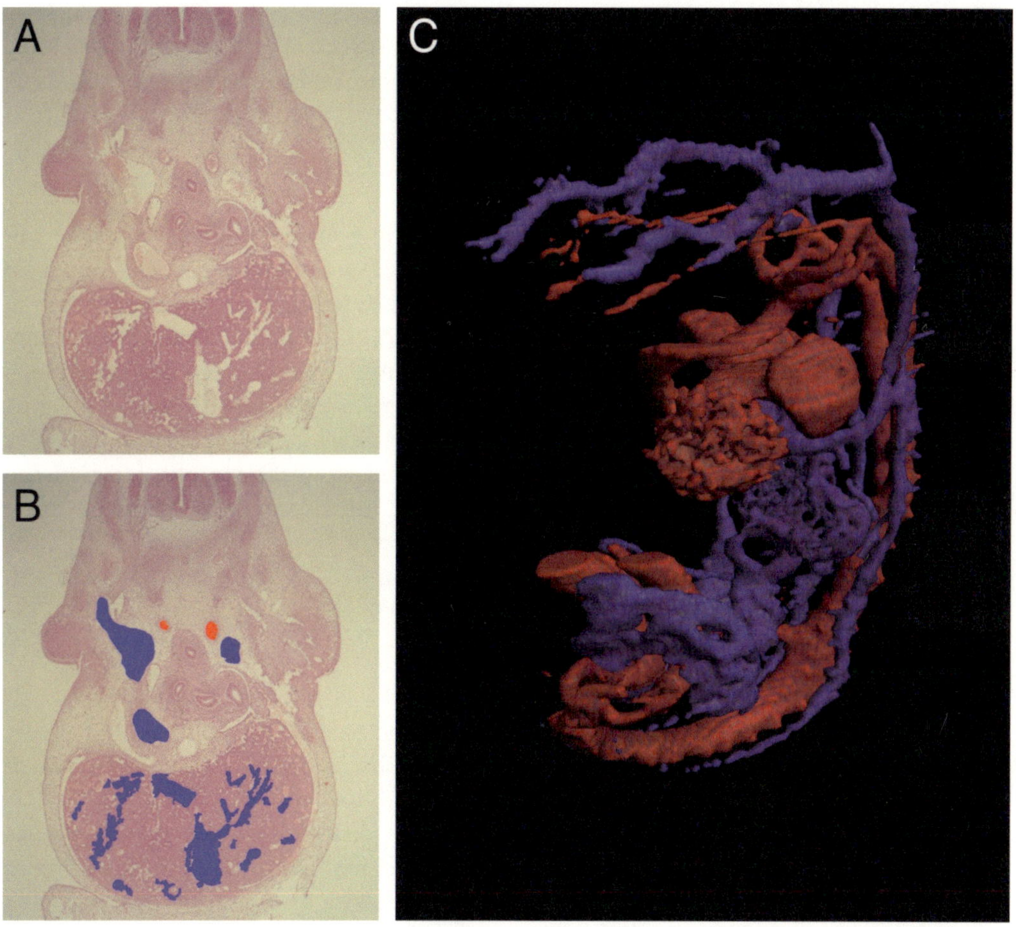

Fig. 2. Three-dimensional reconstruction from serial sections. A,B: Transverse sections of human embryo showing the spinal cord, the root of the upper limb bud, and the liver. The section is digitized (A) and manually segmented (B). C: Three-dimensional reconstruction of the heart and great vessels of human embryo at CS14 using the "DeltaViewer"software.

2.2 3D-imaging

In contrast to serial sections, 3D-imaging allows for rapid 3D rendering such as surface reconstruction and digital resectioning in arbitrary planes. Multiple 3D-imaging modalities have been applied to the human embryos of the Kyoto Collection.

2.2.1 Episcopic fluorescence image capture (EFIC)

Episcopic fluorescence image capture (EFIC) represents a novel 3D-imaging method in human embryology. This imaging technique relies on the embedding of the embryo in paraffin (Weninger and Mohun, 2002), followed by the sectioning of the block using a sliding microtome. Prior to cutting each section, the block face is imaged by capturing tissue autofluorescence. The block is accurately returned to exactly the same photo-position on the microtome, and registered 2D image stacks are automatically generated. EFIC allows for virtual resectioning of the specimen in arbitrary planes (Rosenthal et al., 2004, Weninger et al., 2006), and rapid high-resolution 3D reconstructions (Rosenthal et al., 2004). This method was applied to staged human embryos housed at the Kyoto Collection (Yamada et al., 2010; see Figure 3A).

2.2.2 Magnetic resonance microscopy

Magnetic resonance (MR) imaging applied to the scanning of small samples is called MR microscopy. MR microscopy is a very powerful tool for 3D measurement of chemically-fixed human embryos because of the large amounts of mobile or NMR visible protons present in the formalin preservation fluid (Matsuda et al., 2007). It is a non-invasive and non-destructive imaging process, and has been previously applied to developmental embryology in a number of animal models (Bone et al., 1986, Smith et al., 1992, 1994, 1996). MR imaging offers highly beneficial features (Effmann et al., 1988, Smith et al., 1992, Haishi et al., 2001), reaching a resolution of 40 μm/pixel or higher when scanning the samples for extended periods of time. Imaging of human embryos by MR microscopy was described using superconducting magnets ranging from 1.0T to 9.4T (Smith et al., 1996, Smith et al., 1999, Haishi et al., 2001). The images shown in Fig. 3B and 3C were obtained using MR microscopes equipped with 7T and 2.34T magnets, respectively.

2.2.3 Phase-contrast X-ray computed tomography

X-rays are electromagnetic waves, and are thus, characterized by amplitude and phase. When an X-ray passes through a sample, its amplitude is decreased and its phase is shifted. Conventional X-ray imaging (radiography) is based on absorption-contrast (i.e. amplitude imaging) and represents the mass-density distribution of X-ray inside the sample. Its sensitivity is insufficient to perform detailed analysis of samples consisting of biological soft tissues such as embryos, unless combined with the use of contrast agents or applying higher X-ray doses. Exploiting the phase information of X-rays is a solution. The sensitivity of the phase shift for light elements such as hydrogen, carbon, nitrogen, and oxygen is about 1000 times larger than that of absorption (Momose and Fukuda, 1995). To detect a phase-shift, it is essential to convert the phase shift into a change in X-ray intensity as X-ray intensities are classically measured using current-detecting devices. Conversion methods such as interferometry and diffractometry are used for the generation of 2D and 3D observations using synchrotron radiation. Devices based on this principle have been developed (Becker and Bonse, 1974, Yoneyama et al., 2004), and an image of human embryo at CS 17 obtained using a two-crystal X-ray interferometer (Yoneyama et al., 2011) is featured in Fig. 3D.

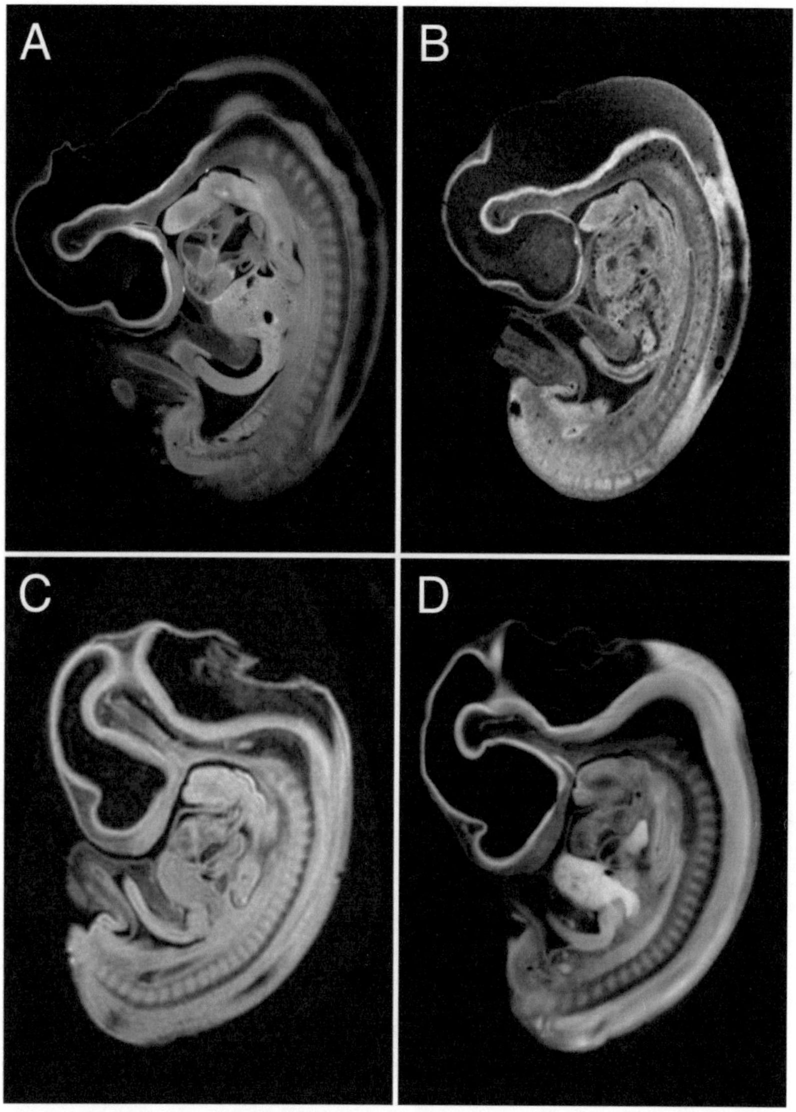

Fig. 3. Images of human embryos obtained using various imaging modalities. CS16 embryo imaging using EFIC (A) and 7T-MRI (B), CS17 embryo imaging using 2.34T MRI (C) and phase-contrast x-ray CT at 17.8keV X-ray energy (D).

3. Analyses of developmental anatomy using 3D-imaging

3.1 MR microscopy project at the Kyoto collection of human embryos

The Kyoto collection counts approximately 45,000 human embryos, and contains historical specimens housed at the Congenital Anomaly Research Center of Kyoto University (Nishimura et al., 1968, Nishimura, 1975, Shiota, 1991, Yamada et al., 2004). Most specimens were obtained from pregnancies terminated during the first trimester due to socioeconomic reasons as legally permitted under the Maternity Protection Law of Japan. Some of the specimens (~20%) are undamaged, well-preserved embryos. When the aborted materials were brought to the laboratory, the embryos were measured, examined, and staged according to the criteria of O'Rahilly and Müller (1987). Further information on the Kyoto Collection of Human Embryos can be found in Chapter 1. In 1999, Kyoto University and the University of Tsukuba initiated a collaborative project aiming to acquire 3D MR microscopic images of thousands of human embryos using a super-parallel MR microscope operated at 2.34T (Matsuda et al., 2003, 2007, Yamada et al., 2006, Shiota et al., 2007). During the course of the project, over 1,200 human embryos were scanned. Further information on the data generated can be found on the web (http://mrlab.frsc.tsukuba.ac.jp/human_embryos/).

3.2 Flow chart: from MR image acquisition to 3D image reconstruction

Approximately 1,200 well-preserved human embryos diagnosed as externally normal at CS13 to CS23 were selected for MR microscopic imaging (Fig. 4A)(Matsuda et al., 2003, 2007,

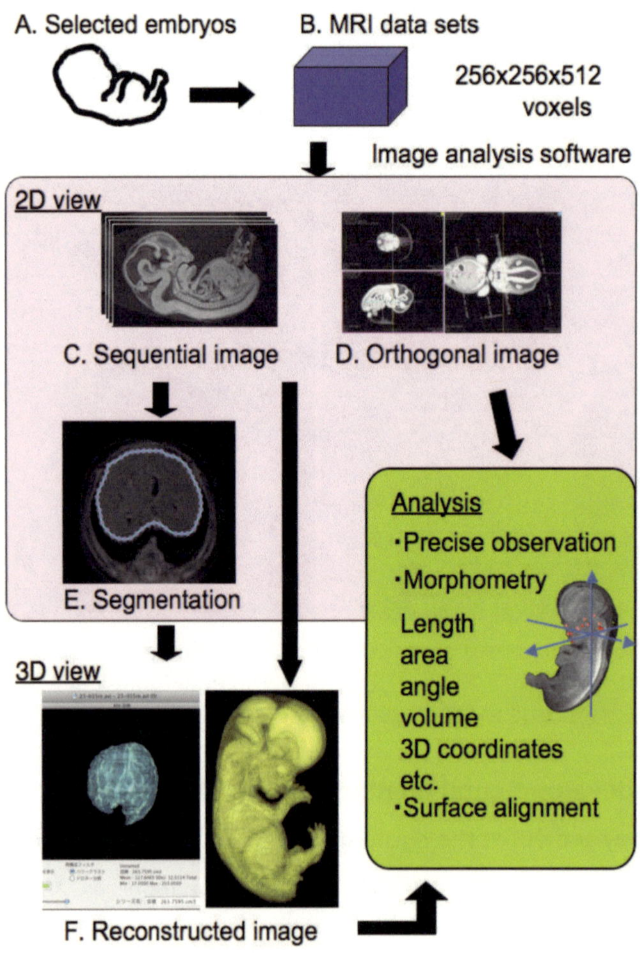

Fig. 4. Flow chart: from MR image acquisition to 3D image reconstruction

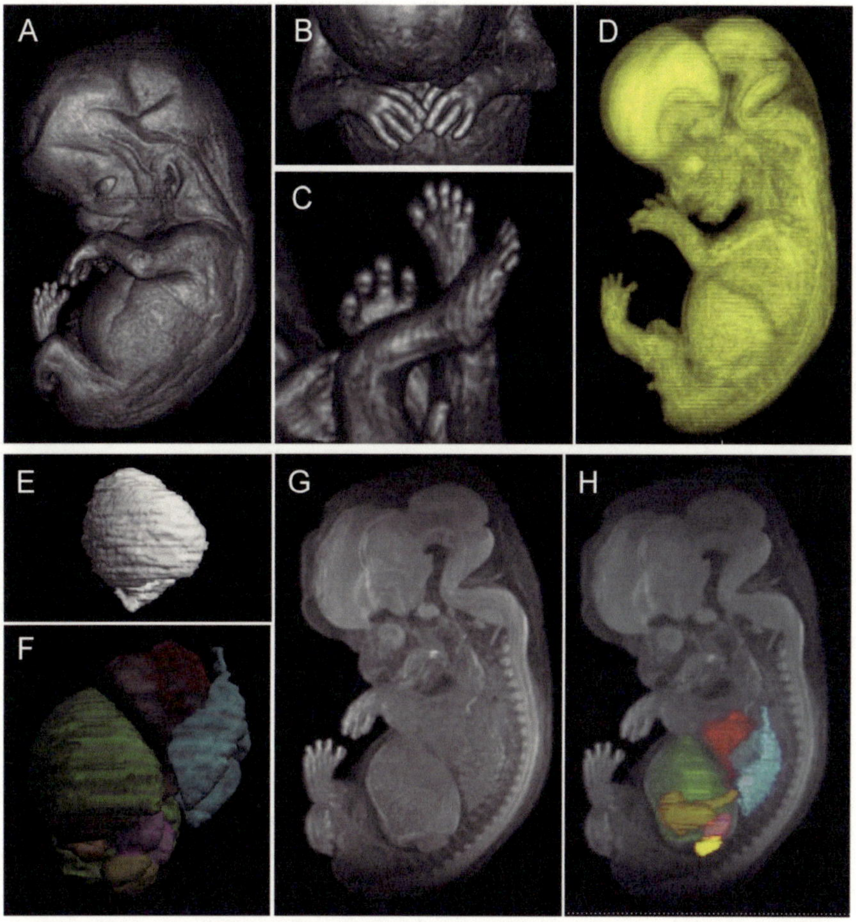

Fig. 5. Samples of 3D reconstructed images. A) 3D images of whole embryo at CS 23 using volume rendering algorithm (Osirix) to observe surfaces. B,C) Magnification of upper and lower extremities, demonstrating fine and detailed reconstruction of embryonic morphology. D) When modifying the volume-rendering settings, both external and internal embryonic structures can be observed. E) 3D-reconstruction of the embryonic liver at CS 23 obtained from segmentation of 2D sequential images. F) Liver (green), lung (blue), heart (red), kidney (yellow), and adrenal glands (purple) were segmented from 2D sequential images and reconstructed in 3D. G) 3D-reconstruction using Maximum intensity projection (MIP) tool (Osirix) in order to generate both surface and internal imaging perspectives. H) Organ images shown in F were overlaid with MIP images shown in G.

Yamada et al., 2006, Shiota et al., 2007). The 3D MR image datasets for each embryo were initially obtained from 256x256x512 voxels (Fig. 4B). Each dataset was subsequently converted into two-dimensional (2D) image stacks (Fig. 4C), which were then digitally resectioned following predefined planes (Fig. 4D). Organs of interest were segmented in series of 2D images (Fig. 4E) and the 3D architectures were computationally reconstructed (Fig. 4F). Images obtained can be freely rotated on the screen, and 3D shapes are easily recognizable and their spatial relationships rapidly determined. The obtained 2D and 3D images obtained can be subjected to further analysis.

3.3 Further processing of reconstructed 3D images using computer software

Recent advances in computer technology have significantly facilitated image rendering on personal computers. A number of algorithms have been developed resulting in multiple 3D reconstruction softwares, many of which are available as open-source. The most popular softwares are summarized in the Appendix section of this chapter. Samples of reconstructed images using such rendering algorithms are represented in Fig. 5.

3.3.1 Imaging using volume rendering techniques (Fig. 5A-D)

Volume rendering techniques are utilized to reconstruct whole embryo images. The display and comparative analysis of 3D images at various developmental stages enables a clearer understanding of embryonic morphogenesis.

Carnegie stages are primarily defined based on external structural features, e.g. cranial facial morphogenesis including eye, nose, pharyngeal arches related organs, posture of the whole embryo, finger and toe development (O'Rahilly and Müller, 1987). The external morphologies obtained by volume rendering have enough quality to determine the developmental stages of the embryos. Because these external morphologies are strictly preserved in this method, the judgment of the staging was identical with that used with original embryo specimens.

3.3.2 Three-dimensional reconstruction from segmentation of 2D sequential images (Fig. 5E, 5F)

Regions of interest (ROI) were segmented from 2D images and then reconstructed using ROI and Osirix reconstruction module. Multiple organs can be individually segmented and combined into 3D images, showing a spatial relationship clearly between adjacent organs. One limitation to 3D image rendering is the lack of information on color and touch sense e.g. pigmentation of the retina, color of superficial arteries or internal organs such as the heart. When modifying the volume rendering settings, external and internal embryonic structures can be observed simultaneously.

3.3.3 Imaging using maximum intensity projection (MIP) method (Fig. 5G, 5H)

Information on both external and internal structures can be acquired using the MIP method (Nakashima et al., 2011). Three-dimensional images obtained by MIP can be superimposed with 3D reconstruction obtained from segmented images, thus creating a see-through effect with internal organs visible from the outside.

3.4 Analysis on 3D reconstructed images

3.4.1 Three-dimensional morphological observation

Three-dimensional reconstruction offers a number of advantages. For instance, the resulting image is amenable to comprehensive examination as the image can be freely rotated on the screen, 3D shapes are easily recognizable and spatial relationships between adjacent organs or tissues become obvious. In Fig. 6, 3D reconstructed images of the embryonic liver (CS18) represented with (Fig. 6A) and without (Fig. 6B) the adjacent heart can be compared and reveal the anatomic relationship between the two organs. Indeed, the recess formed by the left ventricle is a characteristic temporal feature of the cranial surface of the liver between CS17 and CS19.

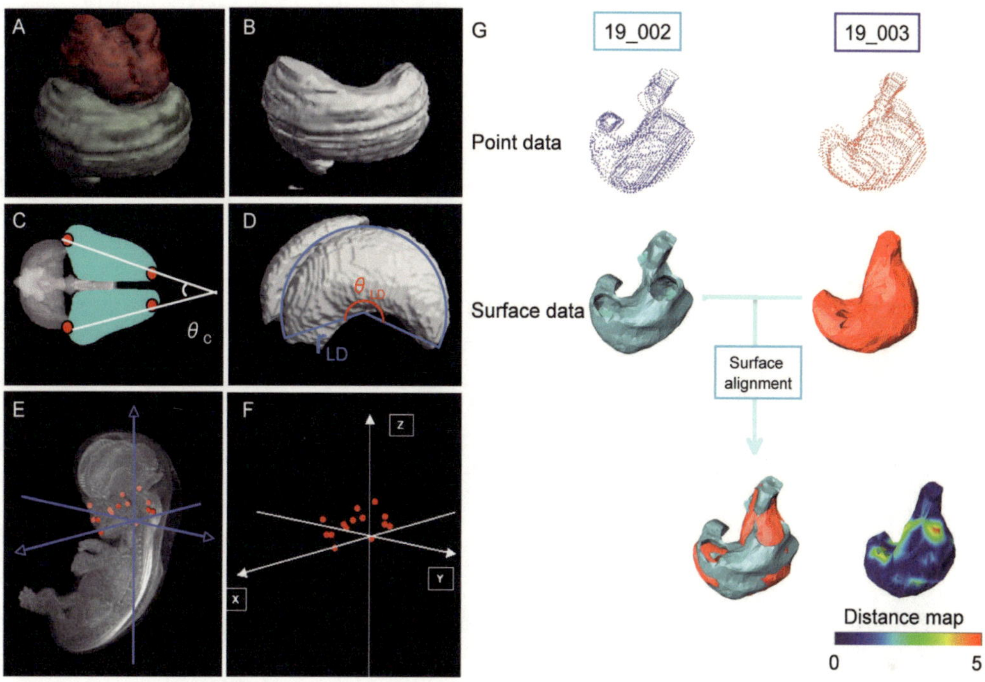

Fig. 6. Analytical methods on 3D reconstructed images.
A,B) Three-dimensional reconstructed image of the embryonic liver (CS18) with (A) and without (B) the heart demonstrate the anatomical relationship between the two organs.
C-D) Morphometry from 3D images of lateral cerebral ventricles (CS22): C) Cranial view. The blue shaded areas represent the lateral ventricles and the angle formed by the bilateral ventricles was measured. D) Lateral view. The viewing perspective was modified allowing measurement of radius and central angles.
E,F) Three-dimensional coordinates of anatomical landmarks are useful for monitoring movements between developmental stages and characterize relationships between anatomical landmarks.
G) Surface alignment provides an averaged view of the organ of interest. Here, the stomachs from two embryos at CS19 were aligned.

3.4.2 Morphometry

Three-dimensional images can be exploited to measure morphological changes in a quantitative manner. Using the image data, not only the total volumes, but also the lengths, angles and areas of the regions and organs of interest can be measured accurately (Fig. 6C, 6D). Morphometric data are useful for evaluating and characterizing developmental features of the embryo, and also for screening for abnormalities.

3.4.3 Three-dimensional coordinates

MRI data sets are provided as cuboid of 256x 256x512 voxels and thus allows for three-dimensional coordinates to be assigned to embryonic landmarks (Fig. 6E, 6F). Three-dimensional coordinates of anatomical landmarks are useful for monitoring the movements of landmarks and define their anatomical relationships during prenatal development.

3.4.4 Surface alignment

Multiple images can be aligned resulting in averaged images and compatibility rates are indicated by color gradients. An embryonic stomach was segmented from 2D sequential images (Fig. 6G) and surface data originating from point datasets of each respective embryo were processed.

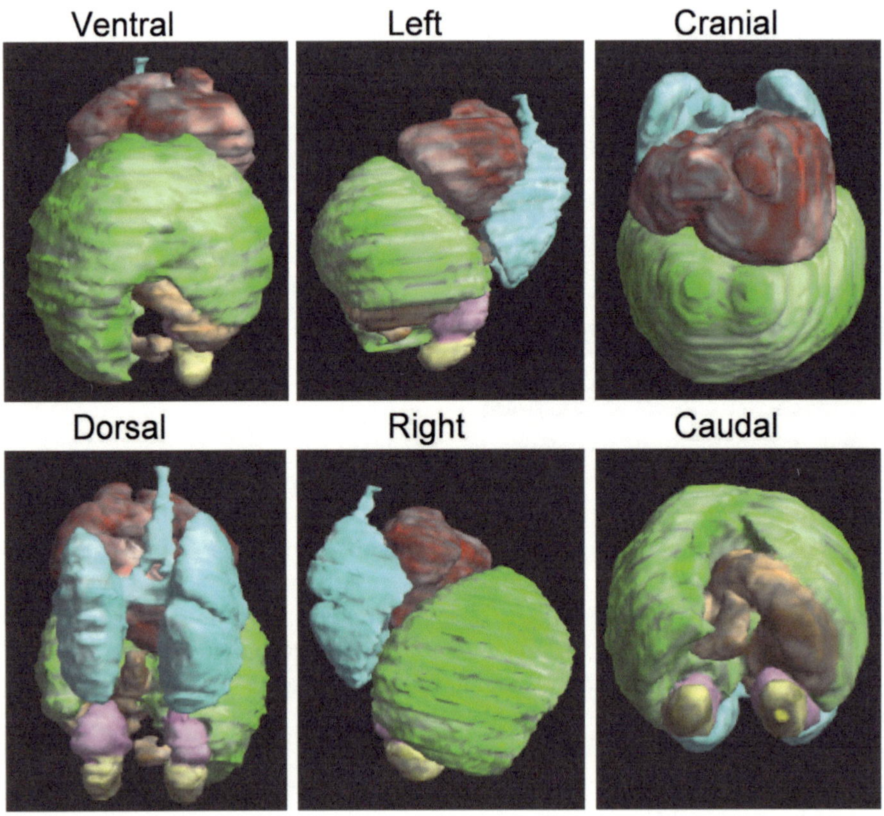

Fig. 7. Representative 3D images of the embryonic liver at CS22 with adjacent organs. Liver (green), lung (blue), heart (red), stomach (brown), kidney (yellow), and adrenal glands (purple) were segmented from 2D sequential images and reconstructed in 3D.

3.5 Representative 3D images of the embryo and fetus organs

Three-dimensional images of various organs in the embryo or the fetus were constructed and representative images of embryonic liver and cerebral ventricles are shown in Fig. 7 and Fig. 8, respectively.

4. Perspective

Recent advances in imaging techniques allow for anatomical analyses of human embryo specimens in earlier stages and for clinical prenatal diagnosis during the first trimester. Current information on normal development during embryonic stages, however, remains insufficient to achieve such clinical evaluation. Further investigations are critical to gain insight into the dynamic and complex events occurring during organogenesis. Dynamic modeling of embryonic structures and 3D digital reconstructions will be valuable tools to elucidate the complex anatomical changes taking place during early embryonic stages. They will serve as useful references to evaluate the appropriate development of embryonic organs, and understand how adjacent organs affect each other's morphology. Now and in the future, this type of information will be indispensable to researchers and to clinicians, and more particularly in respect to the obstetrical ultrasonography conducted in the early gestational weeks.

5. Appendix (softwares)

The use of software is necessary for reconstruction into 3D images and morphometric analysis. The software programs used in this chapter are summarized below. More information is available on the URL of their respective websites.

5.1 OsiriX (http://www.osirix-viewer.com/index.html)

OsiriX is an image processing software dedicated to DICOM images produced by imaging equipment (e.g. MRI, CT, PET, PET-CT, SPECT-CT, Ultrasounds). It is fully compliant with the DICOM standard for image communication and image file formats. OsiriX is able to receive images transferred by DICOM communication protocol from any PACS or imaging modality.

5.2 Image J (http://rsbweb.nih.gov/ij/index.html)

ImageJ is a public domain Java image-processing program inspired from the NIH Image software developed for Macintosh. It runs, either as an online applet or as a downloadable application, on any computer with a Java 1.4 or later virtual machine.

5.3 Delta viewer (http://delta.math.sci.osaka-u.ac.jp/DeltaViewer/index.html)

DeltaViewer is an application program developed for Apple Macintosh. DeltaViewer reads sequences of cross-sectional images of a sample in a manner similar to confocal laser microscopes, CT, MRI, optical or electron microscopes. The computer program then reconstructs the surface of the scanned sample, and displays the image on the screen. The image can then be freely rotated, for characterization of 3D shapes and spatial relationships.

5.4 Avizo (http://www.vsg3d.com/avizo/overview)

Avizo® software is a powerful, multifaceted tool for visualizing, manipulating, and understanding scientific and industrial data. Wherever 3D data sets need to be processed, in materials science, geosciences, environmental or engineering applications, Avizo offers abundant state-of-the-art features within an intuitive workflow and easy-to-use graphical user interfaces.

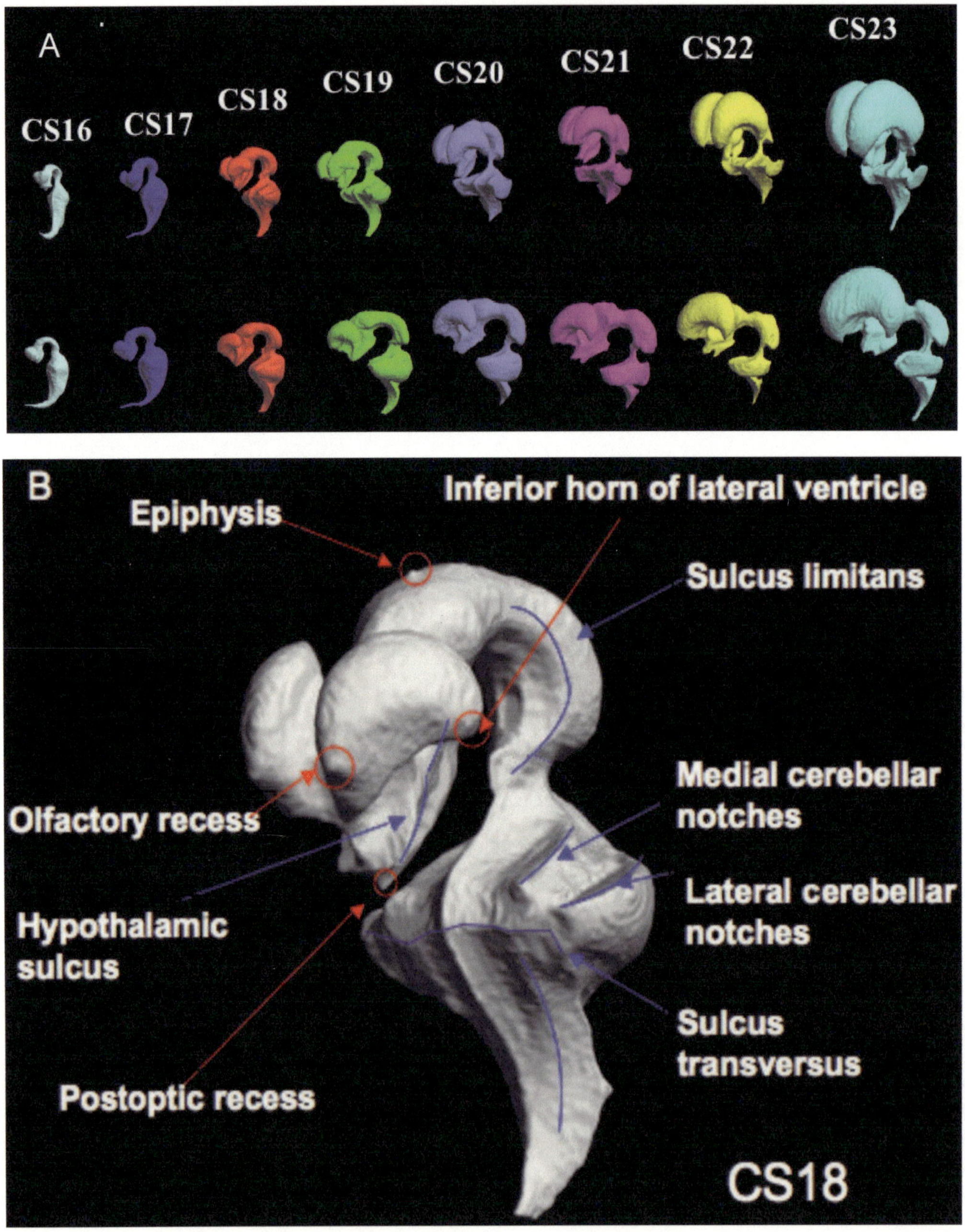

Fig. 8. (A) Representative 3D images of cerebral ventricles between Carnegie stage 16 and stage 23. (B) 3D image illustrating the conservation of anatomic landmarks.

5.5 FMRIB Software Library (FSL) (http://www.fmrib.ox.ac.uk/fsl/index.html)

FSL is a comprehensive library of analytical tools for fMRI (functional magnetic resonance imaging), MRI and DTI (Diffusion tensor imaging) brain imaging data. FSL was mainly developed by members of the Analysis Group at the FMRIB, Oxford, UK. FSL runs on Apple and PCs (Linux and Windows), and is easy to install. Most of the tools can be run either from the command line or as "point-and-click" graphical user interfaces.

5.6 Analyze (http://www.mayo.edu/bir/Software/Analyze/Analyze.html)

Analyze 10.0 is a powerful, comprehensive software package for multi-dimensional display, processing, and measurement of multi-modality biomedical images. Product of more than 25 years of biomedical imaging research and development at Mayo Clinic, this integrated, total solution allows you to significantly enhance your multidimensional biomedical imaging productivity.

6. Acknowledgments

We would like to thank Ms Merumo Ueda, Ms Nami Uematsu, Ms Kyoko Nakajima, and Ms Sayuri Nunomura at the Kyoto University Graduate School of Medicine, Human Health Science, for conducting some of the experiments; Ms Chigako Uwabe at the Congenital Anomaly Research Center for technical assistance in handling human embryos; Prof. Masaaki Wada at the Graduate School of Information Science and Technology at Osaka University for help on the use of the DeltaViewer software; Prof. Katsumi Kose and Dr. Yoshimasa Matsuda at the Institute of Applied Physics at University of Tsukuba and Dr. Stasia A Anderson at the NHLBI Animal MRI Core, National Institutes of Health, for technical help with MR imaging; and Prof. Kohei Shiota, Vice President of Kyoto University, for his support and guidance on the project. The researches were financially supported by Grants #228073, #238058, #21790810 and #22591199 from the Japan Society for the Promotion of Science (JSPS) and the Japan Science and Technology (JST) institute for Bioinformatics Research and Development (BIRD). The researches were also supported by Japan Spina Bifida and Hydrocephalus Research Foundation, and Konica Minolta Science and Technology Foundation. The studies presented in this chapter were approved by the Medical Ethics Committee at Kyoto University Graduate School of Medicine (Kyoto, Japan).

7. References

Becker, B. P. & Bonse, U. 1974. The skew-symmetric two-crystal X-ray interferometer. *Journal of Applied Crystallography*, 7, 593-598.

Bone, S. N., Johnson, G. A. & Thompson, M. B. 1986. Three-dimensional magnetic resonance microscopy of the developing chick embryo. *Invest Radiol*, 21, 782-7.

Born, G. 1883. Die Plattenmodelliermethode. *Archiv für mikroskopische Anatomie*. 22, 584-99.

Effmann, E. L., Johnson, G. A., Smith, B. R., Talbott, G. A. & Cofer, G. 1988. Magnetic resonance microscopy of chick embryos in ovo. *Teratology*, 38, 59-65.

Haishi, T., Uematsu, T., Matsuda, Y. & Kose, K. 2001. Development of a 1.0 T MR microscope using a Nd-Fe-B permanent magnet. *Magnetic resonance imaging*, 19, 875-80.

Heard, O. O. 1951. Section compression photographically rectified. *The Anatomical record*, 109, 745-55.

Heard, O. O. 1953. The influence of surface forces in microtomy. *The Anatomical record,* 117, 725-39.

Heard, O. O. 1957. Methods used by C.H. Heuser in preparing and sectioning early embryos. *Contributions to Embryology,* 36, 1-18.

Matsuda, Y., Ono, S., Otake, Y., Handa, S., Kose, K., Haishi, T., Yamada, S., Uwabe, C. & Shiota, K. 2007. Imaging of a large collection of human embryo using a super-parallel MR microscope. *Magnetic resonance in medical sciences : MRMS : an official journal of Japan Society of Magnetic Resonance.* 6, 139-46.

Matsuda, Y., Utsuzawa, S., Kurimoto, T., Haishi, T., Yamazaki, Y., Kose, K., Anno, I. & Marutani, M. 2003. Super-parallel MR microscope. *Magnetic resonance in medicine : official journal of the Society of Magnetic Resonance in Medicine / Society of Magnetic Resonance in Medicine.* 50, 183-9.

Momose, A. & Fukuda, J. 1995. Phase-contrast radiographs of nonstained rat cerebellar specimen. *Medical physics,* 22, 375-9.

Momose, A., Takeda, T., Itai, Y. & Hirano, K. 1996. Phase-contrast X-ray computed tomography for observing biological soft tissues. *Nature medicine.* 2, 473-5.

Nakashima, T., Hirose, A., Yamada, S., Uwabe, C., Kose, K. & Takakuwa, T. 2011. Morphometric analysis of the brain vesicles during the human embryonic period by magnetic resonance microscopic imaging. Congenital Anomalies. doi: 10.1111/j.1741-4520.2011.00345.x

Nishimura, H. 1975. Prenatal versus postnatal malformations based on the Japanese experience on induced abortions in the human being. . *In:* BLANDEU, R. (ed.) *Aging Gamates.* Basel: S. Karger AG.

Nishimura, H., Takano, K., Tanimura, T. & Yasuda, M. 1968. Normal and abnormal development of human embryos: first report of the analysis of 1,213 intact embryos. *Teratology,* 1, 281-90.

O'Rahilly, R. 1988. One Hundred Years of Human Embryology. *In:* KALTER, H. (ed.) *Issues and Reviews in Terratology* New York: Plenum Press.

O'Rahilly, R. & Müller, F. 1987. *Developmental stages in human embryos: including a revision of Streeter's "horizons" and a survey of the Carnegie Collection.,* Washington, DC, Carnegie Institution of Washington Publication.

Rohlf, F. J. & Bookstein, F. L. 1990. *Proceedings Of The Michigan Morphometrics Workshop,* Ann Arbor, MI, University of Michigan Museum of Zoology.

Rosenthal, J., Mangal, V., Walker, D., Bennett, M., Mohun, T. J. & Lo, C. W. 2004. Rapid high resolution three dimensional reconstruction of embryos with episcopic fluorescence image capture. *Birth defects research. Part C, Embryo today : reviews,* 72, 213-23.

Shiota, K. 1991. Development and intrauterine fate of normal and abnormal human conceptuses. *Congenital Anomalies,* 31, 67-80.

Shiota, K., Yamada, S., Nakatsu-Komatsu, T., Uwabe, C., Kose, K., Matsuda, Y., Haishi, T., Mizuta, S. & Matsuda, T. 2007. Visualization of human prenatal development by magnetic resonance imaging (MRI). *American journal of medical genetics. Part A,* 143A, 3121-6.

Smith, B. R. 1999. Visualizing human embryos. *Scientific American,* 280, 76-81.

Smith, B. R. 2000. Magnetic resonance imaging analysis of embryos. *Methods in molecular biology,* 135, 211-6.

Smith, B. R. 2001. Magnetic resonance microscopy in cardiac development. *Microscopy research and technique,* 52, 323-30.

Smith, B. R., Effmann, E. L. & Johnson, G. A. 1992. MR microscopy of chick embryo vasculature. *Journal of magnetic resonance imaging: JMRI.* 2, 237-40.

Smith, B. R., Huff, D. S. & Johnson, G. A. 1999. Magnetic resonance imaging of embryos: an Internet resource for the study of embryonic development. *Computerized medical imaging and graphics : the official journal of the Computerized Medical Imaging Society,* 23, 33-40.

Smith, B. R., Johnson, G. A., Groman, E. V. & Linney, E. 1994. Magnetic resonance microscopy of mouse embryos. *Proc Natl Acad Sci U S A,* 91, 3530-3.

Smith, B. R., Linney, E., Huff, D. S. & Johnson, G. A. 1996. Magnetic resonance microscopy of embryos. *Computerized medical imaging and graphics: the official journal of the Computerized Medical Imaging Society.* 20, 483-90.

Weninger, W. J., Geyer, S. H., Mohun, T. J., Rasskin-Gutman, D., Matsui, T., Ribeiro, I., Costa Lda, F., Izpisua-Belmonte, J. C. & Muller, G. B. 2006. High-resolution episcopic microscopy: a rapid technique for high detailed 3D analysis of gene activity in the context of tissue architecture and morphology. *Anatomy and embryology,* 211, 213-21.

Weninger, W. J. & Mohun, T. 2002. Phenotyping transgenic embryos: a rapid 3-D screening method based on episcopic fluorescence image capturing. *Nature genetics,* 30, 59-65.

Yamada, S., Itoh, H., Uwabe, C., Fujihara, S., Nishibori, C., Wada, M., Fujii, S. & Shiota, K. 2007. Computerized three-dimensional analysis of the heart and great vessels in normal and holoprosencephalic human embryos. *Anatomical record : advances in integrative anatomy and evolutionary biology,* 290, 259-67.

Yamada, S., Samtani, R. R., Lee, E. S., Lockett, E., Uwabe, C., Shiota, K., Anderson, S. A. & Lo, C. W. 2010. Developmental atlas of the early first trimester human embryo. *Developmental dynamics : an official publication of the American Association of Anatomists,* 239, 1585-95.

Yamada, S., Uwabe, C., Fujii, S. & Shiota, K. 2004. Phenotypic variability in human embryonic holoprosencephaly in the Kyoto Collection. *Birth Defects Res A Clin Mol Teratol,* 70, 495-508.

Yamada, S., Uwabe, C., Nakatsu-Komatsu, T., Minekura, Y., Iwakura, M., Motoki, T., Nishimiya, K., Iiyama, M., Kakusho, K., Minoh, M., Mizuta, S., Matsuda, T., Matsuda, Y., Haishi, T., Kose, K., Fujii, S. & Shiota, K. 2006. Graphic and movie illustrations of human prenatal development and their application to embryological education based on the human embryo specimens in the Kyoto collection. *Developmental dynamics : an official publication of the American Association of Anatomists,* 235, 468-77.

Yoneyama, A., Takeda, T., Tsuchiya, Y., Wu, J., Lwin, T. T., Koizumi, A., Hyodo, K. & Itai, Y. 2004. A phase-contrast X-ray imaging system—with a 60×30 mm field of view—based on a skew-symmetric two-crystal X-ray inteferometer. *Nuclear Instruments and Methods in Physics Research Section A: Accelerators, Spectrometers, Detectors and Associated Equipment,* 523, 217-222.

Yoneyama, A., Yamada, S. & Takeda, T. 2011. Fine Biomedical Imaging Using X-Ray Phase-Sensitive Technique. *In:* Gargiulo, D. G., Mcewan, A. (ed.) *Advanced Biomedical Engineering*. InTech. p107-128.

8

Cardiovascular Development in the First Trimester

Preeta Dhanantwari[1], Linda Leatherbury[2] and Cecilia W. Lo[3]
[1]*Children's Heart Center, Steven and Alexandra Cohen Children's Medical Center of New York, New York,*
[2]*Children's National Heart Institute, Children's National Medical Center, Washington DC,*
[3]*Department of Developmental Biology, University of Pittsburgh School of Medicine, Pittsburgh, USA*

1. Introduction

In current clinical practice of fetal cardiology, rapid advances in medical imaging have opened the door to the diagnosis of human congenital heart disease (CHD) in the first trimester. It is within the first trimester that all of the major cardiac developmental processes that impact congenital heart disease occur, and yet much of our current knowledge of these cardiac developmental events has been extrapolated from research studies in animal models. Given differences in developmental timing and cardiovascular anatomy, data documenting normal first trimester human cardiac development is essential. Data on human cardiac development for accurate fetal diagnosis in the clinical setting is of particular importance given increasing feasibility for in utero surgical intervention. A large dataset was obtained from imaging human embryos donated from the Kyoto collection to the Carnegie collection. The complex morphogenetic changes occurring during human heart development were examined using magnetic resonance imaging (MRI) and episcopic fluorescence image capture (EFIC). This analysis included 52 human embryos and spanned $6^4/_7$-$9^3/_7$ weeks estimated gestational age (EGA), corresponding to Carnegie stages (CS) 13-23. Serial two-dimensional image stacks and three-dimensional reconstructions allowed analysis of external morphology and internal structures of the heart. The developmental timeline of all the major events in human cardiac morphogenesis from 6-10 weeks of gestation was constructed. This includes the temporal profile of atrial and ventricular septation, outflow septation and valvular morphogenesis. This data may ultimately facilitate the assessment and diagnosis of CHD in the clinical setting. A reference guide for these developmental milestones was generated to aid clinical practice. This will be helpful for the early diagnoses of congenital heart disease in the first trimester human fetus. Such early clinical diagnosis will be critically important for appropriate counseling of families, and for the development of in-utero therapy and intervention to improve the prognosis of fetuses with congenital heart disease.

2. Background

With rapid advances in medical imaging, fetal diagnosis of human CHD is now technically feasible in the first trimester. Although the first human embryologic studies were recorded by Hippocrates in 300-400 BC, present day knowledge of normal human cardiac development in the first trimester is still limited. In 1886, two papers by Dr His described development of the heart based on dissections of young human embryos. Free hand wax models were made that illustrated the external developmental anatomy. These wax plate reconstruction methods were used by many other investigators until the early 1900s[1]. Subsequently serial histological sections of human embryos have been used to further investigate human cardiac development[2-6]. Based on analysis of histological sections and scaled reproductions of human embryos, Grant showed a large cushion in the developing heart at 6 6/7 weeks (CS 14) and separate AV valves at 9 1/7 weeks (CS 22)[2]. At the end of the 8th week (CS 8), separate aortic and pulmonary outflows were observed. Orts-Llorca used three dimensional reconstructions of transverse sections of human embryos to define development of the truncus arteriosus and described completion of septation of the truncus arteriosus in 14-16mm embryos, equivalent to EGA 8 weeks (CS18)[5].

Given the complex tissue remodeling associated with cardiac chamber formation and inflow/outflow tract and valvular morphogenesis, the plane of sectioning often limited the information that can be gathered on developing structures in the embryonic heart. These technical limitations in conjunction with limited access to human embryo specimens have meant that much of our understanding of early cardiac development in the human embryo is largely extrapolated from studies in model organisms[7-10]. With possible species differences in developmental timing and variation in cardiovascular anatomy, characterization of normal cardiac development in human embryos is necessary for clinical evaluation and diagnosis of CHD in the first trimester. This will be increasingly important, as improvements in medical technology allow earlier access to first trimester human fetal cardiac imaging and in utero intervention.

Recent studies have shown the feasibility of using magnetic resonance imaging (MRI) to obtain information on human embryo tissue structure[11, 12]. MRI imaging data can be digitally resectioned for viewing of the specimen in any orientation, and three-dimensional (3D) renderings can be obtained with ease. Similarly, episcopic fluorescence image capture (EFIC), a novel histological imaging technique, provides registered two-dimensional (2D) image stacks that can be resectioned in arbitrary planes and also rapidly 3D rendered[10]. With EFIC imaging, tissue is embedded in paraffin and cut with a sledge microtome. Tissue autofluorescence at the block face is captured and used to generate registered serial 2D images of the specimen with image resolution better than MRI. Data obtained by MRI or EFIC imaging can be easily resectioned digitally or reconstructed in 3D to facilitate the analysis of complex morphological changes in the developing embryonic heart. In this manner, the developing heart in every embryo can be analyzed in it entirety with no loss of information due to the plane of sectioning.

Using MRI and EFIC imaging, we conducted a systematic analysis of human cardiovascular development in the first trimester. 2D image stacks and 3D volumes were generated from 52 human embryos from $6^4/_7$ to $9^3/_7$ weeks estimated gestational age (EGA), equivalent to Carnegie stages (CS) 13-23. These stages encompass the developmental window during which all of the major milestones of cardiac morphogenesis can be observed. Using the MRI and EFIC imaging data, we constructed a digital atlas of human heart development. Data from our atlas were used to generate charts summarizing the major milestones of normal human heart development through the first trimester. MRI and EFIC images obtained as part of this study can be viewed as part of an online Human Embryo Atlas. To view the Human Embryo Atlas content, visit http://apps.devbio.pitt.edu/HumanAtlas; guest login ID *Human*, password *Embryo*. This chapter highlights the findings of this landmark evaluation (original article published in Circulation, 2009; 120; 343-351). Permission for reproduction of that original work was obtained from Lippincott Williams & Wilkins (http://lww.com).

3. Specimens

Embryos from the Kyoto collection, at the Congenital Anomaly Research Center at the Kyoto University in Japan, were collected after termination of pregnancies for socioeconomic reasons under the Maternity Protection Law of Japan. Embryos were derived from normal pregnancies without any clinical presentations. The specimens were in fixative for an estimated duration of 30 to over 40 years, making them unsuitable for immunohistochemistry or any molecular/cellular analysis. This collection represents a random sample of the total intrauterine population of Japan[13-16]. During accessioning into the Kyoto collection, the embryos were examined and staged according to the criteria of Carnegie Staging proposed by O'Rahilly[17]. For this study, 52 embryos from the Kyoto collection (see Table 1) were donated to the Carnegie collection of normal human embryos archived at the National Museum of Health and Medicine of the Armed Forces Institute of Pathology (http://nmhm.washingtondc.museum/collections/hdac/Carnegie_collection.htm). Each embryo's age was determined using post conceptional ages previously reported[14], which were then converted to estimated gestational age or menstrual age by adding 14 days, and reported in weeks.

4. Magnetic resonance imaging, episcopic fluorescence image capture, processing, and analysis

High resolution MRI and EFIC images were obtained from 52 human embryos from $6^4/_7$ to $9^3/_7$ weeks of gestation (CS 13-23). These specimens from the Kyoto collection were imaged by MRI and EFIC during preparation for accessioning into the Carnegie collection (Table 1). Human embryos in formalin were treated with 1:20 Magnevist (Berlex, Montville, NJ)/10% formalin solution, rinsed and prepared in 5-30 mm tubes depending on embryo size, with fixative or low melting agar. Samples that diffused gadolinium into the media were further soaked in plain fixative two or more days and re-imaged. Imaging was performed at the NIH Mouse Imaging Facility on a 7.0T Bruker vertical bore MRI system with 150 G/cm gradients (Bruker, Billerica,MA) and 5 to 30 mm microimaging birdcage coils (Bruker, Billerica, MA). Some larger samples were also imaged on a 7.0T, 16mm horizontal bore Bruker Paravision system with 39G/cm gradients and a 38-mm birdcage coil. MRI was acquired with Paravision 3.0.2 operating systems. Samples were imaged using a 3D rapid gradient echo (SNAP) sequence with TR 30-40ms, TE 3.3-4.0ms, 20-90 averages, acquisition time approximately 12 to 50 hours, matrices 256x128x128 to 512x512x512 (see Table 2). Over the whole collection, MRI resolution ranged from 29x35x35 to 117x105x105 μm^3. Resolution was proportionate to the sample size with the smallest embryos having the highest resolution data sets. Individual image data sets are three dimensional and near-isotropic, with all three voxel dimensions being within 10 microns of each other in an individual data set. Most data sets are in the range 35x35x35 to 60x60x60 μm^3. The resolution of each data set is listed in Table 2.

In preparation for EFIC, embryos stored in 10% phosphate buffered formalin were dehydrated and embedded in a mixture of paraffin wax (70.4%), Vybar (24.9%), stearic acid (4.4%) and red aniline dye Sudan IV (0.4%) using techniques previously described[10, 18]. The embedded embryos were then sectioned using a sliding microtome (Leica SM 2500) to obtain sections of 5-8 microns in thickness. The block face was sequentially photographed using epifluorescent illumination with a 100W mercury lamp and a Leica MZ16A stereomicroscope equipped with 425 nm/480 nm excitation/emission filters. Images were captured using an ORCA-ER digital camera (Hamamatsu).

Estimated Gestational Age (weeks)	Carnegie Stage	Total Number Embryos Imaged	Imaging by MRI*	Imaging by EFIC*	EFIC and MRI
6 4/7	13	3	2 (2)	1 (1)	
6 6/7	14	4	3 (3)	2 (1)	1
7 1/7	15	3	1 (1)	2 (2)	
7 3/7	16	8	6 (6)	4 (3)	2
7 5/7	17	4	2 (2)	2 (2)	1
8	18	6	4 (3)	2 (1)	
8 2/7	19	5	3 (3)	2 (0)	
8 4/7	20	5	3 (3)	1 (0)	
8 6/7	21	4	2 (2)	2 (0)	
9 1/7	22	6	5 (3)	1 (0)	
9 3/7	23	4	3 (3)	3 (1)	2
Totals		52 (42)	34 (31)	22 (11)	

*Number of specimen yielding good imaging data indicated in parenthesis.

Table 1. Human Embryo Imaging by MRI and Episcopic Fluorescence Image Capture`

Carnegie Stage	Total Number Embryos	Voxel dimensions acquired by MRI (um)		
13	2	37x35x35	29x35x35	
14	3	29x37x37	33x36x36	37x37x37
15	1	33x35x35		
16	6	39x37x37	47x37x37	39x37x37
		53x52x52	53x52x52	61x43x43
17	2	41x35x35	39x39x39	
18	3	43x60x60	42x44x44	42x54x54
19	3	41x55x55	65x59x59	
		82x87x70		
20	3	45x54x54		
		67x67x62	67x67x63	
21	2	51x56x56	62x51x51	
22	5	57x57x57	60x59x59	64x63x63,
		68x78x78	63x63x63	
23	3	117x105x105	117x105x105	117x105x105

Table 2. MRI Acquisition Resolution

MRI images originally recorded in DICOM were converted into TIFF format using ImageJ (http://rsb.info.nih.gov/ij/). The EFIC 2D image stacks were captured and exported as TIFF files. Both the EFIC and MRI data were processed using OpenLab (Improvision Inc).

3D reconstructions and quick time virtual reality (QTVR) movies were generated using Volocity (Improvision Inc). The 2D image stacks also were digitally resectioned using Volocity (Improvision Inc) to view internal and external cardiac structures in planes similar to standard echocardiographic imaging planes used clinically. In EFIC images, each pixel was a square with length dimensions ranging from 2.34 to13.4 microns/pixel edge. Thus, pixel dimensions ranged from 5.48 μm^2 to 179.56 μm^2. For each embryo, we generated serial 2D image stacks, and 3D reconstructions. From this analysis, we were able to delineate all of the major milestones of human heart development, including chamber formation, septation of the atria, ventricles, and truncus arteriosus, and valvular morphogenesis.

5. Cardiac loop

The cardiac loop or looped heart tube is observed from EGA $6^4/_7$ to $7^5/_7$ weeks (CS13 to CS17). 3D reconstruction of the heart at $7^5/_7$ weeks (CS17) reveals internal structures of the cardiac loop (Fig.1). The only exit for blood from the left sided inflow limb, consisting of the atrial cavity, atrioventricular junction, and the presumptive left ventricle, is the interventricular foramen (also known as primary foramen, primary interventricular foramen, bulboventricular foramen or embryonic interventricular foramen) (double arrow in Fig.1); while the only exit for blood from the right sided outflow limb, consisting of the

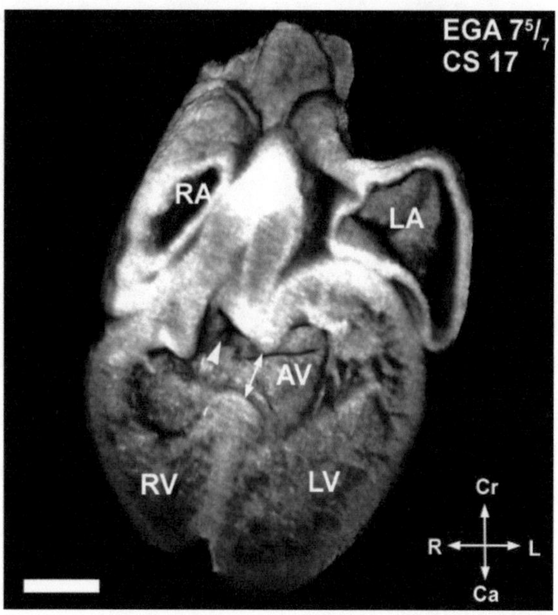

For all figures, compass shown correspond to: A=anterior P=posterior, R=right, L=left, Cr=cranial, Ca=caudal.

2D EFIC image stacks were reconstructed in 3D to show the looped heart tube in a EGA $7^5/_7$ weeks (CS17) embryo. The double headed arrow indicates the interventricular foramen. The orifice of the developing atrioventricular junction is seen as a horizontal line above the label AV. The truncus arteriosus (arrowhead) is also seen. Endocardial cushion tissue surrounding the atrioventricular junction is adjacent to the truncus arteriosus.

RA: right atrium, LA: left atrium, RV: presumptive right ventricle, LV: presumptive left ventricle. Scale bar = 0.6 mm.

Fig. 1. 3D view of the cardiac loop in a GA $7^5/_7$ weeks (CS17) embryo.

presumptive right ventricle is the truncus arteriosus (arrowhead in Fig.1). Also of note, the atrioventricular junction (AV in Fig.1) is surrounded by endocardial cushion tissue, which is contiguous with the truncus arteriosus.

The developmental changes seen in the cardiac loop are shown in more detail in Figure 2, with images from embryos at $6^4/_7$ (CS13) (Fig.2A-E) and $7^5/_7$ weeks (CS17) (Fig.2F-I). As the looped heart tube matures, the atrial and ventricular chambers expand in size, giving rise to distinct

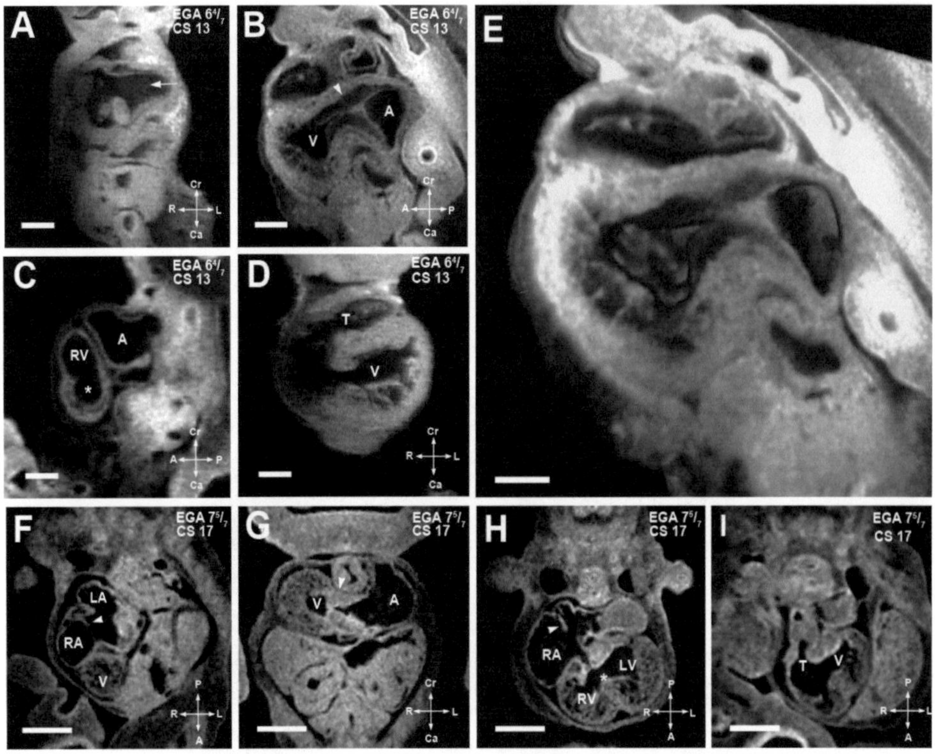

(A-E). EFIC and MRI images of EGA $6^4/_7$ weeks (CS13) embryos shown in various imaging planes. Imaging in the frontal plane (A) shows the common cardinal veins or the open venous confluence (arrow), while sagittal view (B) shows primitive endocardial cushions at the atrioventricular junction (arrowhead). A 3D model of the same embryo (E) shows the extent of the interventricular foramen as well as the contour of the endocardial cushions. MRI image of another embryo in the sagittal plane (C) shows the presumptive right ventricle (**RV**), atrial chamber (**A**), and a nondistinct interventricular foramen (*), while the ventricular chamber (**V**) and a single, undivided truncus arteriosus (**T**) can be seen in an frontal section of a third embryo (D).
Scale bars: (A-D)=0.4 mm, (E)=0.25 mm
(F-I). MRI images of EGA $7^5/_7$ weeks (CS17) embryo. Image from an oblique transverse plane (F) shows the right and left atrial (**RA, LA**) chambers as septation is progressing (arrowhead). The developing ventricle (**V**) is seen. Viewed in the transverse plane in (G), well formed dense endocardial cushion tissue is seen at the atrioventricular junction (arrowhead). Another section in the transverse plane in (H) shows the right and left ventricular cavities with a more distinct interventricular foramen (*). Septum primum can be seen as atrial septation progresses (arrowhead). The single undivided truncus arteriosus (**T**) and interventricular foramen communicating with the presumptive left ventricle (**V**) can be seen in an oblique transverse plane (I). Scale bar: (E-H) = 1.250 mm.
LV: presumptive left ventricular chamber, **T:** truncus arteriosus .

Fig. 2. Defining structures of the cardiac loop.

subdivisions recognizable as the primitive left and right atria and presumptive left and right ventricles (Fig.2H). At $6^4/_7$ weeks (CS13), the endocardial cushions seen lining the atrioventricular junction appear thin with little apparent cellular content. As development progresses, they become filled with dense material (Fig.2B,E,G). The interventricular foramen also shows striking changes during this developmental period. It is a wide and open communication at $6^4/_7$ weeks (CS13) (asterisk in Fig.2C), but as the chambers grow, it becomes a narrow and more distinct opening (foramen), by $7^3/_7$ to $7^5/_7$ weeks (CS16-17) (asterisk in Fig.2H,3C). The superior atrioventricular cushion can be seen (Fig.2G). The inflow consisting of the venous confluence or primitive atrium (Fig.2A) is observed to communicate with the ventricular chamber via the atrioventricular junction (Fig.2B,E,G). The presumptive left ventricle communicates with the presumptive right ventricle via the interventricular foramen (asterisk in Fig. 2C,H). The outflow from the cardiac loop comprises the yet undivided truncus arteriosus (T in Fig. 2D,I) arising from the presumptive right ventricle.

6. Atrial septation (EGA $6^6/_7$-8 weeks)

The process of atrial septation is thought to begin with a thin septum primum growing from the posterior wall of the atrium, from a location cranial to the pulmonary vein orifice. It grows towards and eventually fuses with the endocardial cushions[19]. At 6 $^6/_7$ weeks gestation (CS 14), the mesenchymal cap of the primary atrial septum could be seen in contact with the superior atrioventricular cushion. The atrial spine, a mesenchymal structure, was also observed. The atrial spine fuses with the inferior atrioventricular cushion (6 6/7 weeks (CS 14)) (Fig.3A,B), and plays an important role in closure of the primary foramen. Although the pulmonary vein orifice was not seen by our imaging, it can be inferred from previous studies that it lies to the left of the atrial spine[20]. Septum primum can be observed at 6 $^6/_7$ weeks of gestation and its developmental progression through 7 $^5/_7$ weeks can be seen in Figures 2H, 3A,B, and E. Later, septum secundum develops as an infolding of the dorsal wall of the right atrium, completing atrial septation with fenestrations forming the foramen ovale. Both atrial septum primum and secundum were present by 8 weeks (CS18). At this stage, the mesenchymal cap can be seen fused with the now divided superior atrioventricular cushion (Fig.3F). This is consistent with developmental timing suggested by others[21, 22].

7. Ventricular septation (EGA 7 $^3/_7$-$9^1/_7$ weeks)

Towards the end of the looped heart tube stages of development ($7^3/_7$ and $7^5/_7$ weeks, CS16,17), distinct separation of presumptive LV and RV chambers is evident. The beginning of the muscular interventricular septum can be seen at these stages, but ventricular septation is not yet complete (Fig.2H,3C,D). By 8 weeks (CS18), the muscular ventricular septum can be seen extending from the floor of the ventricular chamber towards the crux of the heart (Fig.3F). This leaves open a relatively large interventricular foramen which allows communication between the ventricles. Recent lineage tracing experiments in mice have suggested that the muscular interventricular septum is comprised of cells originating from the ventral aspect of the primitive ventricle, with closure of the ventricular foramen mediated by dorsal migration of this precursor cell population; these cells likely represent a subpopulation of cells derived from the secondary heart field[23]. Immunohistochemical analysis of human fetal cardiac tissue showed myocytes expressing G1N2 antigen localized in a ring around the junction between the future right and left ventricles[24]. In later developmental stages, G1N2 expressing cells are found in the area clinically termed the inlet ventricular septum, but not in the subaortic outflow septum.

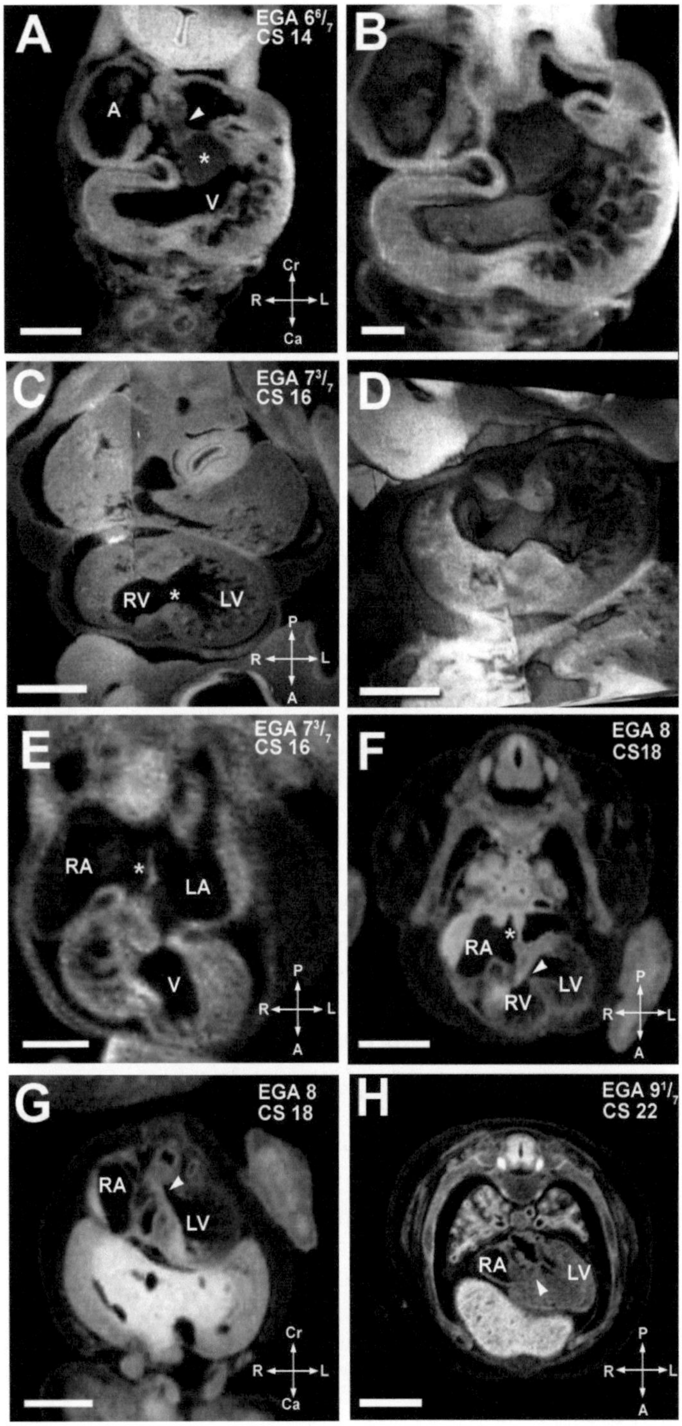

(A,B). EFIC image of EGA $6^6/7$ weeks (CS14) embryo in the transverse plane (A) shows the atrial spine (arrowhead) attached to the inferior cushion (asterisks). 3D reconstruction (B) highlights the endocardial cushions and trabeculation in the ventricular chamber. Scale bar = 0.515 mm in (A), 0.272mm in (B).

(C,D). An EFIC image of EGA $7^3/_7$ weeks (CS16) embryo in the oblique plane (C) showing right and left ventricular chambers connected by an interventricular foramen (*). 3D reconstruction of the same embryo (D) delineates the contour of the interventricular foramen and the orifices of the atrioventricular canal and the truncus arteriosus. Scale bar = 0.5mm for (C), and 0.900mm for (D).
(E) MRI image of an embryo at EGA $7^3/_7$ weeks (CS16) also in the transverse plane. It shows the formation of septum primum (*) between the right and left atria (RA, LA). Scale bar = 0.5 mm.
(F,G) MRI image of an EGA 8 weeks (CS18) embryo in an oblique transverse plane (F) shows a complete atrial septum (*). The most caudal portion of the septum primum, the mesenchymal cap, has fused to the superior cushion. The growth of the muscular ventricular septum into the ventricular cavity is also shown. The crest of the muscular interventricular septum is present with an incomplete inlet ventricular septum (arrowhead) immediately above it. Panel G, another MRI image of the same embryo in an oblique coronal plane, shows the formed outlet ventricular septum (arrowhead). Together these two images show that outlet ventricular septation is completed before inlet ventricular septation. Scale bars in (F,G) = 1.5 mm.
(H). MRI image of embryo at EGA $9^1/_7$ weeks (CS22) in an oblique coronal plane shows a completed inlet ventricular septum (arrowhead). Scale bar = 2mm.
A: primitive atrium/venous confluence, **RA**: right atrium, **LA**: left atrium, **V**: ventricular chamber, **LV**: left ventricular chamber, **RV**: right ventricular chamber.

Fig. 3. Major events of atrial and ventricular septation.

At 8 weeks (CS 18), the ventricular septum at the level of the left ventricular outflow is closed (Fig.3G), but part of the inlet ventricular septum at the level of the atrioventricular valves remains open (arrowhead in Fig.3F). The inlet and membranous portions of the ventricular septum are fully closed at $9^1/_7$ weeks (CS22), completing ventricular septation (Fig.3H). The area clinically termed the inlet ventricular septum has been shown in prior studies to originate from the embryonic right ventricle[25]. In agreement with previous reports on human development, our data showed the final portion of the ventricular septum to close included what likely comprises a combination of the membranous and inlet ventricular septum. These findings suggest that an arrest in development of the ventricular septum could result in ventricular septal defects similar to those observed clinically.

8. Formation of the atrioventricular valves (EGA $7^3/_7$-8weeks)

Atrioventricular valve morphogenesis begins at the looped heart tube stages, with large endocardial cushions prominently seen at the center of the cardiac loop (asterisks in Fig.3A,4A). The atrioventricular canal is divided by the endocardial cushions, which form on the posterior (dorsal) and anterior (ventral) walls of the atrioventricular canal. These cushions eventually divide the atrioventricular canal into right and left atrioventricular orifices[2, 19]. A well delineated atrioventricular junction can be seen at $7^3/_7$ weeks gestation (CS16) (Fig.4B,C). At 7 $^3/_7$ and 7 $^5/_7$ weeks (CS16 and CS17), the atrioventricular junction was still undivided. A few days later, by 8 weeks gestation (CS18), separate atrioventricular valves can be seen (arrowheads in Fig.4D,E), with left sided mitral and right sided tricuspid valves forming. An embryo at 8 weeks (CS18) is approximately 10 mm in size, correlating well with the embryonic stage at which fusion of the endocardial cushions is thought to occur[26]. The valve leaflets however appear thick at this stage. By $9^1/_7$ weeks (CS22), the atrioventricular valve leaflets are thinner and more mature in appearance (Fig.3H). At $7^3/_7$ weeks (CS16), distinct posterior and anterior cushions are not observed, the inferior atrioventricular cushion is observed and this timing is consistent with previous reports of human embryonic development.[22]

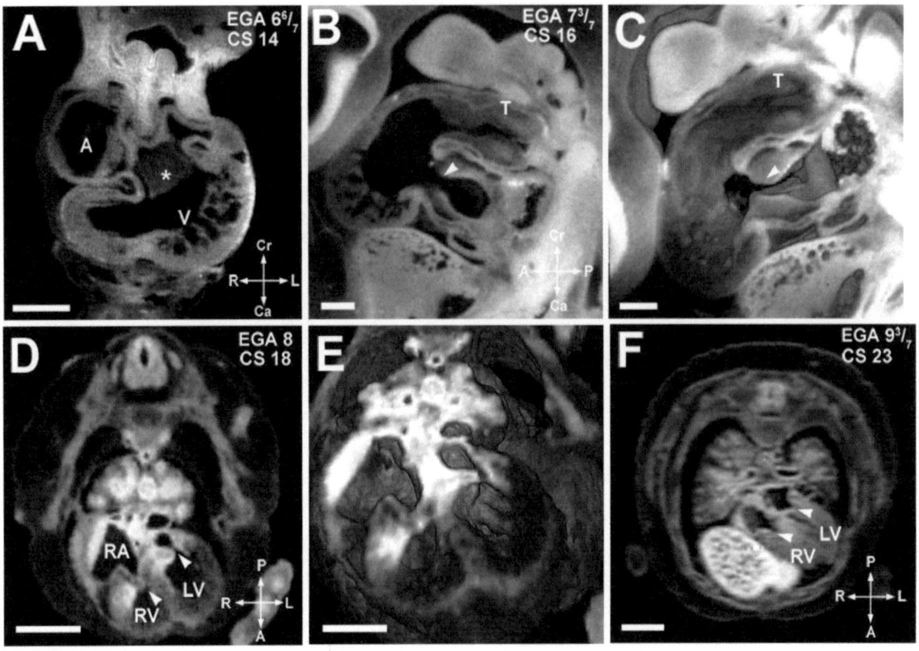

(A). EFIC image of an embryo at EGA $6^6/_7$ weeks (CS 14) in the transverse plane shows a large endocardial cushion (*) in the center of the cardiac loop. Scale bar = 0.515 mm
(B,C). EFIC image of an embryo at EGA $7^3/_7$ weeks (CS16) in a sagittal plane (B) shows a tight, well formed atrioventricular junction (arrowhead) and the truncus arteriosus (**T**). 3D volume of the same embryo (C) shows exquisite detail of the contour and shape of the endocardial cushions and the truncus arteriosus (T). Scale bar in (B,C)=0.389mm.
(D,E). MRI image in an oblique transverse plane (D) of an embryo at EGA 8 weeks (CS 18) shows separate atrioventricular valves. The valve leaflets appear thick at this stage. Note right and left atrioventricular valves denoted by arrowheads. 3D volume of the same embryo (E) shows indentation associated with the opening in the inlet ventricular septum. Scale bar for (D)=1.5 mm, (E)=1.1mm.
(F) MRI image in an oblique transverse plane of a more mature EGA $9^3/_7$ weeks (CS 23) embryo. It shows separate atrioventricular valves with thinner valve leaflets (arrowheads). The inlet septum is closed. Scale bar = 2 mm.
A: primitive atrium, **RA:** right atrium, **V:** ventricular chamber, **RV:** right ventricular chamber, **LV:** left ventricular chamber

Fig. 4. Major milestones of atrioventricular valve morphogenesis.

9. Outflow septation and semilunar valve morphogenesis (EGA 7 3/7 to 8 weeks)

The major developmental processes occurring at the level of the truncus arteriosus consist of septation into two separate arterial channels, and semilunar valve morphogenesis. The truncus arteriosus is formed largely from cells derived from the secondary heart field[27]. Septation of the truncus arteriosus is dependent on activity of the secondary heart field and migrating neural crest cells[28, 29], and is achieved with in growth of ridges. In the proximal truncus arteriosus, we observed truncal cushions in the form of swellings at $7^1/_7$ weeks (CS15) (arrowhead in Fig.5A). This forming aorticopulmonary septum undergoes a gradual spiraling course that ultimately completes truncus arteriosus septation into separate aorta and pulmonary arteries[28]. At $7^3/_7$ weeks (CS16), this spiraling course of the forming aorticopulmonary septum is evident as a spiraling in the orientation of the lumen along the proximodistal axis of the truncus arteriosus (Fig.5D-F). The truncus arteriosus remains as a single channel proximally (Fig.5D-E), but distally, it divides into two separate channels (Fig.5F). Smooth muscle derived from the secondary heart field and from cardiac neural crest cells plays a crucial role in the septation and alignment of the truncus arteriosus[28].

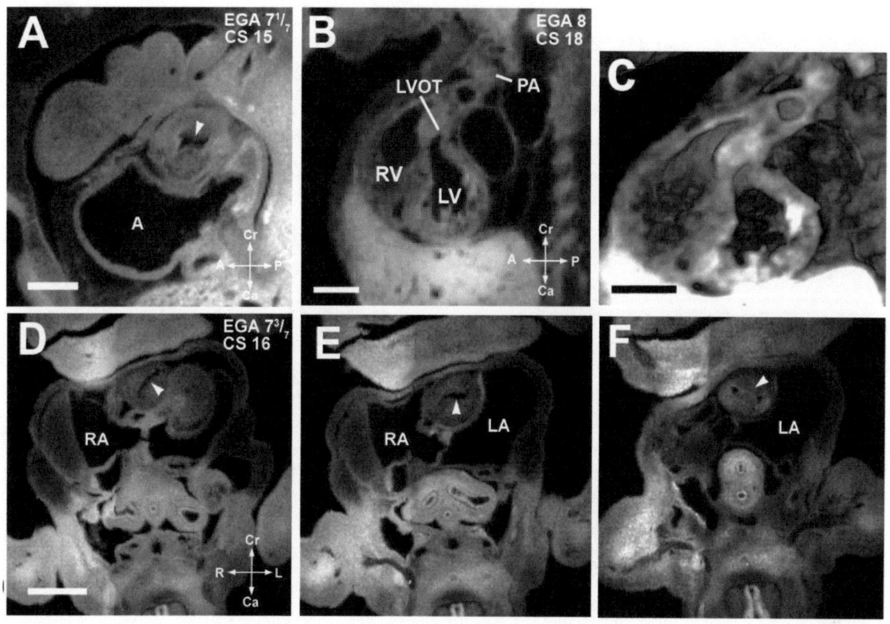

(A). EFIC image of an embryo at EGA $7^1/_7$ weeks (CS 15) in the sagittal plane shows a single orifice of the truncus arteriosus with inward swelling of the aorticopulmonary septum (arrowhead) which precedes septation of the truncus arteriosus. Scale bar = 0.622 mm.
(B,C) EFIC image of an EGA 8 (CS 18) embryo (B) show a distinct pulmonary artery (**PA**) emerging from the right ventricle (RV) and a left ventricular outflow tract (**LVOT**) or aorta emerging from the left ventricle (LV). 3D volume of the same embryo (C) shows crossing of the great arteries. Scale bar in (B,C)=1.35 mm.
(D-F). EFIC images of a embryo at EGA $7^3/_7$ weeks (CS 16) in oblique transverse planes showing the truncus arteriosus. Note changing orientation of the lumen (D,E) indicative of spiraling of the cushions (see arrowheads). In (F), the aorticopulmonary septum (arrowhead) has divided the distal portion of the truncus arteriosus into two separate arterial channels to the right and left of the aorticopulmonary septum. Scale bar = 0.9 mm.
A: primitive atrium, **RA:** right atrium, **LA:** left atrium, **RV**: right venetricle, **LV:** left ventricle.

Fig. 5. Septation of the truncus arteriosus.

Bartelings and Gittenberger de Groot[6] suggested that in $7^3/_7$ weeks (CS16) embryos septation begins at the ventriculo-arterial junction and progresses proximal to distal in the truncus arteriosus. However, our findings show septation of the truncus arteriosus occurring in the opposite direction, being complete distally in the $7^3/_7$ week (CS16) embryo, at a time when the proximal truncus arteriosus is still undivided. This would suggest that the direction of septation is distal to proximal. This is supported by Kirby[28], who described the proximal truncus arteriosus closing zipper-like from distal to proximal towards the ventricles. Our data also support both the timing and direction of septation proposed by

Anderson et al[29]. They described septation of the truncus arteriosus initiating distally and progressing proximally with the presence of distal septation and the absence of proximal septation at $7^{3}/_{7}$ week (CS 16). Moore[19] described bulbar ridges at the fifth week post conception, equivalent to 7 weeks gestation. Assuming the bulbar and truncal cushions are forming at the same time, our finding of truncal cushions in the outflow at $7^{1}/_{7}$ weeks (CS15) also corroborates these investigators' timeframe.

The process of semilunar valve morphogenesis, similar to atrioventricular valve morphogenesis, began earlier with the formation of truncal cushion tissue which was observed in the outflow starting at $7^{1}/_{7}$ weeks (CS15). At 8 weeks (CS18), distinct pulmonary and aortic valves can be seen (Fig.5B,C). These valve leaflets, as well as atrioventricular valve leaflets, are initially thick. They undergo a process of thinning as the valve leaflets continue to form and mature; a process that continues well after the formation of distinct valve leaflets (Fig. 6). By $9^{1}/_{7}$ weeks (CS22), all of the major structures of the heart are formed, with the last developmental milestone being completion of the inlet ventricular septum (see above).

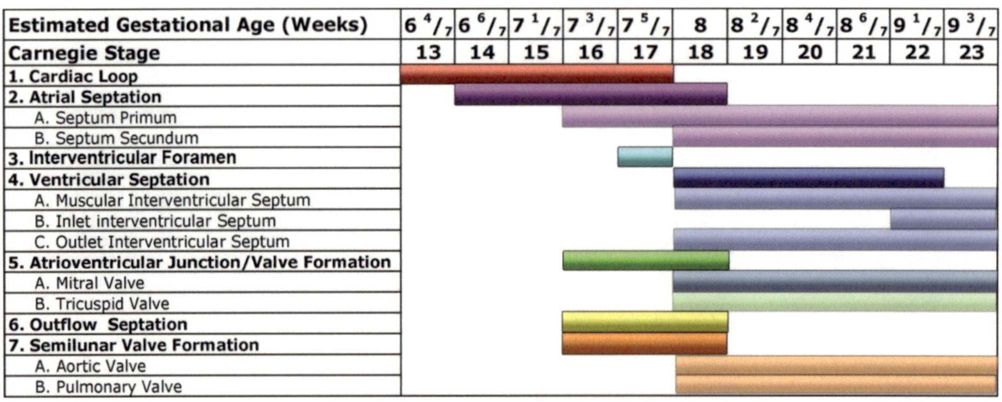

Fig. 6. Developmental time course of human cardiac morphogenesis.

10. Summary

As rapid advances in technology provide first trimester human fetal cardiac imaging and opportunities for in utero intervention continue to advance, there is increasing need for data documenting human cardiac development in the first trimester. Using a large data set generated by MRI and EFIC imaging, the major developmental milestones of human cardiac morphogenesis were delineated spanning EGA $6^{4}/_{7}$-$9^{3}/_{7}$ weeks. A summary timeline is provided in Figure 6 for the temporal profile of atrial and ventricular septation, outflow septation and valvular morphogenesis. In addition, Figures 7 and 8 were generated as reference guides to aid clinical practice. They contain thumbnail images of cardiac structures seen at each developmental milestone of cardiac morphogenesis. Full size images and Quicktime movies of the 2D serial image stacks of these embryos can be viewed and the web based Human Embryo Atlas (http://apps.devbio.pitt.edu/HumanAtlas) using guest login *Human* and password *Embryo*. A deeper understanding of human cardiovascular development, including this large dataset and the reference guides generated, may ultimately aid in clinical practice and facilitate prenatal diagnosis of CHD and appropriate counseling of families.

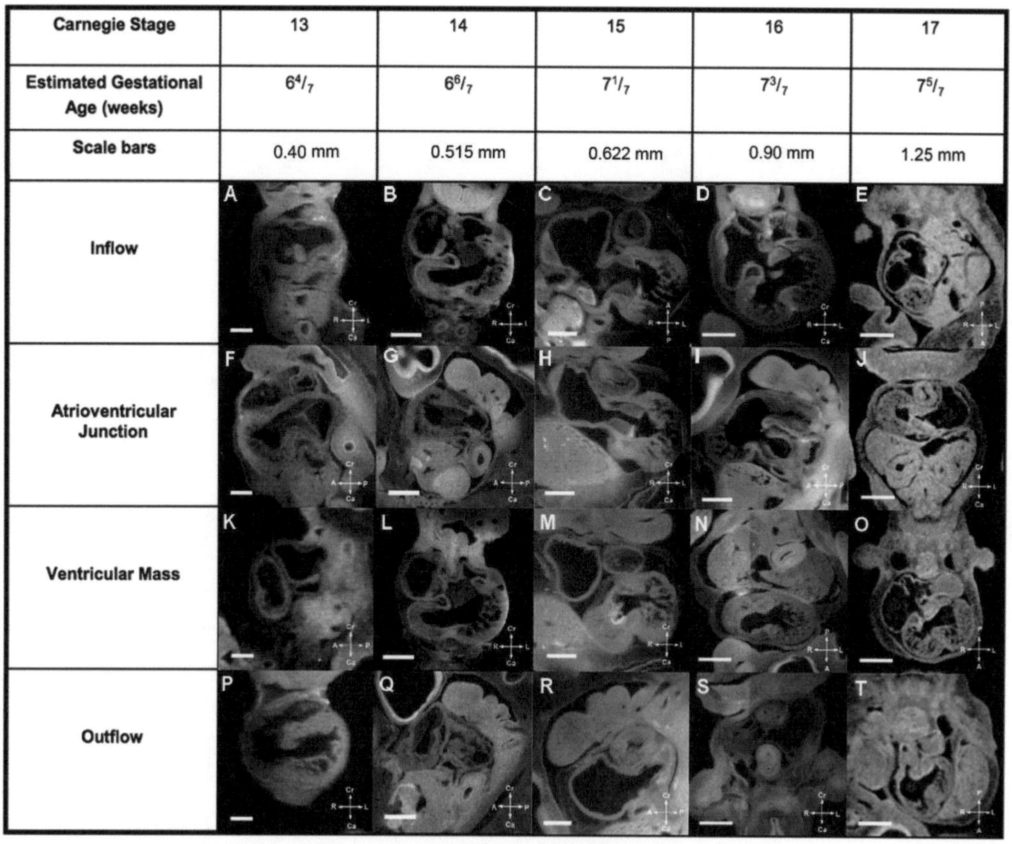

Fig. 7. Summary of Human Cardiac Developmental Milestones

Outlined in the chart is the timing for major cardiac morphogenetic events and the presence of various cardiac structures in the human embryo. The timeline indicated for Atrioventricular Junction/Valve Formation (green bar) refer to when a distinct atrioventricular junction is observed before atrioventricular valve leaflets are evident. The timelime indicated for Semilunar Valve Formation (orange bar) refer to when distinct truncal cushion tissue is observed and before semilunar valve leaflets are evident. The demarcation of Mitral Valve, Tricuspid Valve, Aortic Valve and Pulmonary Valve delineate the developmental stages when distinct valve leaflets are observed and the stages when the valve leaflets continue to undergo maturation and thinning. The timeline indicated for Interventricular Foramen refer to when any communication is present between the right and left ventricular chambers.

Major cardiac developmental structures present in EGA $6^4/_7$ weeks to $7^5/_7$ weeks (CS13-17) embryos are summarized in Figure 7, while Figure 8 shows the major developmental structures present in EGA 8 weeks to $9^3/_7$ weeks (CS18-23) embryos. One can look at a developmental structure at a specific estimated gestational age to determine what normal development is for that structure at that age in human cardiac development. The compass orients the observer to the plane of section.

Carnegie Stage	18	19	20	21	22	23
Estimated Gestational Age (weeks)	8	$8\frac{2}{7}$	$8\frac{4}{7}$	$8\frac{6}{7}$	$9\frac{1}{7}$	$9\frac{3}{7}$
Scale Bars	1.50 mm	1.50 mm	1.50 mm	1.75 mm	2.00 mm	2.00 mm

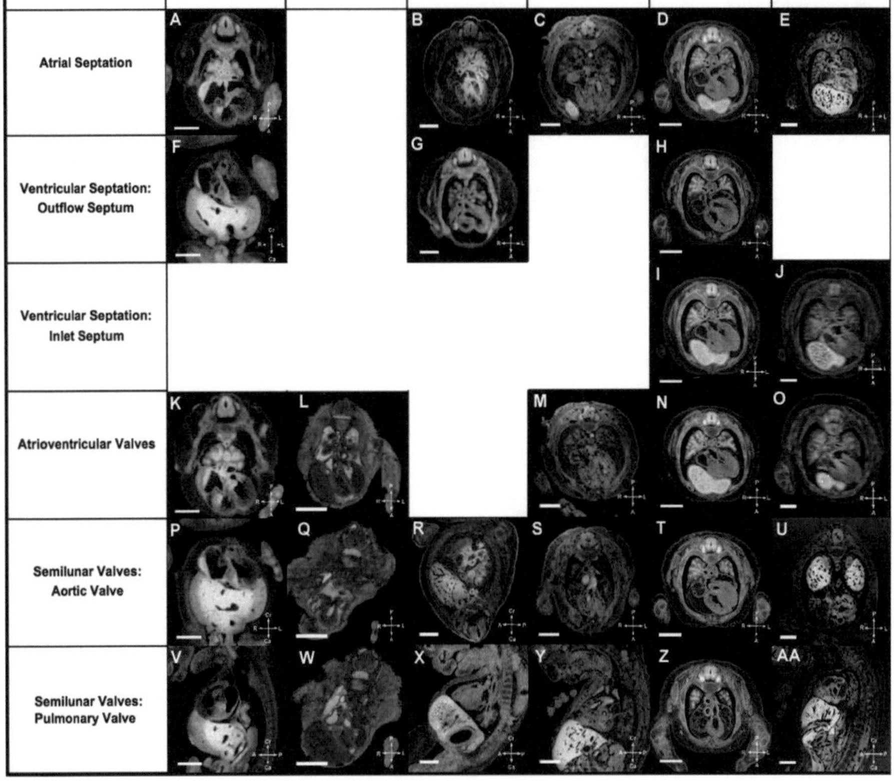

Fig. 8. Summary of Human Cardiac Developmental Milestones

The FIGURE NUMBER and PANEL LABELS correspond to panel labels of the individual thumbnails in Figures 7 and 8.

Figure 7A-E: Inflow
Figure 7F-J: Atrioventricular Junction
Figure 7K-O: Ventricular Mass
Figure 7P-T: Outflow
Figure 8A-E: Atrial septation
Figure 8F-H: Ventricular septation: Outflow Septum
Figure 8I,J: Ventricular septation: Inlet Septum
Figure 8K-O: Atrioventricular valves
Figure 8P-U: Semilunar valves: Aortic Valves
Figure 8V-AA: Semilunar valves: Pulmonary Valve

11. Acknowledgements

This work was supported by NIH grant ZO1-HL005701. The Kyoto collection was supported by Japanese Ministry of Education, Culture, Sports, Science and Technology

(Grant 19390050); Japanese Ministry of Health, Labor and Welfare (Grant: 17A-6) and Japan Science Technology Agency (BIRD grant). We would like to thank the research team at the National Institutes of Health. Their contribution was essential to the original work. Members of the team include Mary T Donofrio, MD, Elaine Lee BA, Anita Krishnan MD, Rajeev Samtani, Shigehito Yamada MD PhD , Stasia Anderson PhD and Elizabeth Lockett MA. Shigehito.Yamada was supported by Kyoto University Foundation.

12. Disclosures

Preeta Dhanantwari: None; Cecilia Lo: None; Linda Leatherbury: Research Grant: Comparison of Human Cardiac Development in the First Trimester with Mouse: Analysis with High Resolution MRI and EFIC.

13. References

[1] Kramer T. The partitioning of the truncus and conus and the formation of the membranous portion of the interventricular septum in the human heart. *Am J Anat.* 1942; 71:343-370.

[2] Grant RP. The embryology of ventricular flow pathways in man. *Circulation.* 1962; 25:756-779.

[3] Goor DA, Edwards JE, Lillehei CW. The development of the interventricular septum of the human heart; correlative morphogenetic study. *Chest.* 1970; 58(5):453-467.

[4] Anderson RH, Wilkinson JL, Arnold R, Lubkiewicz, K. Morphogenesis of bulboventricular malformations. I. Consideration of embryogenesis in the normal heart. *Br Heart J.* 1974; 36(3):242-255.

[5] Orts-Llorca F, Puerta Fonolla J, Sobrado J. The formation, septation and fate of the truncus arteriosus in man. *J Anat.* 1982; 134(Pt 1):41-56.

[6] Bartelings MM, Gittenberger-de Groot AC. The outflow tract of the heart--embryologic and morphologic correlations. *Int J Cardiol.* 1989; 22(3):289-300.

[7] Tonge M. Observations on the development of the semilunar valves of the aorta and pulmonary artery of the heart of the chick. *Phil Trans Roy Soc (London).* 1869; 159:387-411.

[8] Hamburger V HH. A series of normal stages in the development of the chick embryo. *Journal of Morphology.* 1951; 88:49-92.

[9] DeHaan RL. Development of form in the embryonic heart. An experimental approach. *Circulation.* 1967; 35(5):821-833.

[10] Rosenthal J, Mangal V, Walker D, Bennett M, Mohun TJ, Lo CW. Rapid high resolution three dimensional reconstruction of embryos with episcopic fluorescence image capture. *Birth Defects Res C Embryo Today.* 2004; 72(3):213-223.

[11] Smith BR, Linney E, Huff DS, Johnson GA. Magnetic resonance microscopy of embryos. *Comput Med Imaging Graph.* 1996; 20(6):483-490.

[12] Shiota K, Yamada S, Nakatsu-Komatsu T, Uwabe C, Kose K, Matsuda Y, Haishi T, Mizuta S, Matsuda T. Visualization of human prenatal development by magnetic resonance imaging (MRI). *Am J Med Genet A.* 2007; 143A(24):3121-3126.

[13] Nishimura H. *Prenatal versus postnatal malformations based on the Japanese experience on induced abortions in the human beingAging Gametes: Their Biology and Pathology* Seattle, WA: Karger, AG and Basel; 1975.

[14] Nishimura H, Takano K, Tanimura T, Yasuda M. Normal and abnormal development of human embryos: first report of the analysis of 1,213 intact embryos. *Teratology.* 1968; 1(3):281-290.

[15] Shiota K. Development and intrauterine fate of normal and abnormal human conceptuses. *Congenit Anom Kyoto* 1991; 31:67-80.

[16] Yamada S, Uwabe C, Fujii S, Shiota K. Phenotypic variability in human embryonic holoprosencephaly in the Kyoto Collection. *Birth Defects Res A Clin Mol Teratol.* 2004; 70(8):495-508.

[17] O'Rahilly R MF. Developmental stages in human embryos: including a revision of Streeter's "Horizons" and a survey of the Carnegie collection. *Washington DC: Carnegie Institution of Washington publication.* 1987.

[18] Weninger WJ, Mohun T. Phenotyping transgenic embryos: a rapid 3-D screening method based on episcopic fluorescence image capturing. *Nat Genet.* 2002; 30(1):59-65.

[19] Moore K, Persaud T. *The developing human clinically oriented embryology.* 8th ed. Philadelphia: WB Saunders; 2007.

[20] Lamers WH, Moorman AF. Cardiac septation: a late contribution of the embryonic primary myocardium to heart morphogenesis. *Circ Res.* 2002; 91(2):93-103.

[21] Wessels A, Anderson RH, Markwald RR, Webb S, Brown NA, Viragh S, Moorman AF, Lamers WH. Atrial development in the human heart: an immunohistochemical study with emphasis on the role of mesenchymal tissues. *Anat Rec.* 2000; 259(3):288-300.

[22] Anderson RH, Webb S, Brown NA, Lamers W, Moorman A. Development of the heart: (2) Septation of the atriums and ventricles. *Heart.* 2003; 89(8):949-958.

[23] Stadtfeld M, Ye M, Graf T. Identification of interventricular septum precursor cells in the mouse embryo. *Dev Biol.* 2007; 302(1):195-207.

[24] Wessels A, Vermeulen JL, Verbeek FJ, Viragh S, Kalman F, Lamers WH, Moorman AF. Spatial distribution of "tissue-specific" antigens in the developing human heart and skeletal muscle. III. An immunohistochemical analysis of the distribution of the neural tissue antigen G1N2 in the embryonic heart; implications for the development of the atrioventricular conduction system. *Anat Rec.* 1992; 232(1):97-111.

[25] Lamers WH, Wessels A, Verbeek FJ, Moorman AF, Viragh S, Wenink AC, Gittenberger-de Groot AC, Anderson RH. New findings concerning ventricular septation in the human heart. Implications for maldevelopment. *Circulation.* 1992; 86(4):1194-1205.

[26] Van Mierop LH, Kutsche LM. Development of the ventricular septum of the heart. *Heart Vessels.* 1985; 1(2):114-119.

[27] Waldo KL, Hutson MR, Ward CC, Zdanowicz M, Stadt HA, Kumiski D, Abu-Issa R, Kirby ML. Secondary heart field contributes myocardium and smooth muscle to the arterial pole of the developing heart. *Dev Biol.* 2005; 281(1):78-90.

[28] Kirby M. *Cardiac development.* New York: Oxford University Press; 2007.

[29] Anderson RH, Webb S, Brown NA, Lamers W, Moorman A. Development of the heart: (3) formation of the ventricular outflow tracts, arterial valves, and intrapericardial arterial trunks. *Heart.* 2003; 89(9):1110-1118.

9

Development, Differentiation and Derivatives of the Wolffian and Müllerian Ducts

Monika Jacob, Faisal Yusuf and Heinz Jürgen Jacob
Department of Anatomy and Molecular Biology, Ruhr-University Bochum, Germany

1. Introduction

The Wolffian ducts (pro- and mesonephric ducts) are the most important and earliest structures formed during the development of the urogenital system in vertebrates including humans. The Wolffian ducts originate in the prospective cervical region of the young embryo but later migrate caudally inducing the development of the pronephric and mesonephric tubules along their migratory route. In addition to being the inducers of the first two generations of the kidney, namely the pronephros and mesonephros, the Wolffian ducts also give rise to the ureteric buds which drive the growth and differentiation of the permanent kidneys, the metanephroi. The paired ureteric bud arises as outpouching from the caudal end of the Wolffian duct and induces the epithelialisation of the metanephric blastema leading to the formation of the renal corpuscles and tubular part of the nascent metanephric kidney, while the entire collecting system consisting of the ureter, the renal pelvis, the calyces and the collecting ducts take their origin from the ureteric bud.

Gender specific contributions of the Wolffian ducts amount to the induction and development of the Müllerian (paramesonephric) ducts, the anlagen of the female genital ducts, while in males, the Wolffian ducts elongate to form the epididymal ducts and the vasa deferentia. The seminal vesicles are formed during regression and transformation of the mesonephroi.

The developmental significance of the Wolffian duct for the development of the excretory and genital system can be drawn from the extirpation experiments in vertebrate embryos where the absence of Wolffian ducts showed that neither kidneys, nor male or female genital ducts develop.

Human embryos shown in this article were collected by the late Prof. K.V. Hinrichsen during the years 1970 till 1985. They are from legally terminated pregnancies in agreement with the German law and following the informed consent of the parents. For the description of human embryos the Carnegie stages (CS) are used.

2. Wolffian ducts

The Wolffian ducts are named after the German anatomist Caspar Friedrich Wolff (1733-94) who first described the paired mesonephros, also called Wolffian body and its duct. The mesonephroi represent the second kidney generation of vertebrates. The first generation, the pronephroi precede the mesonephroi in a temporal and spatial sequence. The pronephric ducts are continuous caudally with the mesonephric ducts. Therefore, we use the term Wolffian ducts for the common pro- and mesonephric ducts.

2.1 Development of the Wolffian ducts

The Wolffian duct anlagen arise from the right and left intermediate mesoderm between somites and somatopleure. They first appear as continuous ridges caudal to the sixth pair of somites at CS 10 in embryos with ten somites. Since the developmental steps are comparable with other vertebrates one can see how the Wolffian duct anlage shown here as a mesenchymal ridge in the scanning micrograph of a chick embryo (Fig. 1a) segregate from the dorsal part of the intermediate mesoderm.

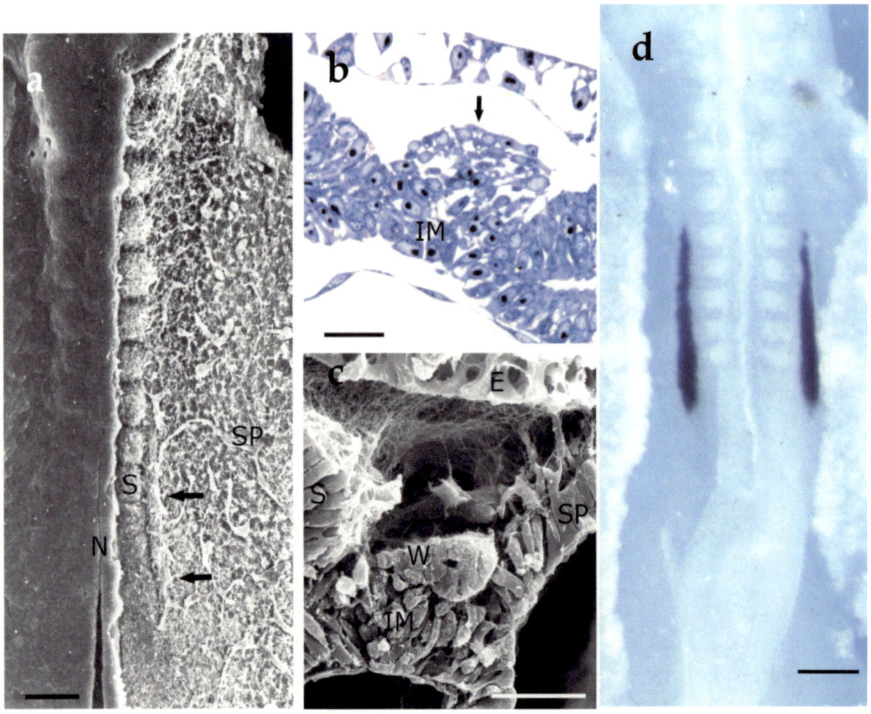

Fig. 1. Formation of the Wolffian ducts
a) Dorsal view of the Wolffian duct at stage 10 HH after extirpation of the ectoderm on the right side. Note the anlage of the Wolffian duct (arrows) adjacent to the last somite (S) and the anterior part of segmental plate. N, neural tube; SP, somatopleure. Bar = 100 µm.
b) Transverse semithin section through the mesenchymal anlage of the Wolffian duct (arrow). IM, intermediate mesoderm. Bar = 25 µm c) Canalized epithelial duct (W) on the ventral part of the intermediate mesoderm (IM). E, ectoderm; S, somite; SP, somatopleure; Bar = 25 µm. d) *Pax2* expression in the Wolffian duct anlagen in a stage 10 HH chick embryo (ten somites) as shown by *in situ* hybridization; Bar = 0.3 mm.

The mesenchymal ridges segregate from the dorsal part of the intermediate mesoderm (Fig. 1b). In human embryos at CS 11, the Wolffian ducts undergo mesenchymal-epithelial transitions and form two epithelial canalized ducts (Fig. 1c), on either side of the somites and segmental plate, however, their caudal tips maintain their mesenchymal identity and help them to migrate caudad on the intermediate mesoderm to join the cloaca at CS 12 (3 to 5 mm, 26 days, 26-28 somites).

The Wolffian duct anlagen can be identified by the expression of the *Pax2* gene (Fig. 1d), a transcriptional regulator of the paired-box gene family (see Torres et al., 1995) that controls the development of the different kidney generations. During urogenital development of vertebrates, *Pax2* appears at first within the Wolffian duct anlagen and in successive order in the other kidney generations and even in the Müllerian ducts. *Pax2* seems to induce the mesenchymal-epithelial transformation of the intermediate mesoderm (Dressler et al., 1990). Pax8 has synergistic effects, but knockout animals reveal no kidney defects.

Other genes have also been found to be important in early kidney development. Kobayashi et al. (2004) documented the expression of the LIM- class homeodomain transcription factor *Lim1* in the Wolffian ducts and knockout animals fail to develop Wolffian ducts. The homeobox gene *Emx2* was proposed to regulate the epithelial function of Pax2 and Lim1 (Miyamoto et al., 1997).

2.1.1 Migration of the Wolffian ducts

Experimental and morphological data suggest that the extension of the Wolffian ducts along their caudal path is not only the result of proliferation, but of active migration of the cells at their posterior tips (Jacob et al., 1992). Furthermore, experiments performed in chicken embryos (Grünwald, 1937; Jacob and Christ, 1978) show the significance of the mesenchymal tip of the Wolffian duct: as following its extirpation, migration of the duct stops and the mesonephros fails to develop on the operated side (Fig. 2). The metanephros

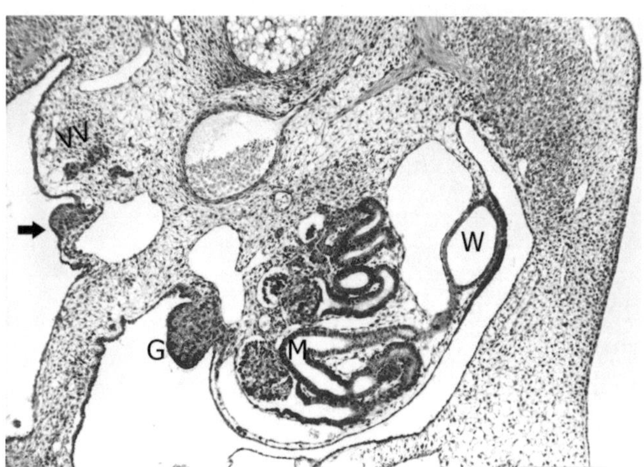

Fig. 2. Extirpation of the caudal tip of the Wolffian duct.
Transverse section through a chicken embryo sacrified two days after extirpation of the caudal part of the Wolffian duct. Control side with well developed mesonephros (M), Wolffian duct (W), and gonadal anlage (G). On the operated side (left) the mesonephros shows only rudimentary tubules (vv) and a smaller gonadal anlage (arrow). Bar = 100 μm.

and the genital ducts of both genders eventually fail to develop. The gonad although appearing normal, is considerably reduced in size on the manipulated side.

The cells at the duct tip extend long cell processes, which are in contact with the extracellular matrix (Fig. 3a). Also required for the caudally directed migration of the Wolffian duct are the special properties of the extracellular matrix through which the duct migrates. Epithelial parts of ducts implanted at the place of the tip cells were able to migrate towards the cloaca even if their cranial end was rotated. Only the intermediate mesoderm caudal to the duct tip induces and guides this migration. Matrix molecules like fibronectin are supposed to be an important component of the special substrate needed for the migration of the Woffian ducts (Jacob et al., 1991). Although fibronectin may be a prerequisite for cell migration, its nearly ubiquitous occurrence rules out a specific role in directed cell migration of this molecule in this context (see also Bellairs et al., 1995). It is suggested that polysialic acid plays a more specific role in the migration of chicken Wolffian ducts. NCAM polysialic acid had a similar distribution as fibronectin, and treatment of the living embryo with Endo-N specifically degrades polysialic acid and stops the caudal extension of the duct.

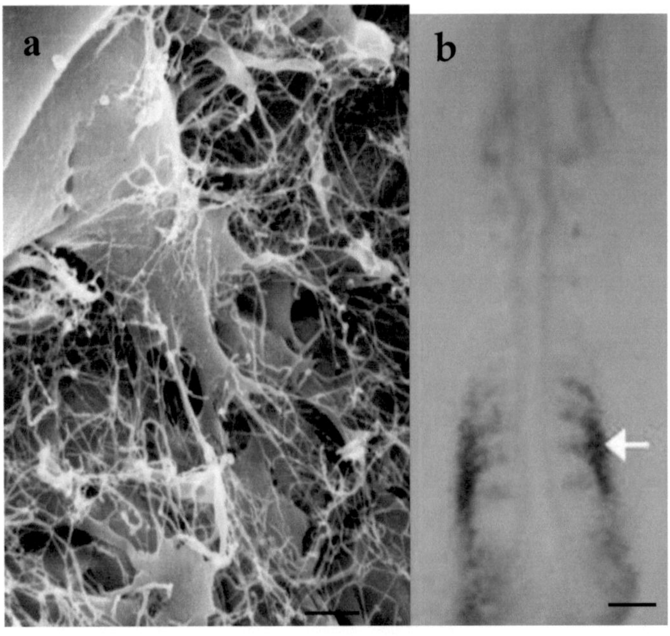

Fig. 3. Migration of Wolffian ducts.
a) Scanning electron micrograph of the tip region from a stage 13 HH (Hamburger, Hamilton) chick embryo Wolffian duct. Note the cell processes, which are in contact with the extracellular matrix. Bar = 10 µm. b) In situ hybridization of a stage 9 HH chick embryo showing *CXCR4* expression domain in the posterior half of the most caudal somites and in the intermediate mesoderm (*white arrow*). Bar = 0.2 mm.

Since the migration of the Wolffian ducts is a crucial step in the development of the urogenital system the search for the molecules that guide migration and regulate insertion of the ducts is still ongoing. Research over the years has brought some molecules to light that may be involved in guidance of this migration either by adhesion gradients or chemotaxis. A guidance cue identified in Axolotl is GDNF, which activates signaling through the c GFRα1-Ret receptor (Drawbridge et al., 2000). In the chicken embryos, the receptor CXCR4 was shown (Fig. 3b and Yusuf et al., 2006) to be expressed in the region of the developing mesonephros anlage. Furthermore Grote et al. (2006) suggested that Pax2/8 regulated Gata3, which itself controls Ret expression is necessary for Wolffian ducts guidance.

2.2 Development of pro- and mesonephros

During the caudad extension and migration of the Wolffian ducts they induce the formation of nephric tubules within the right and left intermediate mesoderm starting with the pronephros in the cervical region. The characteristics of the pronephroi are that they form

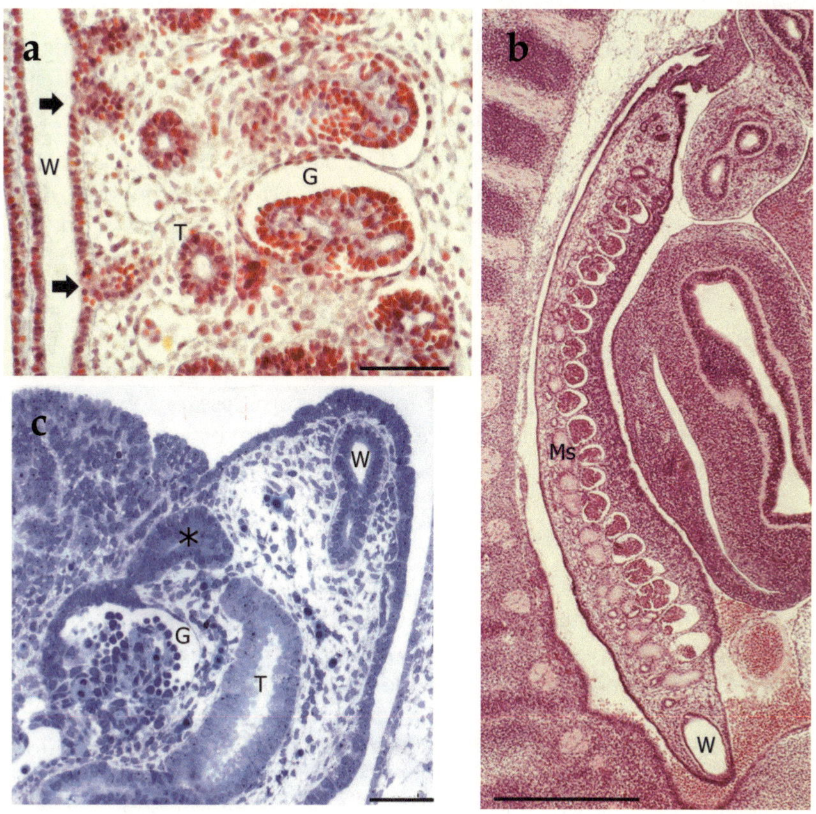

Fig. 4. Development of mesonephros
a) Sagittal section through the cranial part of the mesonephros of a 7.5 mm (CS 14/15) embryo with the longitudinal Wolffian duct (W) on the left side. Arrows, openings of tubules (T) into the duct; G, glomerulus. Azan staining. Bar = 50 μm. b) Sagittal section of the whole mesonephros (Ms) of a 10 mm (CS 16) embryo. Note the serially arranged nephrons with tubules and mesonephric corpuscles. W, caudal dilated part of the Wolffian duct. HE staining. Bar = 500 μm. c) Transverse semithin section of a 14.8 mm (CS 18) embryo W, Wolffian duct; asterisk, secretory part of a tubule; T, collecting part; G, glomerulus; Bar = 50 μm.

external glomerula and their tubules drain into the coelomic cavity via openings called nephrostomata. These structures exist also in human embryos though in higher vertebrates, the pronephroi are only rudimentary with no significant excretory function.

Early in the fourth week follows the successive induction of mesonephric tubules extending from the thoracal to the lumbal region. These tubules drain into the Wolffian ducts (Fig. 4a) and their blind ends form typical renal corpuscles with Bowman's capsule and glomerulus (Fig. 4a-c). Each tubule may be divided in a secretory and a more faintly stained collecting part (Fig. 4c). The secretory part resembles the proximal tubule of the permanent kidney with well-established microvilli.

The formation of tubules is terminated by CS 14 with a total number ranging between 35 to 38.

2.3 Development and differentiation of the ureteric buds

The permanent kidneys, the metanephroi develop by interaction of the ureteric bud with the metanephric blastema in the lumbosacral region of the intermediate mesoderm.

Early in the fifth week (CS 14) ureteric buds branch from the posterior ends of the Wolffian ducts at the level of the first sacral segment (Fig. 5a). According to Chi et al. (2009) the epithelium in the caudal part of the Wolffian duct convert prior to budding from a simple epithelium into a pseudostratified. The exact position and outgrowth in dorso-cranial direction of the ureteric buds is critical to join the metanephric blastema and thus for the development of the permanent kidneys.

The ampulla-like blind end of each ureteric bud is surrounded by a cap of dense mesenchyme, forming the metanephric blastema (Fig. 5a and b). Reciprocal interactions between ureteric bud and metanephric mesenchyme are necessary for the outgrowth and branching of the ureteric bud on one hand and the mesenchymal-epithelial transformation and tubulogenesis of the metanephric blastema on the other hand (Fig. 5b and c).

2.3.1 Branching of the ureteric buds

The contact point of the ureteric bud and the metanephrogenic blastema represents the coming together of two functionally distinct kidney parts, namely the urine conducting and the urine producing system respectively. An appropriate out pouching site of ureteric bud from the Wolfian duct followed by its dichotomic patterning enable not just a formation of a functional urinary tract, but also ensure the viability of the metanephric kidney. Extensive research over the last decades in this field underlines the significance of appropriate ureteric bud outgrowth and patterning as urinary tract malformations are amongst the most common congenital defects accounting to around 1% of all congenital defects. Further impact of faulty ureteric bud branching also affects the absolute nephron number in the kidney which may play out as a predisposition to chronic renal failure.

The correct outgrowth of the ureteric buds and their dichotomic budding is controlled by a network of genes (see for review Constantini and Kopan, 2010) with GDNF/RET signaling as a main factor. GDNF is expressed in the metanephric mesenchyme and the Ret receptor tyrosine kinase and its co-receptor Gfrα1 in the tip of the ureteric bud. It has been experimentally shown that it is not the expression, but the activity of the RET that is decisive for the site of ureteric bud out pouching selection. Wnt signaling transducter β-catenin (Marose et al., 2008) and Gata3 (Grote et al., 2008), a zinc finger transcription factor, act together and are pivotal in modulating the RET activity at the prospective ureteric bud formation site in the caudal Wolffian duct.

The mode of branching was shown by Osathanondh and Potter (1963) using microdissection. At CS 16 the ampullated tip divides into two branches determing the cranial and caudal pole of each metanephros.

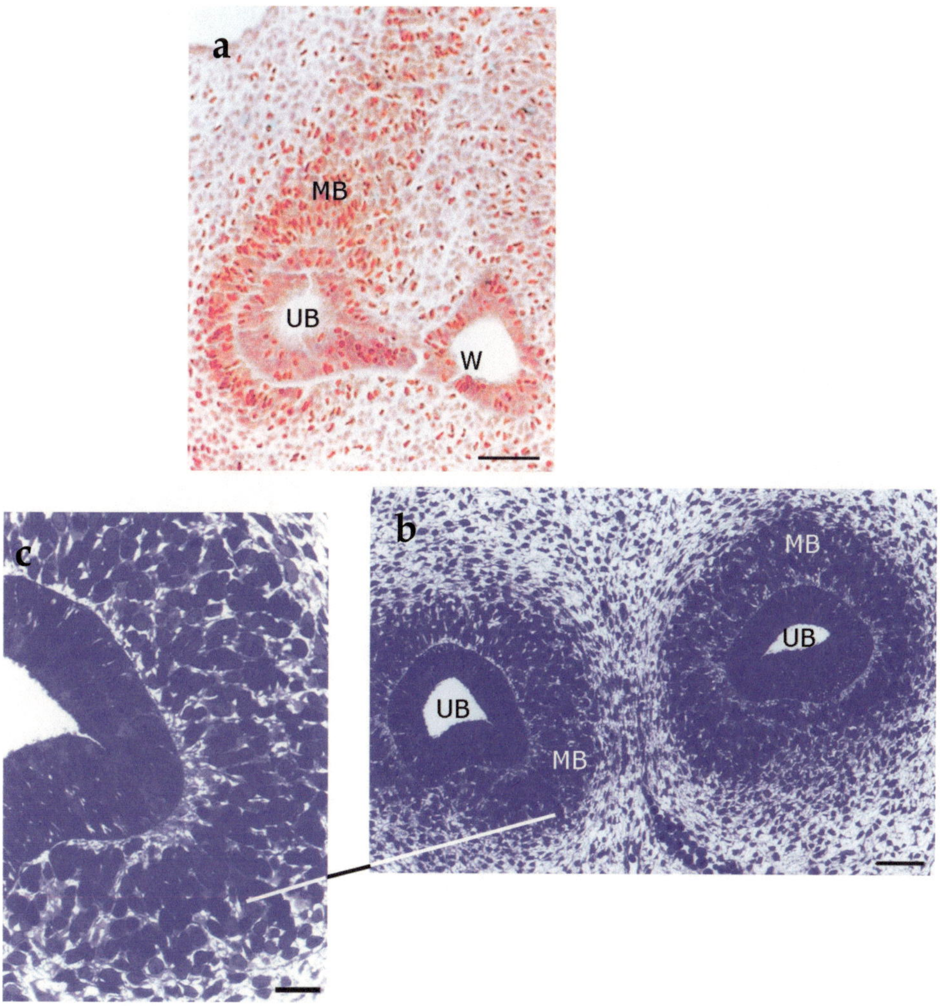

Fig. 5. Ureteric buds and metanephrogenic blastemata
a) Sagittal section from a 6.5 mm (CS 14) embryo with outgrowing ureteric bud (UB). W, Wolffian duct; MB, metanephrogenic blastema. Azan staining. Bar = 50 μm. b) Horizontal section from a 10.5 mm (CS 16) embryo. The tip of ureteric bud (UB) is dilated and starts branching induced by the metanephrogenic blastema (MB). Bar = 50 μm. c) Detail from b marked by the line. The cells of the dense metanephrogenic blastema connect the dividing tip of the ureteric bud with multiple cell processes. Bar = 20 μm.

The mode of branching is unique to the kidney with lateral and terminal bifid branches (Al-Awqati and Goldberg, 1998). The terminal branch can no longer divide since it induces the formation of nephrons.

At CS 19 four to six generations of branching can be observed. Within the metanephrogenic blastema adjacent to the ampulla vesicles form. Each vesicle eventually differentiates into a tubule and the glomerulus (Fig. 6).

The first three generations of division dilate and fuse to form the renal pelvis, the fourth and fifth form the calyces. The further divisions - 6 to approximately 15 - generate the collecting ducts. By the 22nd to 23rd weeks of gestation branching is completed.

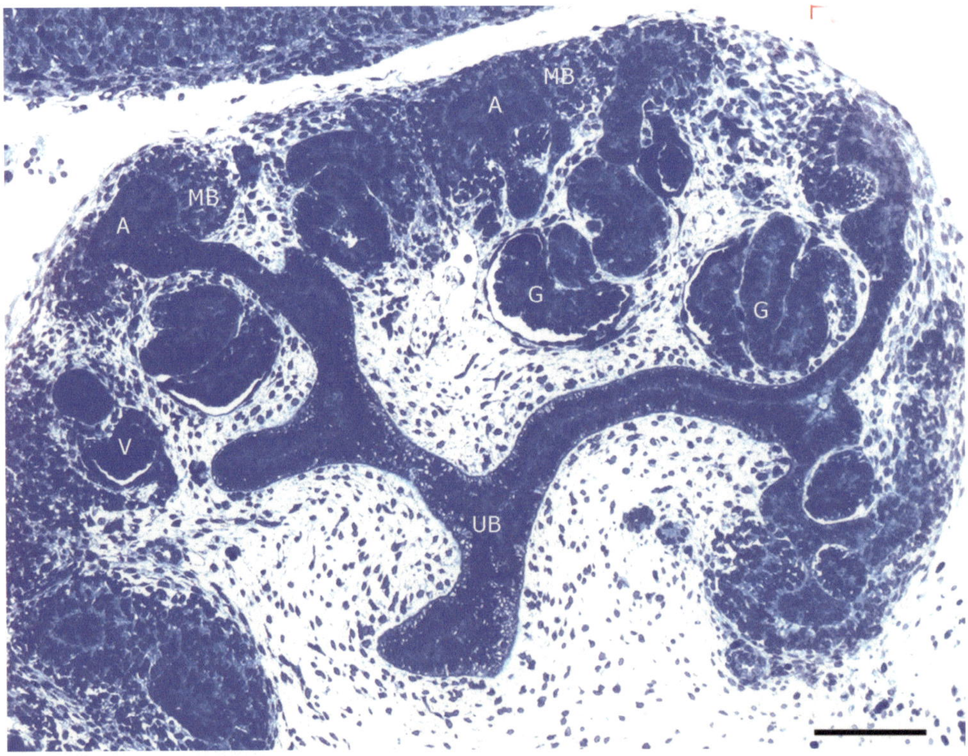

Fig. 6. Branching of ureteric bud.
Semithin-section through the metanephros of a 25 mm (CS 22) embryo. Dichotom branching of the ureteric bud (UB). The ampulla-like blind end (A) induces the formation of vesicles (V) within the metanephrogenic blastema (MB). The vesicles differentiate into tubules and glomeruli (G). Bar = 100 μm.

2.4 Differentiation of the Wolffian ducts in male fetuses

The stabilization and further growth of the Wolffian ducts depend on androgen that is produced in the testes of male embryos starting from the eighth week of gestation. An active stimulation is necessary to prevent regression of the ducts and the mesonephric tubules and to induce the differentiation of epididymides and vasa deferentia. The androgen receptor is first found in the mesenchyme surrounding the duct epithelium and interacts with different growth factors like EGF (epidermal growth factor) (see for review Hannema and Hughes, 2007). Expression of EGF and its receptor can be increased by androgen treatment and vice versa. EGF modulates sexual differentiation by enhancement of AR-mediated transcriptional activity and not enhancement of AR gene expression receptor (Gupta, 1999).

2.4.1 Development of the epididymis

Epididymal development depends on a cascade of molecular and morphological events controlling transformation and regression of mesonephric nephrons and the persistence of the Wolffian duct (Kirchhoff, 1999). In the male, some of the mesonephric tubuli eventually form the ductuli efferentes located in the caput epididymidis, while the Wolffian ducts differentiate into the right and left ductus epididymidis and the vas (ductus) deferens. During the transformation of the mesonephroi into the paired epididymis, two waves of regression are observed. The first wave of regression occurs in the most cranial nephrons and starts before the caudal parts of the mesonephroi are fully developed and is correlated with an inner descent of mesonephroi and gonads. Felix (1911) found this wave to be terminated in 21mm embryos (about CS 20). The second wave of regression includes the caudal part of the mesonephroi persisting as rudimental paradidymis. In the third month, the surviving mesonephric tubuli unite with the anlage of the rete testis.

The process of transformation from nephrons into ductuli efferentes remains poorly understood. In some vertebrates, a special mode involves the *de novo* formation of ductuli efferentes from the Bowman's capsules in the chicken (Budras and Sauer, 1975) or from the dorsal part of the giant nephric corpuscle of the bovine embryo (Wrobel, 2001). The appearance of the apoptotic p53 proteins and the antiapoptotic bcl-2 in the mesonephros from the seventh week on (Carev et al., 2006) coincide with the regression on one hand and the survival of some tubules on the other hand.

We investigated the development of the epididymis in human embryos from 14,8 mm (CS 18) to a 170 mm fetus. The CS 18 embryo reveals well-developed mesonephroi (Fig. 4c). The structure of the glomeruli is similar to those of the metanephroi with a thin capillary endothelium and podocytes. The structure of the proximal tubules resembles that of the proximal tubules of the permanent kidney, however the distal parts of the mesonephric tubules seem to have only collecting function.

Shortly later, already in the first wave of regression or at the beginning of the second period, degeneration of glomeruli and proximal tubuli starts. According to Felix (1911) only the distal parts of the tubuli adjacent to the testis (epigenital tubules) survive. They elongate to form coiled ductuli, which eventually join the rete testis. In our 26 mm embryo (eighth week) long and straight tubules are found near the developing rete testis. More medial sections (Fig. 7a) show nephric corpuscles with fused or degenerating glomeruli and thickened Bowman's capsule at the testicular side.

The 32 mm fetus (ninth week) exhibits condensed and small glomeruli. Near the anlage of the testicular rete, tubules with narrow or obliterated lumina are visible (Fig. 7b). However their morphological features do not elucidate whether they belong to remnants of degenerating proximal tubules or are new outgrowths from Bowman's capsules. A mesenchymal sheath forms around the wide Wolffian ducts, a prerequisite for the subsequent elongation and coiling of the Wolffian ducts since androgens are supposed to act via mesenchymal androgen receptors.

In a 45 mm embryo the paired Wolffian duct had increased in length and transformation into the ductus epididymidis starts in the proximal region with the characteristic coiling. During the enormous elongation up to six meters in the adult epididymis, the duct twists into another direction and folds onto itself. Constraints of the surrounding mesenchymal tissue are the supposed forces for the coiling and the narrow space which forces the duct to compact in the anterior region especially in the later corpus of epididymis (Joseph et al., 2009).

In a 68 mm fetus, the epididymal duct assumes an increasingly coiled arrangement. The blind ends of the prospective ductuli efferentes are dilated.

The 88 mm fetus, 13th week, shows the rete testis on either side fused with the ductuli efferentes. The epididymal duct is highly convoluted, but the distal part remains straight (Fig. 7c). It is lined by a non-specific cylindrical epithelium and is surrounded by many concentric layers of mesenchyme.

In the 170 mm fetus, 21th week, in the anterior region a dense coiling and an increased mesenchymal sheath are found. The mesenchyme is essential for the maturation of the ducts and especially for the formation of the vasa deferentia. At this stage, testis and epididymis establish contact with the jelly gubernaculum (Barteczko and Jacob, 2000).

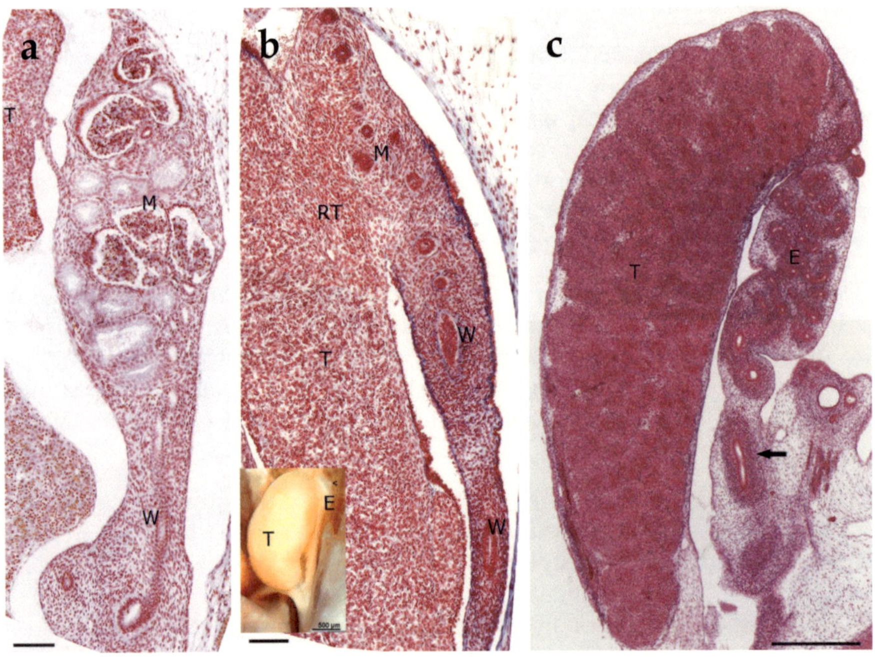

Fig. 7. Development of epididymis
a) Sagittal section of a 26 mm (eighth week) male embryo. In the epigenital part of the mesonephros (M) fused glomeruli and tubules are visible; W, Wolffian duct; T, testis. Azan staining. Bar = 100 µm. b) Sagittal section of a 32 mm (ninth week) male fetus. Tubules of mesonephros (M) with narrow or obliterated lumina are found near the rete testis (RT). T, testis; W, Wolffian duct. Azan staining. Bar = 100 µm. Inset: Testis and epididymis of a 68 mm about 11 weeks, fetus. Asterisk, appendix epididymidis. c) Sagittal section through testis (T) and epididymis (E) of a 88 mm (13th week) male fetus. Note the coiled ductus epididymidis and the straight vas deferens (arrow). HE staining. Bar = 500 µm.

The differentiation of the specific sections of the Wolffian ducts is regulated by the regional expression of Hox genes. In mouse embryos *Hoxa9* and *Hoxd9* are expressed in the epididymis and vas deferens, *Hoxa10* and *Hoxd10* in the caudal epididymis and the vas deferens, *Hoxa11* in the vas deferens, and *Hoxa13* and *Hoxd13* in the caudal portion of the WD and seminal vesicles (Hannema and Hughes, 2007).

2.4.2 Differentiation of the distal part of the Wolffian duct

The secretion of testosterone stimulates also the differentiation of the distal parts of the Wolffian ducts into the vasa (ductus) deferentia and the seminal vesicles. As already mentioned, the regional differentiation of the Wolffian duct is related to Hox genes. E.g. *Hoxa-10* domain of expression in male mice embryos has a distinct anterior border at the junction of the cauda epididymidis and the ductus deferens and extends to the sinus urogenitalis (Podlasek et al., 1999).

The development of the straight ductus deferens is characterized by the formation of the thick coat of circular smooth muscle cells.

The seminal vesicles sprout out of the Wolffian duct close to its entrance into the urethral part of the urogenital sinus between the tenth and twelfth week. The common ducts of vasa deferentia and seminal vesicles are called ductus ejaculatoria.

At around the ninth week of gestation, the ureteric buds have separated from the Wolffian ducts and their openings lie superior to those of the Wolffian ducts into the bladder part of the sinus urogenitalis. The common view that the Wolffian ducts are incorporated into the posterior bladder wall to form the trigone is now questioned and lineage studies have shown that the trigone mesenchyme derives from the bladder musculature (Viana et al., 2007). Apoptosis seems to play a role in ureter transposition. Regulation of the different growth and insertion of ureteric bud and distal Wolffian duct (vas deferens) is unknown.

2.5 Differentiation of the Wolffian ducts in female fetuses

In the female, the Wolffian ducts degenerate due to the absence of testosterone. Only rudiments persist as Gartner's ducts or cysts running in the broad ligament to the wall of the vagina.

3. Müllerian ducts

The Müllerian (paramesonephric) ducts are named after the German physiologist Johannes Peter Müller (1801-58). The formation of the human Müllerian ducts starts in the sixth week when other organs are already functional. They develop in close proximity and by induction of the Wolffian ducts. In male embryos they regress shortly after their formation under the influence of the anti-Müller-hormone produced by the Sertoli cells of the testes. In female embryos they further differentiate and form the oviducts (uterine tubes), the uterus and the vagina.

3.1 Development of the Müllerian ducts

The formation of the human Müllerian ducts starts in the sixth week (CS 16) as drop-like aggregations of cells beneath the cranial part of the Müllerian or tubal ridges corresponding to the thickened stripes of coelomic epithelium located near the Wolffian ducts (Jacob et al., 1999). Here, at the transition zone between pro- and mesonephros a discrete population of cells within the coelomic epithelium gives rise to the epithelium of the paired Müllerian duct as shown by lineage tracing studies (Guioli et al., 2007). In the 11,5 mm embryo ostium-like indentations of the coelomic epithelium were observed determining both so-called funnel-regions. Placode-like thickenings and deepenings of the coelomic epithelium form the anlagen of the Müllerian ducts. In some vertebrates including humans, these cranial parts of the Müllerian duct are supposed to contain remnants of nephrostomes from the last pronephric and the first mesonephric tubules (see for discussion Jacob et al., 1999; Wrobel and Süß, 2000). A solid cord of cells forms from each ostium or funnel region and rapidly grows caudally in close vicinity to the Wolffian ducts. It has been experimentally shown that in vertebrates the Wolffian ducts are required for the induction of Müllerian duct formation and in their absence no Müllerian duct can develop.

Labeling dividing cells with BrdU in chick and mouse embryos provide evidence that high cell proliferation of the Müllerian duct epithelium and the coelomic epithelium of the funnel region can be regarded as the motor of the caudal extension of the Müllerian ducts (Jacob et al., 1999; Guioli et al., 2007) ranging from 330 μm length in a 12.5 mm embryo and between 1440 and 1220 μm in a 17 mm embryo (Felix, 1911). Interestingly, in chick and human embryos two to four accessory openings into the coelomic cavity were observed in the cranial part of the Müllerian ducts (Felix, 1911; Jacob et al., 1999). Since these accessory funnels exist only during the robust expansion phase of the Müllerian ducts development, they probably supply more cells from the coelomic epithelium at the funnel field. Whether they are remnants of pronephric tubules has to be elucidated.

The major part of each Müllerian duct anlage canalizes (Fig. 8a) with the exception of the caudal tip. In 17 to 21 mm human embryos, at the point where the ducts are in close contact no basal lamina is present between each Müllerian and Wolffian duct (Fig. 8b). In this way the Wolffian ducts guide the Müllerian ducts to the lumbal region. However, Müllerian and Wolffian duct epithelium can be distinguished because of their distinctive morphological features (Laurence et al., 1992). The Müllerian ducts are more pseudostratified and reveal

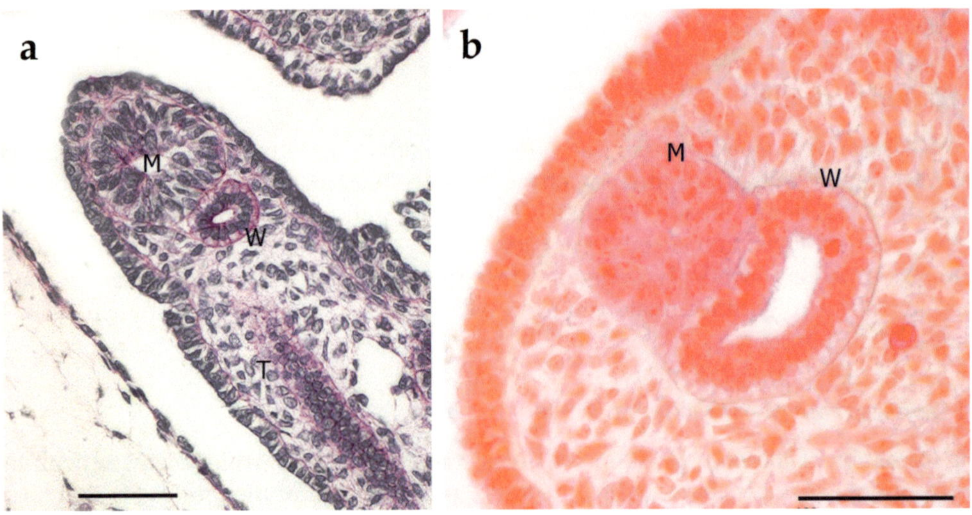

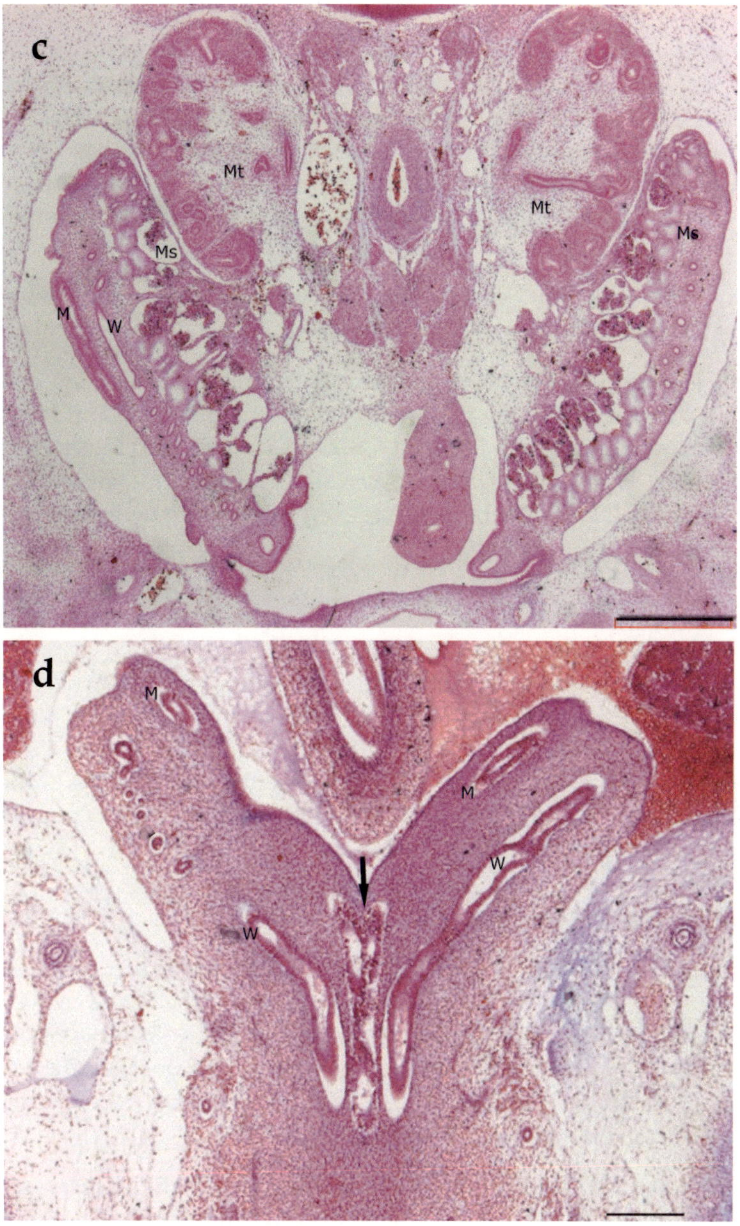

Fig. 8. Formation of the Müllerian ducts
a) Frontal section from a 16 mm (CS 18) embryo. Cranial part of the Müllerian duct (M) adjacent to the Wolffian duct (W). PAS staining. Bar = 50 µm. b) Sagittal section through a 21 mm (CS 20, eighth week) embryo. Note the close relation of müllerian (M) and Wolffian duct (W). Azan staining. Bar = 50 µm. c) Frontal/horizontal section of a 26 mm (CS 22) eighth week with both mesonephroi (Ms) and the developing metanephroi (Mt). W, Wolffian duct; M, Müllerian duct. Azan staining. Bar = 500 µm. d) Frontal section through a 29 mm (CS 23). The Müllerian ducts (M) are fused in the midline (arrow). W, Wolffian duct. Azan staining. Bar = 200 µm.

a larger number of elaborate microvilli at their luminal surfaces. Wolffian ducts exhibit abundant intracytoplasmatic glycogen. Furthermore, immunohistochemical investigations in chick and mouse embryos have also shown that the Müllerian ducts differ from the Wolffian ducts in their expression of the mesenchymal marker vimentin characterizing them as mesothel while the Wolffian ducts are true epithelial tubes expressing cytokeratin (Jacob et al., 1999; Orvis and Behringer, 2007). From this and other experimental and molecular data available any cell contributions from the Wolffian ducts to the Müllerian ducts could be excluded (Jacob et al., 1999; Guioli et al., 2007; Orvis and Behringer, 2007).

While the Müllerian ducts grow caudally, their cranial parts are separated from the Wolffian ducts by circular mesenchymal layers (Fig. 8c) derived from the dissolved tubal ridges.

In the 22 mm embryo (CS 21), the Müllerian ducts cross the Wolffian ducts to extend medially and join each other. In the midline the two Müllerian ducts run caudally and fuse to a single tube, the uterovaginal canal. At CS 22 to 23 this canal inserts at the separated anterior part of the cloaca, the sinus urogenitalis. Here the mesenchyme of the ducts proliferates and protrudes the wall of the sinus urogenitalis forming the Müllerian tubercle.

At first the fusion of the Müllerian ducts is only external with the formation of a common basal lamina, because a septum still separates the fused ducts. A single lumen was found at CS 23 (Hashimoto, 2003).

Genes that are required for Müllerian duct formation are also found in kidney development: *Lim1* specifies cells in the coelomic epithelium (Kobayashi et al., 2004) and *Wnt-4* induces the invagination of these cells (Vainio et al., 1999). The Wolffian duct also induces the expression of *Pax2* in the Müllerian duct although the anterior part of the Müllerian ducts is initially formed in Pax2 mutants (Torres et al., 1995), indicating an autonomy of the funnel region (for review see also Massé et al., 2009).

3.2 Regression of the Müllerian ducts in male fetuses

Regression of the Müllerian ducts in males is due to the production of anti-Müllerian hormone (AMH), also named Müllerian-inhibiting substance (MIS), by the Sertoli cells of the testes. A hormone for development of male reproductive duct different from testosterone was first postulated by Jost (1953). Secretion of AMH, a member of the transforming growth factor-β (TGF-β) family, starts in the eighth week of gestation and provokes the irreversible regression of the Müllerian duct in the eighth and ninth week (Rey, 2005).

AMH induces apoptosis within the Müllerian duct epithelium through a paracrine mechanism binding to the AMH type2 receptor (AMHRII) expressed in the mesenchyme around the epithelial tube. Allard et al. (2000) found a cranio- caudal gradient of AMHRII in the peritubal mesenchyme followed by a wave of apoptosis. They furthermore suggest that β-catenin, playing a role in the Wnt signaling, mediates apoptosis. They also described that beside apoptosis, an epithelio-mesenchymal transformation is important for regression. Apoptosis needs the disruption of the basal lamina correlating with the loss of fibronectin and expression of the metalloproteinase 2 gene (*Mmp2*) (see for review Massé et al., 2009).

The Müllerian ducts do not completely disappear. The most cranial parts are supposed to persist as appendices testis (see below) and the caudal parts as prostatic utricles. However,

Shapiro et al. (2004) concluded from their immunohistochemical studies that the utricle forms as an ingrowth of specialized cells from the dorsal wall of the sinus urogenitalis.

3.3 Differentiation of the Müllerian ducts in female fetuses

In the female, where AMH is lacking, the uniform Müllerian ducts differentiate in very specific segment to give rise to the uterine tubes (oviducts), the uterus, cervix and the vagina. These specification along the antero-posterior axis is due to a specific *Hox*-code. As during the differentiation of the Wolffian duct in male fetuses, Hox genes are expressed according to a spatial and temporal axis. In the female reproductive tract the *HOXA/hoxa* genes 9, 10, 11 and 13 are expressed (Taylor et al., 1997) and their pattern is highly conserved between the murine and the human. Furthermore members of the Wnt family are necessary for a correct pattern and differentiation of the female reproductive tract. e.g. Loss of function of *Wnt-7a* was reported to result in a partial posteriorization of the female reproductive tract, specifically, the oviduct had acquired characteristics of the uterus and the uterus characteristics of the vagina (Miller and Sassoon, 1998).

3.3.1 Differentiation of the uterine tubes

The non-fused cranial part of the Müllerian ducts form the uterine tubes (oviducts) reaching from the abdominal ostium with anlage of fimbria to the insertion of the gubernacula Hunteri (later round ligaments) (Fig. 9a). During the twelfth week of gestation, the simple columnar epithelium grows more than the surrounding mesenchyme thus forming the characteristic folding of the epithelium lining a stellate lumen (Wartenberg, 1990). The paratubal mesenchyme proliferates and differentiates into the smooth muscle layers and the lamina propria.

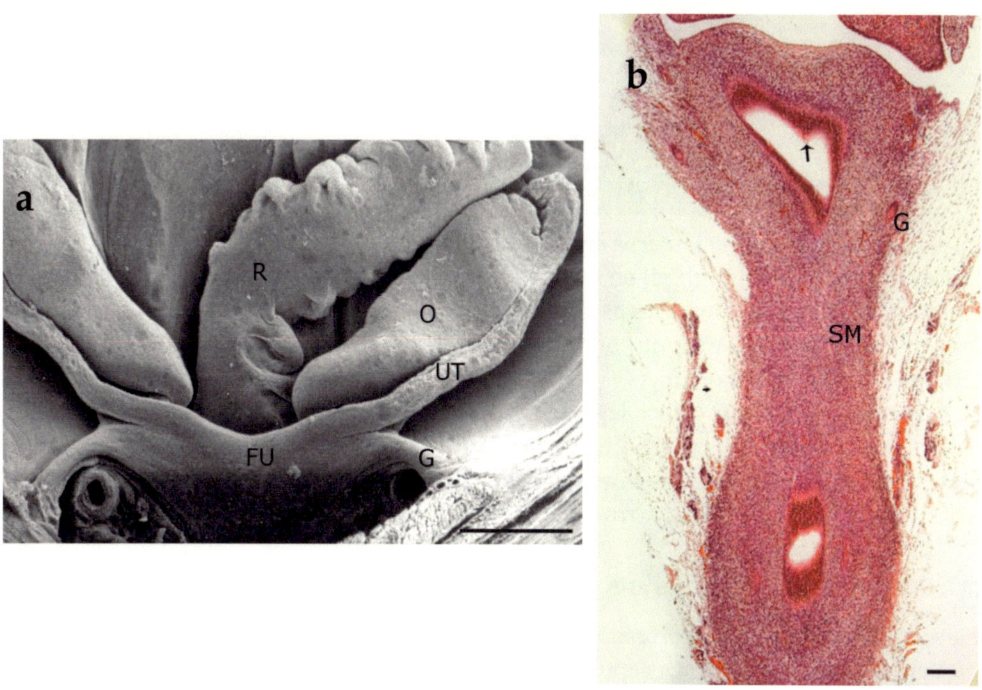

c

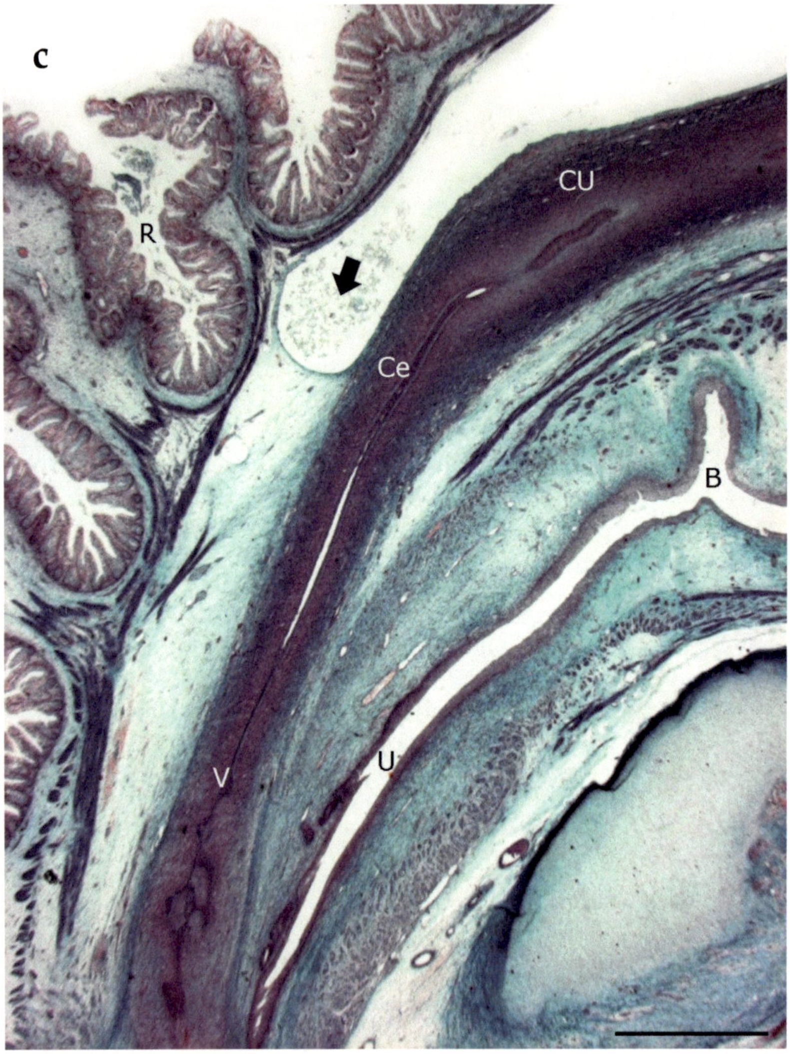

Fig. 9. Formation of oviduct, uterus and vagina
a) Scanning electron micrograph on the broad ligament of a 78 mm CRL (crown-rump length, about 12 weeks) female fetus. The upper border of the ligament is formed by the uterine tubes (UT) and the fundus of the uterus (FU). The insertions of the gubernacula (G) mark the transition from oviducts to uterus. O, ovar; R, rectum. Bar = 1mm. b) Uterus anlage of a 4 month fetus. Note the thick layer of smooth musculature (SM) and the remnant of the septum (arrow). Gartner ducts (G) are found within the uterus wall. Bar = 100 µm. c) Uterus and vagina anlage of a 150 mm (4 month) fetus. CU, corpus uteri; Ce, cervix; V, vagina; R, rectum; B, bladder; U, urethra; arrow, excavatio rectouterina. Bar = 1mm.

3.3.2 Differentiation of uterus and cervix

The uterus develops from the fused upper parts of the Müllerian ducts but the fusion is at first not complete since a thick septum is formed at the fundus of the uterus between week

13 and 20 of gestation (Figs. 9a and b). According to Muller et al. (1967), fusion of the ducts and resorption of the septum begins at the region of the isthmus and proceeds simultaneously in cranial and caudal direction. Incomplete fusion of the Müllerian ducts or incomplete resorption of the septum gives rise to many malformations. Any form of duplicity of the uterovaginal canal may be found from uterus bicornis to complete duplication of uterus and vagina, uterus didelphys with double vagina.

The differentiation of the mesenchymal wall of the uterus into smooth muscle starts as in the uterine tubes during the third months (Fig. 9b and c). Initially the epithelium reveals not as high proliferation as the oviduct epithelium and the uterus lumen is lined by a smooth surface without folds.

The region specific differentiation of the epithelium within oviducts (uterine tubes), uterus, cervix and vagina seems to occur perinatally also under the influence of the above-mentioned hox genes. The last step in differentiation of the epithelium is the formation of uterine glands. According to studies of Meriscay et al. (2004) in the mice, *Wnt5a* from stromal cells provides a specific signal that permits the luminal epithelium to form glands.

3.3.3 Differentiation of vagina

The development of the vagina is a matter of controversy and is under discussion. The solid caudal end of the uterovaginal canal inserts at the sinus urogenitalis between the openings of the Wolffian ducts and forms the Müllerian tubercle. Within this tubercle, the tissue of Wolffian and Müllerian ducts intermingle and make it difficult to define their genesis. Since the classic study of Koff (1933) on the development of the human vagina it is generally believed that the cranial part of the vagina is derived from the Müllerian ducts and the caudal part is formed from the sinus urogenitalis. Morphological studies of Forsberg (1965) argue for this view since the so-called Müllerian vagina has initially a pseudostratified columnar epithelium. Furthermore human males with complete androgen insensitivity syndrome but with functional AMH develop a shortened vagina. New genetic and experimental studies contradict this view (see for review Cai, 2009). In case of the shortened vagina it has been shown that the caudal part of the Müllerian duct is insensitive to AMH and under influence of androgen contributes to prostate development (Cai, 2009). Analysis of the vagina in testicular feminization mutated mice by Drews et al. (2002) demonstrated in male embryos, that the entire vagina arises from the Müllerian ducts growing caudal along the sinus urogenitalis together with the Wolffian ducts. In the male embryo, androgens binding to androgen receptors in the mesenchyme of the caudal Wolffian duct soon stop this caudal migration. Cai (2009) reviewed morphological, genetic and molecular studies and presented a model of the formation of the caudal vagina. The caudal ends of the Müllerian ducts insert into the sinus urogenitalis wall in which BMP4 is strongly expressed after induction by Shh (Sonic hedgehog). BMP4 mediates caudal extension of the uterovaginal canal.

The distal part of the uterovaginal canal, which extends caudad is at first a more or less solid cell plate known as vaginal plate. However Terruhn (1980) has found by injection technique that already at 14th week of gestation, the vagina as well as the uterus revealed a lumen (compare Fig. 9c). Later at the 26th week of gestation a functional plugging of the endocervical canal was observed presumably due to a secretory activity of the epithelium.

4. Remnants of the Müllerian or Wolffian ducts (hydatids) in adults

Hydatids of genital organs were first discovered by Morgagni. They are remnants of the cranial part of the Müllerian ducts and Wolffian ducts. In males, the frequent appendices of the testes develop from the funnel region of the Müllerian ducts. Due to a cranial crossing-over of Müllerian and Wolffian ducts, the Müllerian ducts come close to the upper poles of the testes (see Fig. 11a). They are not pedunculated and contain connective tissue and many blood vessels.

Different types of appendices epididymides are found. They all arise from the cranial ampullated ends of the Wolffian ducts and are in most cases pedunculated (Jacob & Barteczko, 2005). They may be vesicular or solid and often reveal a twisted stalk (Fig. 10a).

Likewise, in females, hydatids are found that are often pedunculated. They may occur at the fimbriae of the Fallopian tubes deriving from the Müllerian ducts, or as paratubular appendices vesiculosae or hydatids of Morgagni deriving their origin from the Wolffian ducts or mesonephric tubules (Fig. 10b).

The clinical relevance of these structures is torsion of pedicle with acute syndrome within scrotum or abdomen. Tumors deriving from these vestigial structures are also described.

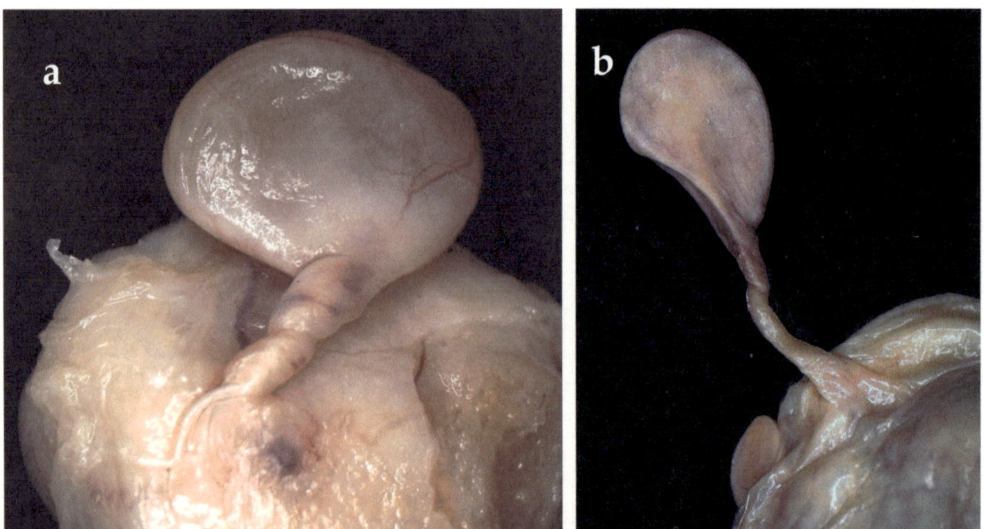

Fig. 10. Remnants of Müllerian or Wolffian ducts in adults
a) Pedunculated twisted hydatid (appendix epididymidis) as remnant of the ampullated blind cranial end of the Wolffian duct. 10.1 x 9 mm
b) Paratubular hydatid with torsion of pedicle. Length with pedicle 12.5 mm.

5. Summary and conclusion

The Wolffian ducts are the first appearing structures of the urogenital system and their migration and inductive properties are critical for the development of the permanent kidneys and the genital ducts in males and females. The development of the gonads, however, occurs independent of the Wolffian ducts.

Shortly after the onset of somite differentiation, the Wolffian duct anlagen separate from the intermediate mesoderm. During caudal migration they induce the pro- and mesonephroi within the ventral part of the intermediate mesoderm. Near the caudal entrance into the cloaca (sinus urogenitalis) an ureter bud sprouts out from each Wolffian duct and grows dorso-cranially to join the metanephric blastema (Fig. 11a). Each ureter bud divides in a special dichotomy manner and forms ureter, pelvis, calyces and collecting ducts of the permanent kidney (Fig 11 b and c).

The Wolffian ducts need androgens for further differentiation. In males, each duct forms a coiled ductus epididymidis and the straight vas deferens (Fig. 11b). Sprouting of the seminal vesicles occurs near the urogenital sinus.

The ductus epididymidis together with some persisting tubules of the mesonephros differentiates into the epididymis, which via the rete testis is in close connection with the testis enabling transport and maturation of spermatozoa. Shortly before birth, the epididymis descends into the scrotum together with the testis.

In females, the Wolffian ducts do not differentiate further, but persists as rudimentary Gartner's ducts in the broad ligament lateral to the uterus. The Gartners's ducts are found generally lateral to the uterus, but might also reach down to the wall of the vagina and can give rise to cysts (Fig. 11c).

a

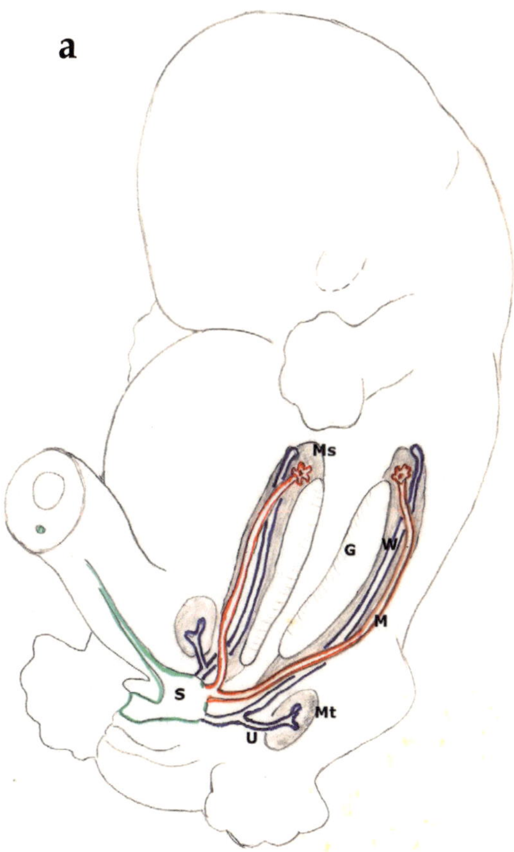

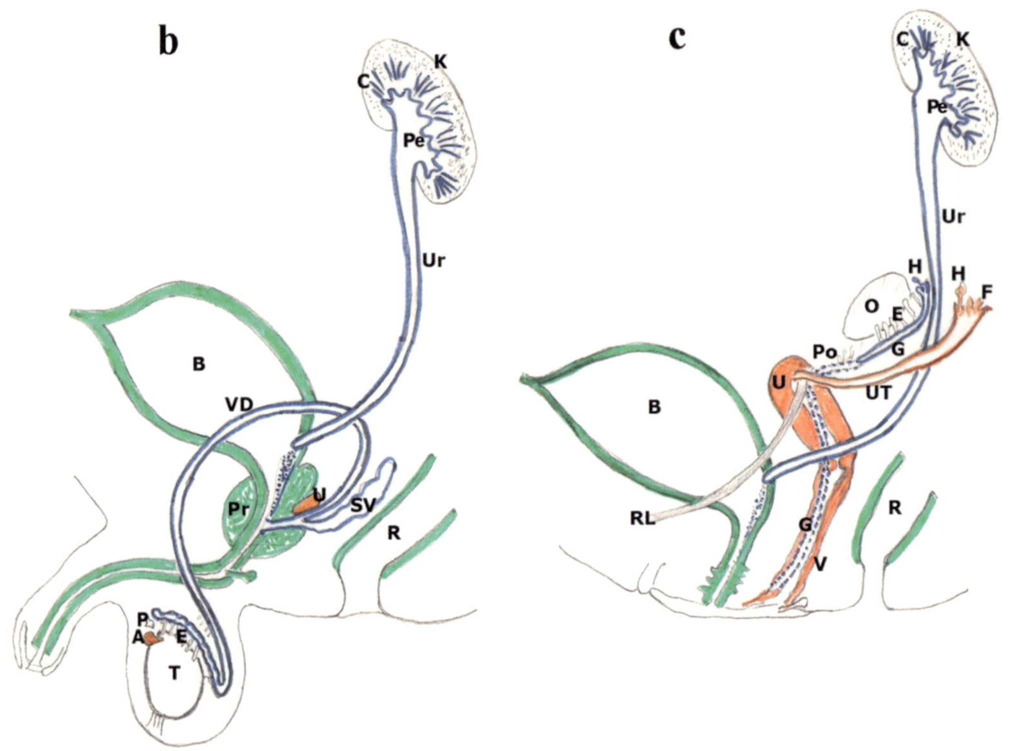

Fig. 11. Schematic drawings of genital ducts
a) Indifferent stage with Müllerian and Wolffian ducts in both genders. G, gonad; M, Müllerian duct; Ms, mesonephros, Mt, metanephros; S, sinus urogenitalis; U, ureter bud; W, Wolffian duct. Modified after Larsen b) Male differentiation of Wolffian duct (blue color). Red, remnants of Müllerian duct = Appendix testis (A) and utriculus prostaticus (U); dotted area, trigonum vesicae, according to classical view of Wolffian ducts origin. Green, derivatives of endoderm. B, bladder; C, collecting ducts; E, Epididymis; K, kidney; P, paradidymis; Pe, pelvis of kidney with calyces; Pr, prostata; R, rectum; SV, seminal vesicle; T, testis; Ur, ureter; VD, vas deferens. c) Female differentiation of Müllerian ducts (red). Differentiation and vestigial structures of Wolffian ducts blue. Green, Derivatives of endoderm. B, bladder; C, collecting ducts E, epoophoron; F, fimbriae; G, Gartner's duct; H, hydatids; K, kidney; O, ovar; Pe, pelvis of kidney with calyces; Po, paroophoron; R, rectum; RL, round ligament; U, uterus; Ur, ureter; UT, uterine tube; V, vagina. b) and c) modified after Hamilton , Boyd, Mossman.

The Müllerian ducts appear later in organogenesis but like the Wolffian ducts they develop at first in a similar manner in male and female embryos (Fig. 11a). The Müllerian ducts need induction of the Wolffian ducts with exception of the most cranial funnel region, which is supposed to include some nephrostomata from the regressing pronephros. The cells of the Müllerian ducts derive from the splanchnopleure exactly from the bilateral thickened stripes of coelomic epithelium, the Müllerian ridges. No cellular contribution from the Wolffian ducts was observed. The Müllerian ducts use the Wolffian ducts as guide to grow caudad, but in the lumbal region they cross the Wolffian ducts in the midline to form the uterovaginal canal (Fig. 11a). In females, they than differentiate into uterine tubes and the fused part forms uterus and vagina (Fig. 11c). New concepts of vaginal development contradict the classic view that the caudal part of the vagina derives its origin from the urogenital sinus, but is supportive of the view that origin of the vagina can be traced solely back to the Mullerian duct.

In males, AMH induces apoptosis and epithelio-mesenchymal transformation of the Müllerian ducts. Only the most cranial and the most caudal parts frequently persist as appendix testis and utriculus prostaticus (Fig. 11b), demonstrating special properties of these regions.

The differentiation of the indifferent ducts into their special structures in adults is listed in table 1. From this it becomes clear that all anlagen of the urogenital system are identical in the indifferent stage of development. The female differentiation is more passive while male differentiation needs genetic and hormonal factors. Early developing structures leave their trace in the adults as a vestigial organ which might be of clinical interest.

A better understanding of the organogenesis of the genital ducts under their well orchestrated genetic control during critical period of development would greatly help in diagnosing congenital malformations early and would serve as a guideline for designing therapeutic modalities for the treatment of disorders of the urogenital system.

indifferent	male	female
Wolffian duct	Ductus epididymidis	Gartner's duct
	Vas deferens	(Appendix vesiculosa)
	Seminal vesicle	
	(Appendix epididymidis)	
	Ureter	Ureter
	Renal pelvis and calyces	Renal pelvis and calyces
	Collecting ducts	Collecting ducts
Müllerian duct	(Appendix testis)	Tuba uterina
	(Utriculus prostaticus)	Uterus
		Vagina
		(Appendix vesiculosa)
Sinus urogenitalis	Bladder	Bladder
	Urethra	Urethra
	Prostata	Caudal part of vagina?
Tubules of mesonephros	Ductuli efferentes	Epoophoron
	Paradidymis	Paroophoron

Table 1. Anlagen of genital ducts and their differentiation in male and female organs and vestigial structures in parenthesis.

6. References

Allard, S.; Adin. P; Gouédard. L; di Clemente, N; Josso, N; Orgebin-Crist. M.C; Picard, J.Y & Xavier, F. (2000). Molecular mechanisms of hormone-mediated Müllerian duct regression: involvement of beta-catenin. *Development,* Vol.127, No.15, pp. 3349–3360

Al-Awqati, Q. &Goldberg, M. (1998). Architectural patterns in branching morphogenesis in the kidney. *Kidney International,* Vol.54, No.6, pp. 1832-1842

Barteczko, K.J. & Jacob, M.I. (2000). The testicular descent in human. *Advances in Anatomy Embryology and Cell Biology,* Vol. 156, pp. 1-96, ISBN 3-540-67315-6

Bellairs, R; Lear, P; Yamada, K.M; Rutishauser, U. & Lash, J.W. (1995). Posterior extension of the chick nephric (Wolffian) duct: the role of fibronectin and NCAM polysialic acid. *Developmental Dynamics,* Vol.202, No.4, pp. 333- 342

Budras, K.D. & Sauer, T. (1975). Morphology of the epididymis of the cock (Gallus domesticus) and its effect upon the steroid sex hormone synthesis. I. Ontogenesis, morphology and distribution of the epididymis. *Anatomy and Embryology,* Vol.148, No.2, pp. 175-96

Cai, Y. (2009). Revisiting old vaginal topics: conversion of the Müllerian vagina and origin of the "sinus" vagina. *The International Journal of Developmental Biology,* Vol.53, No.7, pp. 925-934

Carev, D., Krnic, D., Saraga, M., Sapunar, D. & Saraga-Babic, M. (2006). Role of mitotic, pro-apoptotic and antiapoptotic factors in human kidney development. *Pediatric Nephrology,* Vol.21, No.5, pp. 627-636

Chi, X; Michos, O; Shakya, R; Riccio, P; Enomoto, H; Licht, J.D; Asai, N; Takahashi, M; Ohgami, N; Kato, M; Mendelsohn, C. & Constantini,F.(2009). Ret-dependent cell rearrangements in the Wolffian duct epithelium initiate ureteric bud morphogenesis. *Developmental Cell, Vol.*17, No.2, pp.199–209

Constantini, F. & Kopan, R. (2010). Patterning a complex organ: branching morphogenesis and nephron segmentation in kidney development. *Developmental Cell,* Vol.18, No.5, pp. 698-712

Drawbridge, J; Meighan, C.M. & Mitchell, E.A. (2000). GDNF and GFRalpha-1 are components of the axolotl pronephric duct guidance system. *Developmental Biology,* Vol.228, No.1,pp. 116-24

Dressler, G.R; Deutsch, U; Chowdhury, K; Nornes, H.O. & Gruss, P. (1990). Pax2, a new murine paired-box-containing gene and its expression in the developing excretory system. *Development,* Vol.109, No.4, pp. 797- 809

Drews, U.; Sulak, O. & Schenck, P.A. (2002). Androgens and the development of the vagina. *Biology of Reproduction,* Vol.67, No.4, pp.1353-1359

Felix, W. (1911) Die Entwicklung der Harn- und Geschlechtsorgane. In: *Handbuch der Entwicklungsgeschichte des Menschen,* Vol. 2 (eds. F. Keibel & F.P. Mall), pp. 732-955, Hirzel, Leipzig

Grote, D; Souabni, A; Busslinger, M. & Bouchard, M. (2006). Pax2/8-regulated Gata3 expression is necessary for morphogenesis and guidance of the nephric duct in the developing kidney. *Development,* Vol.133, No.1, pp. 53-61

Grote, D; Boualia, S.K; Souabni, A; Merkel, C; Chi ,X; Costantini, F; Carroll, T. & Bouchard, M. (2008). Gata3 acts downstream of beta-catenin signaling to prevent ectopic metanephric kidney induction. *PLoS Genetics,* Vol.4, No.12, e1000316

Grünwald, P. (1937). Zur Entwicklungsmechanik des Urogenitalsystems beim Huhn. *Wilhelm Roux' Archiv für Entwicklungsmechanik der Organismen,* Vol.136, pp. 786-813

Guioli, S.; Sekido, R. & Lovell-Badge, R. (2007). The origin of the Mullerian duct in chick and mouse. *Developmental Biology*, Vol.302, No.2, pp. 389-398

Gupta, C. (1999). Modulation of androgen receptor (AR)-mediated transcriptional activity by EGF in the developing mouse reproductive tract primary cells. *Molecular Cell Endocrinology*, Vol.152, No.1-2, pp. 169-178

Hannema, S.E. & Hughes, I.A. (2007). Regulation of Wolffian duct development. *Hormone Research*, Vol.67, No.3, pp. 142-151

Hashimoto, R. (2003). Development of the human Müllerian duct in the sexually undifferentiated stage. *The Anatomical Record Part A*, Vol.272, No.2, pp. 514-519

Jacob, H.J., & Christ, B. (1978). Experimentelle Untersuchungen am Exkretionsapparat junger Hühnerembryonen. *XIXth Morphological Congress Symposia Charles. University Prague, pp. 219-225.*

Jacob, M., Christ, B., Jacob, H.J., &Poelmann, R. (1991). The role of fibronectin and laminin in the develpoment and migration of the avian Wolffian duct with reference to somitogenesis. *Anatomy and Embryology*, Vol.183, No. 4, pp.385-395.

Jacob, M.; Jacob. H.J. & Seifert, R. (1992). On the differentiation and migration of the Wolffian duct in avian embryos. In *Formation and Differentiation of Early Embryonic Mesoderm* (eds Bellairs R, Sanders EL, Lash JW)) *NATO ASI Series, Series A: Life Sciences*, Vol.231, pp. 77-86. New York: Plenum Press

Jacob, M.; Konrad, K. & Jacob, H.J. (1999). Early development of the Müllerian duct in avian embryos with reference to the human. *Cells Tissue Organs*, Vol.164, No.2, pp.63-81

Jacob, M. & Barteczko, K. (2005). Contribution to the origin and development of the appendices of the testis and epididymis in humans *Anatomy and Embryology*, Vol.209, No.4, pp. 287-302

Joseph, A.; Yao, H.; Hinton, B.T. (2009). Development and morphogenesis of the Wolffian/epididymal duct, more twists and turns. *Developmental Biology*, Vol.325, No.1, pp. 6-14

Jost, A. (1953). Problems of fetal endocrinology: the gonadal and hypophyseal hormones. *Recent Progress in Hormone Research*, Vol.8, pp.379–418

Kirchhoff, C.. (1999). Gene expression in the epididymis. *International Review of Cytology*, Vol.188, pp.133-202

Kobayashi, A ; Shawlot, W. ; Kania, A. & Behringer, R.R. : (2004). Requirement of *Lim1* for female reproductive tract development. *Development*, Vol.131, No.3, pp. 539-49

Koff, A.K. (1933). Development of the vagina in the human fetus. *Contribution to Embryology*, Vol.24, pp.61-90.

Laurence, W.D.; Whitaker, D.; Sugimura, H.; Cunha, G.R.; Dickersin, R. & Robboy, S.J. (1992). An ultrastructural study of the developing urogenital tract in early human fetuses. *American Journal of Obstetrics and Gynecology*, Vol.167, No.1, pp. 185-189

Marose, T.D.; Merkel, C.E.; McMahon, A.P. & Carroll, T.J. (2008) Beta-catenin is necessary to keep cells of ureteric bud/Wolffian duct epithelium in a precursor state. *Developmental Biology*, Vol.314, No.1, pp..112–126

Massé, J.; Watrin, T.; Laurent, A.; Deschamps, S.; Guerrier, D. & Pellerin, I. (2009). The developing female genital tract: from genetics to epigenetics. *International Journal of Developmental Biology*, Vol.53, No.2, pp. 411-424

Meriscay, M.; Kitajewski, J. & Sassoon, D. (2004). *Wnt5a* is required for proper epithelial-mesenchymal interaction in the uterus. *Development*, Vol.131, No.9, pp. 2061-2072

Miller, C & Sassoon, D.A. (1998). Wnt-7a maintains appropriate uterine patterning during the development of the mouse female reproductive tract. *Development*, Vol.125, No.6, pp. 3201-3211

Miyamoto, N ; Yoshida, M ; Kuratani, S ; Matsuo, I . & Aizawa, S. (1997). Defects of urogenital development in mice lacking *Emx2*. *Development,* Vol.124, No.9, pp. 1653-1664

Muller, P.; Musset, R.; Netter, A.; Solal, R.; Vinourd, J-C. & Gillet, J-Y. (1967). Etat du haut appareil urinaire chez les porteuses de malformations *utérines. Etude de 132 observations. II. Essai* d'interprétation. *La Presse Medicale,* Vol.75, No.26, pp. 1331-1336

Orvis, G.D. & Behringer, R.R. (2007). Cellular mechanisms of Müllerian duct formation in the mouse. *Development,* Vol.306, No.2, pp. 493-504

Osathanondh, V. & Potter, E.L. (1993). Development of human kidney as shown by microdissection. II. Renal pelvis, calyces and papillae. *Archives of Pathology,* Vol.76, pp. 277-289

Podlasek, C.A.; Seo, R.M.; Clemens, J.Q.; Ma, L.; Maas, R.L. & Bushman, W. (1999). *Hoxa-10* deficient male mice exhibit abnormal development of the accessory sex organs. *Developmental Dynamics,* Vol.214, No.1, pp. 1–12

Rey, R. (2005). Anti-Müllerian hormone in disorders of sex determination and differentiation. *Arquivos Brasileiros de Endocrinologia & Metabologia,* Vol.49, No.1, pp. 26-36

Shapiro, E.; Huang, H., McFadden, D.E.; Masch, R.J.; Ng, E.; Lepor, H. & Wu, X.R. (2004). The prostatic utricle is not a Müllerian duct remnant: immunohistochemical evidence for a distinct urogenital sinus origin. *Journal of Urology,* Vol.172, No.4pt2, pp. 1753-1756

Taylor, H.S. ; Vanden Heuvel, G.B. & Igarashi, P. (1997). A conserved *Hox* axis in the mouse and human female reproductive system: late establishment and persistent adult expression of the *Hoxa* cluster genes. *Biology of Reproduction,* Vol.57, No.6, pp. 1338-1345

Terruhn, V. (1980). A study of impression moulds of the genital tract of female fetuses. *Archives of Gynecology and Obstetrics,* Vol.229, No.3, pp. 207-217

Torres, M ; Gomez-Pardo, E ; Dressler G.R. & Gruss, P. (1995). *Pax-2* controls multiple steps of urogenital development. *Development,* Vol.121, No.12, pp. 4057-4065

Viana, R.; Batourina, E.; Huang, H.; Dressler, G.R.; Kobayashi, A.; Behringer, R.R.; Shapiro, E.; Hensle, T.; Lambert, S. & Mendelsohn, C. (2007). The development of the bladder trigone, the center of the anti-reflux mechanism. *Development,* 134, No.20, pp. 3763-3769

Vainio, S.; Heikkilä, M.; Kispert,A.; Chin, N. & McMahon, A.P. (1999). Female development in mammals is regulated by Wnt-4 signalling. *Nature,* Vol.397, No.6718, pp. 405-409

Wartenberg, H. (1990). Entwicklung der Genitalorgane und Bildung der Gameten, In: *Humanembryologie,* K.V. Hinrichsen, (Ed.) pp. 745-822, Springer ISBN 3-540-18983-1 Berlin, Heidelberg, New York

Wrobel, K.H. (2001). Morphogenesis of the bovine rete testis: extratesticular rete, mesonephros and establishment of the definitive urogenital junction. *Anatomy and Embryology,* Vol.203, No.4, pp. 293-307

Wrobel, K.H. & Süß, F. (2000). The significance of rudimentary nephrostomial tubules for the origin of the vertebrate gonad. *Anatomy and Embryology,* Vol.201, No.4, pp. 273-290

Yusuf, F., Rehimi, R., Dai, F.& Brand-Saberi, B. (2006). Expression of chemokine receptor CXCR4 during chick embryo development. *Anatomy and Embryology,* 210, No.1, pp. 35-41

10

Cytogenetic Analysis of Spontaneous Miscarriage

Nobuaki Ozawa
Department of Obstetrics and Gynecology,
National Hospital Organization Tokyo Medical Center, Tokyo,
Japan

1. Introduction

Approximately 15% of all clinically recognized pregnancies end in spontaneous miscarriage. The most frequent cause of spontaneous miscarriage is fetal chromosome abnormalities such as autosomal trisomy, monosomy X and polyploidy. In this chapter, cytogenetic abnormalities associated with spontaneous miscarriage are reviewed based on the latest studies. Molecular cytogenetic technique has been introduced in the genetic analysis of miscarriages in addition to the conventional karyotyping and provides new insights into this field.

2. Cytogenetic abnormalities of miscarriage

The considerable proportion of all conceptions fails to reach a live birth in humans. Approximately 15% of all clinically recognized pregnancies end up with miscarriage, and the total pregnancy loss is estimated to be 30-50% of all conceptions (Rai & Regan, 2006; Stephenson & Kutteh, 2007). The most important etiology of pregnancy loss is cytogenetic factor, namely chromosome abnormality. About 50-60 % of spontaneous miscarriages are etiologically attributed to chromosome abnormalities (Kajii, et al., 1980; Rai & Regan, 2006; Stephenson & Kutteh, 2007; Simpson, 2007; The ESHRE Capri Workshop Group [ESHRE], 2008). The proportion of chromosome abnormality in chemical abortion, defined as demise before clinical recognition by ultrasound examination, is unclear, but the proportion is expected to be higher than clinical miscarriage, as the incidence of chromosome abnormality is reported to be inversely proportional to gestation (Stephenson & Kutteh, 2007; Simpson, 2007).

The most common chromosome abnormality in miscarriage is autosomal trisomy, followed by ployploidy such as triploidy or tetraploidy, monosomy X and structural abnormality (Stephenson & Kutteh, 2007). Trisomies are generally the results of meiotic errors leading to the appearance of chromosomally abnormal gametes, which is strongly associated with maternal age (Simpson, 2007). All autosomal trisomies except trisomies 13, 18, 21 miscarry at early stage of gestation (ESHRE, 2008). Although there should be a corresponding monosomy for each trisomy, monosomy is rarely detected in clinical miscarriage except chromosome X, suggesting that autosomal monosomies are unlikely to be compatible with survival (ESHRE, 2008). Polyploidy mainly originates from fertilization by polyspermy or postzygotic division error (Simpson, 2007). In monosomy X, the lack of X chromosome mostly derives from paternal meiotic division error of sex chromosomes (Simpson, 2007). Structural rearrangements and chromosomal mosaicism due to postzygotic errors are occasionally detected in miscarriages. In case of balanced structural rearrangements, either parent usually has the same rearrangement and the cytogenetic cause for miscarriage is deniable, whereas *de novo* occurrence of balanced structural rearrangements might be associated with abnormal phenotype owing to possible gene interruption (Bui, et al., 2011). On the other hand, unbalanced structural rearrangements are always connected with abnormal phenotype, and naturally selected as miscarriage when the imbalance is too severe for embryos to survive. Mosaicism occurs as the result of postzygotic or mitotic errors. If abnormal cell lines persist during the preimplantation stage, embryos will be candidates for fetal or confined placental mosaicism, leading to miscarriage or impaired fetal development (Bielanska, et al., 2002; Vorsanova, et al., 2005). Although the consequence is unclear, the high incidence of mosaicism is demonstrated in miscarriage specimens (Vorsanova, et al., 2005).

3. Cytogenetic investigation of miscarriage

The identification of genetic cause of miscarriage is not necessarily performed as routine clinical work, as most of them are untreatable and unavoidable due to sporadic occurrence. However, it is highly recommended to identify karyotype and establish the cause of miscarriage in cases with recurrent miscarriages (RM) (Stephenson, et al., 2002). RM affects 1-5% of women, and the etiologies are multiple and at times even multifactorial (Rai & Regan, 2006; Stephenson & Kutteh, 2007). The estimated causes of RM include genetic, anatomical, endocrinologic, immunologic and thrombophilic disorders (Rai & Regan, 2006; Stephenson & Kutteh, 2007), although most of them have not yet be fully clarified. In fact, no credible explanation can be given for more than half of the cases, and about half of miscarriages are attributed to fetal chromosome abnormalities even in RM (Stephenson, et al., 2002).

When abnormal karyotype is the cause of miscarriage in RM patients, it is possible to avoid unnecessary testing or treatments for RM (Stephenson, et al., 2002), and abnormal karyotype results reportedly have a better prognosis for future pregnancies (Ogasawara, et al., 2000), although there might be an increased recurrence risk for another trisomy pregnancy in cases with gonadal mosaicism or genetic tendency to non-disjunction (ESHRE, 2008). On the other hand, the further investigation and alteration of current treatments would become necessary in case of miscarriage with normal karyotype in RM patients. When unbalanced structural abnormality is detected in miscarriage, ascertainment of carrier status in the parents is important to offer accurate information about the possibility of having another miscarriage or abnormal offspring and preimplantation genetic diagnosis (PGD) should be considered for the carrier couples (ESHRE, 2008). Thus, cytogenetic investigation of miscarriage specimens is crucial for the management of RM patients and provides valuable information for future pregnancies (Stephenson, et al., 2002; Diego-Alvarez, et al., 2005; ESHRE, 2008; Jobanputra et al., 2011). In addition, the identification of the possible cause of miscarriage is generally very comforting for RM patients, as they usually have psychological distress such as self-blame, anxiety, depression and grief (Nikcevic, et al., 1999).

4. Cytogenetic analytic methods for miscarriage specimens

4.1 Classical cytogenetics

Traditionally, cytogenetic analysis of miscarriage has been performed by G-banding method for metaphase spread after culture of villous cells (Kajii, et al., 1980). This standard cytogenetic methodology needs living cells to culture and the quality of metaphase is crucial for analysis. Thus, the fresh miscarriage specimens are desirable for analysis (Stephenson, et al., 2002). In fact, the success rates for culture and karyotyping of miscarriages vary among laboratories, ranging from 60 to 90% (Kajii, et al., 1980; Stephenson, et al., 2002; Jobanputra, et al., 2011). It has also been speculated that conventional karyotyping may detect only abnormal karyotypes that permit cell proliferation *in vitro* and the miscarriage specimens that fail to grow might have the rare abnormalities that do not sustain culture growth (Benkhalifa, et al., 2005; Jobanputra, et al., 2011). Another serious concern on classical cytogenetics is that overgrowth of maternally-derived cells or microorganisms contaminated in the specimen is not uncommon (Bell, et al., 1999; Jarrett, et al., 2001; Vorsanova, et al., 2005; Jobanputra, et al., 2011), because the complete removal of maternal decidua/blood cell is not always possible. As a result, karyotype could be falsely categorized as normal female, and skewed sex ratio in favor of females is often recognized in karyotype analysis of miscarriage specimens. In addition, incorrect interpretation such as tetraploidy could occur by tissue culture artifact (Doria, et al., 2010). Subtle abnormalities such as microdeletion are also overlooked due to the limited resolution in banding. Furthermore, microscopic chromosome analysis of cultured cells is time-consuming and labor intensive.

In recent years, several new genetic methods have been introduced in cytogenetic analysis of miscarriage to overcome the above-mentioned drawbacks of conventional karyotyping. In classical banding method, direct or semidirect analysis is attempted to reduce tissue culture effect by minimizing culture time. This technique allows a rapid analysis of all kinds of chromosome abnormalities (Morales, et al., 2008), although there is still a possibility of culture failure.

4.2 Interphase fluorescence in-situ hybridization (FISH)

Fluorescence in-situ hybridization (FISH) on the interphase nucleus of uncultured cells has been performed not only for prenatal samples obtained by amniocentesis or chorionic villus sampling (Shaffer & Bui, 2007), but also spontaneous miscarriage samples (Jobanputra, et al., 2002; Vorsanova, et al., 2005; Doria, et al., 2010; Jobanputra, et al., 2011). This procedure enables rapid identification of common aneuploidies using relatively small amounts of cells, avoiding major drawbacks of classical cytogenetics such as culture failure, overgrowth of maternal cells and tissue culture artifact (Vorsanova, et al., 2005; Doria, et al., 2010; Jobanputra, et al., 2011). The accurate diagnosis of polyploidy (Fig. 1) or the frequency of abnormal cell line in low-grade mosaicism cases is possible only by this method. Multiplex probe sets for analysis are selected based on knowledge about the frequencies of autosomal trisomies detected in spontaneous miscarriage and the availability of commercial probe sets (Jobanputra, et al., 2002). The limitation of this technique is that information of chromosomes not included in probe sets is lacking and structural abnormality is undetectable unless specific probes are applied. In addition, this relatively labor-intensive technique may have technical problems such as hybridization failure or cross-hybridization of probes to different chromosomes.

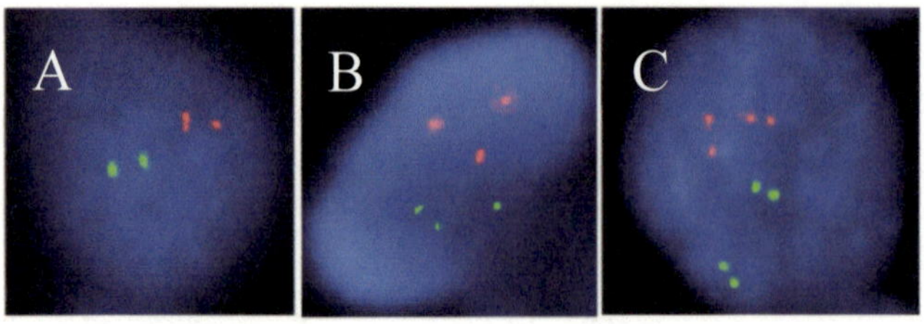

Fig. 1. The representative results of FISH analysis.
FISH analysis was performed by AneuVysion Prenatal Set (Abbott Japan) for the villous cells dispersed from the miscarriage specimens. Green fluorescence; DNA probe corresponding to the RB1 gene (13q14) labeled with SpectrumGreenTM, orange fluorescence; DNA probe corresponding to loci D21S529, D21S341 and D21S342 (21q22.13-q22.2) labeled with SpectrumOrangeTM. A; Diploid, B; Triploid, C; Tetraploid.

4.3 Molecular cytogenetic methods

With the development of new molecular techniques for chromosome analysis (Shaffer & Bui, 2007; Bui, et al., 2011), DNA-based analysis has been introduced in cytogenetic analysis of miscarriage. DNA-based analysis is divided into two groups; PCR-based analysis such as quantitative fluorescent polymerase chain reaction (QF-PCR) and multiplex ligation-dependent probe amplification (MLPA), and microarray-based comparative genomic hybridization (aCGH). Compared to conventional karyotyping, these methods require only a few amounts of specimens, especially PCR-related methods, avoiding analysis failure due to inadequate amounts of samples. In addition, they are applicable for non-dividing or non-viable cells that fail to grow *in vitro* or archived tissue such as formalin-fixed or paraffin-embedded tissues, enabling retrospective investigation when the need for karyotype analysis is recognized later.

4.3.1 Quantitative fluorescent polymerase chain reaction (QF-PCR)

Polymorphism markers are used widely in molecular cytogenetic studies as well as forensic medicine. In recent years, the diagnostic efficacy of quantitative fluorescent polymerase chain reaction (QF-PCR) assay has been demonstrated in prenatal testing using fetal DNA derived from amniocentesis or chorionic villus sampling (Shaffer & Bui, 2007). Also in miscarriage analysis, several reports have indicated that QF-PCR assay is a rapid, low-cost and reliable tool to diagnose aneuploidies (Diego-Alvarez, et al., 2005; Diego-Alvarez, et al., 2006; Zou, et al., 2008). Besides, it can provide information about both parental and meiotic origin of aneuploidy and detect uniparental disomy (UPD) by additional parental testing (Diego-Alvarez, et al., 2005). Generally, short tandem repeats (STR) markers in the chromosomes where aneuploidies are commonly found in miscarriages, namely 13, 15, 16, 18, 21, 22 and sex chromosomes, are used. The PCR products amplified using the labeled primers with a fluorescent dye are visualized by capillary electrophporesis and fluorescent intensity (peak area/height) and size of the amplified products are quantitatively evaluated. In normal heterozygous pattern, two peaks of fluorescent activities are observed with the ratio of 1:1 (disomic diallelic), whereas only one fluorescent peak is detected in homozygous pattern. In a trisomic case, the STR markers can be detected either as three fluorescent peaks, 1:1:1 (completete heterozygote), or two fluorescent peaks, 2:1 (trisomic diallelic) (Diego-

Alvarez, et al., 2005; Zou, et al., 2008). Triploidy is also detected when all markers present trisomic patterns (Fig. 2), while postzygotic tetraploidy is difficult to detect. Low grade of mosaicism could also be recognized. On the other hand, the cytogenetic analysis could result in uninformative results when all STR markers of a chromosome show monoallelic patterns, and the aneuploidies not associated with the chromosomes examined are not detectable. Balanced chromosome rearrangements are also missed.

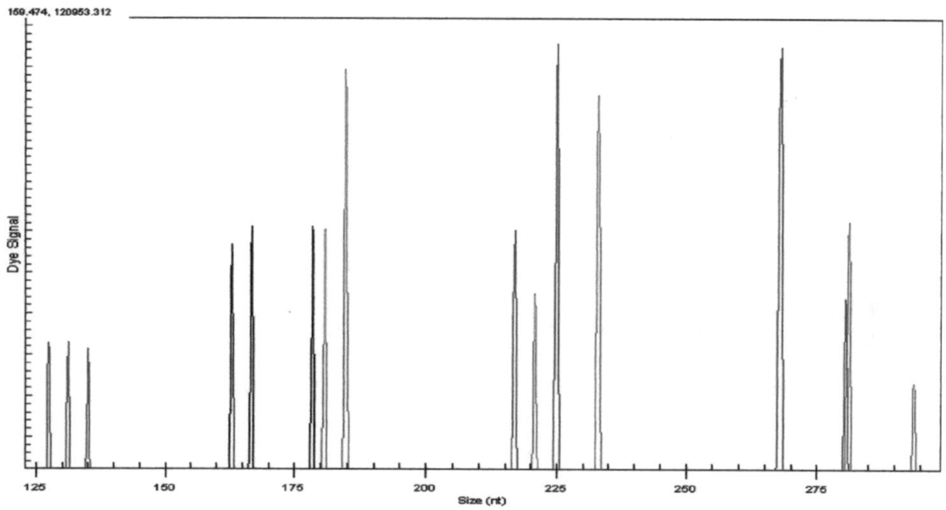

Fig. 2. The representative result of STR analysis.
STRs were analyzed by GenomeLab Human STR Primer Set (Beckman Coulter) for the miscarriage specimen. The PCR product has three distinct peaks or two peaks with the ratio of 1:2, suggesting triploidy.

4.3.2 Multiplex Ligation-Dependent Probe Amplification (MLPA)

Multiplex Ligation-Dependent Probe Amplification (MLPA) is an efficient genetic diagnostic technique based on polymerase chain reaction (PCR) amplification to detect copy-number changes (Schouten, et al., 2002). MLPA permits the relative quantification of more than 40 sequences in a single multiplex assay using only 20ng of sample DNA (Diego-Alvarez, et al., 2006). Denatured genomic DNA is hybridized with a set of two probes, which consist of a target specific sequence and a universal forward or reverse PCR primer binding site (Schouten, et al., 2002). One probe has a stuffer sequence to generate various PCR products with different sizes (Fig. 3). After ligation of the two parts of hybridized probes, the products are amplified by PCR using only one fluorescent-labeled primer pair. The multiplex-fluorescent products are separated by capillary electrophoresis and the peak height/areas are quantified. The relative amounts of amplified products depend on the quantity of target DNA present in the sample (Schouten, et al., 2002; Slater, et al., 2003), enabling the detection of copy number changes such as deletion, duplication or whole chromosome aneuploidy In prenatal testing, MLPA has been carried out as a rapid, flexible, sensitive and robust assay to screen aneuploidy such as trisomy 13, 18, 21 in a single experiment using a small amount of genomic DNA (Slater, et al., 2003; Shaffer & Bui, 2007).

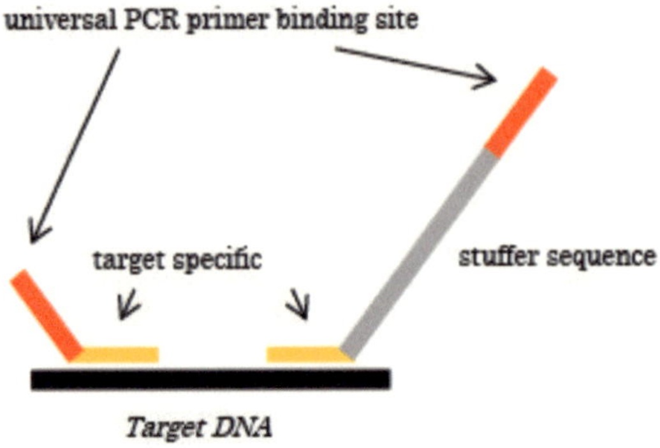

Fig. 3. The probe sets for MLPA analysis.

A set of two probes are used for MLPA analysis. Each probe has a target specific sequence and a universal forward or reverse PCR primer binding site. One probe has a stuffer sequence to generate various PCR products with different sizes (Schouten, et al., 2002).

Since almost all of cytogenetic abnormalities of miscarriage involve gains or/and losses of subtelomere copy numbers, MLPA targeted for every subtelomere region is applicable for miscarriage analysis (Bruno, et al., 2006; Diego-Alvarez, et al., 2007; Donaghue, et al., 2010; Carvalho. et al., 2010). Whole chromosome aneuploidies are indicated if the increased or decreased copy number dosages at both arms of one individual chromosome are recognized (Fig. 4). The increased or decreased dosage of only one chromosome end indicates a segmental aneuploidy, and unbalanced structural abnormalities are indicated when the dosage change of another chromosome end is also present. The favorable aspect of this method in the clinical setting is low cost and reduced turn round time for analysis as well as high accuracy and robustness (Bruno, et al., 2006; Diego-Alvarez, et al., 2007; Donaghue, et al., 2010; Carvalho. et al., 2010). It can be easily implemented in standard laboratories and facilitate laboratory work by simultaneous analysis of large number of samples or automated system.

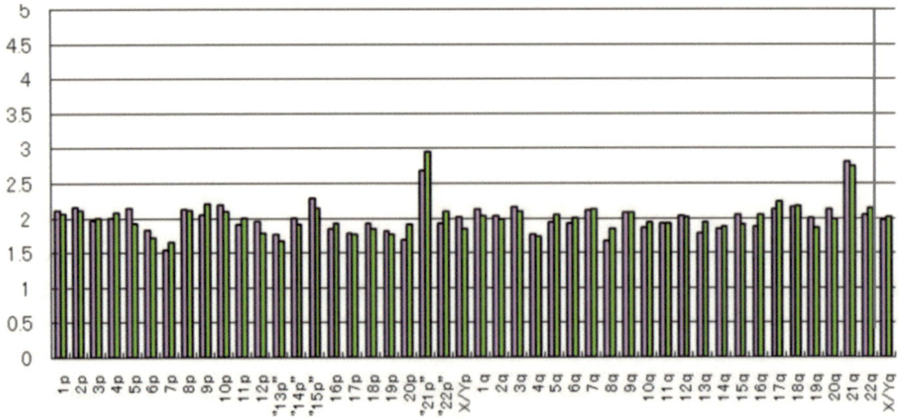

Fig. 4. The representative result of MLPA analysis.
MLPA assay was performed using SALSA MLPA KIT P036-E1 (MRC-Holland). Both arms of chromosome 21 showed increased copy number dosages, suggesting trisomy 21.

Since aneuploidies are diagnosed by the results of only one or a few PCR products, the discordant results attributed to the inherent copy number polymorphism could occur when two probe sets are utilized (Ahn, et al., 2007). Moreover, this method has a limitation in miscarriage analysis in that polyploidy or balanced structural abnormalities remain undetectable (Bruno, et al., 2006; Diego-Alvarez, et al., 2007; Donaghue, et al., 2010; Carvalho. et al., 2010).. Unbalanced Robertsonian translocation could be misdiagnosed as single chromosome aneuploidy. The detection of mosaicism would also be limited depending on the proportion of aneuploid cell line.

4.3.3 Microarray-based comparative genomic hybridization (aCGH)

Microarray-based comparative genomic hybridization (aCGH) is a powerful genetic tool for the comprehensive analysis of DNA copy number gains and losses throughout the whole genome at high resolution in a single experiment. In recent years, this technique has been vigorously applied in the clinical setting such as investigation of mental retardation, developmental delay and dysmorphism, especially in cases with normal karyotypes (Hayashi, et al., 2011). In addition, the identification of pathogenic copy number variations could lead to the discovery of genes responsible for various conditions/disease and the elucidation of specific gene function (Inzawa, et al., 2004; de Ravel, et al., 2007; Hayashi, et al., 2011). Array platforms are composed of a large number of genomic DNA clones such as bacterial artificial chromosomes or oligonucleotides. Test genomic DNA and reference genomic DNA are differently labeled with different fluorescent dye, and mixed together with blocking DNA to intercept repetitive sequences in the genome. After hybridization of this mixture to an array of genomic clones, the fluorescence ratio of two fluorochromes is measured for each spot (Snijders, et al., 2003; de Ravel, et al., 2007). of arrayed clones (Fig. 5) (Snijders, et al., 2003; de Ravel, et al., 2007).

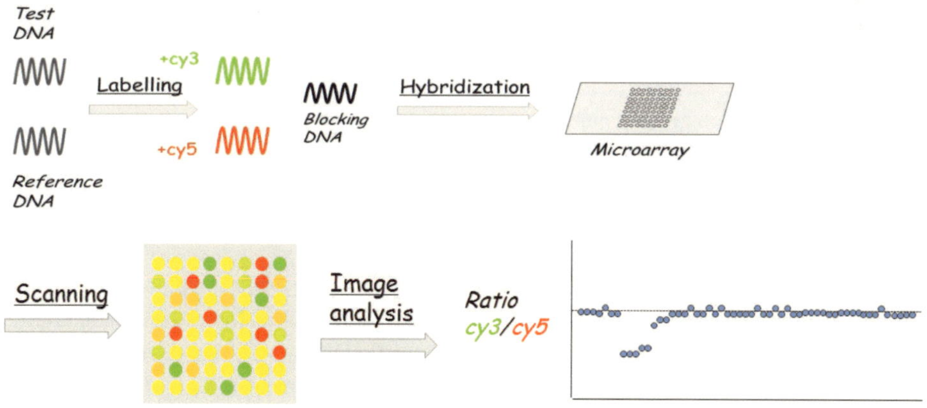

Fig. 5. Schematic diagram of aCGH technique.
Test and reference genomic DNA are differently labeled with different fluorescent dye, and mixed together with blocking DNA. This mixture is hybridized to an array of genomic clones, and the fluorescence ratio of two fluorochromes is measured for each spot.

Although structural status of chromosome aberrations is not recognized, DNA copy-number changes are detected at high-throughput and high-resolution manner. Since most of all observed chromosome abnormalities in spontaneous miscarriage involve coy-number changes in one or more subtelomere regions, this technique can apply miscarriage analysis, like MLPA with subtelomere probe sets (Schaeffer, et al., 2004). The increased or decreased copy number changes of all spots of any individual chromosome indicate a whole chromosome aneuploidy. The increased or decreased dosages of not all spots of a chromosome indicate a segmental aneuploidy, and unbalanced structural abnormalities are indicated when the terminal dosage change is present in two different chromosomes (Fig. 6).

As DNA-based analysis, aCGH can overcome some drawbacks of conventional karyotyping including culture failure, overgrowth of maternal cells and tissue culture effect (Schaeffer, et al., 2004). In addition, the spectrum of cytogenetic abnormalities detected is broader compared to MLPA and the resolution of analysis is more detailed than conventional karyotyping, allowing the detection of cryptic deletion or duplication (Schaeffer, et al., 2004; Shimokawa, et al., 2006), which might lead to the identification of new regions or genes that play a role in early embryonic development or demise. In fact, the recent studies have shown the involvement of submicroscopic abnormalities in miscarriages (Table 1), although it is unclear whether these subtle imbalances could cause miscarriage.

	Time of miscarriage	**Submicroscopic abnormalities (bp)**
Schaeffer et al. (2004)	≤20 wks	del 9p21, dup 15q11-q13, dup 10qtel
Benkhalifa et al. (2005)*	9-11 wks	del 22q13, dup 1pter
Shimokawa et al. (2006)	5-12 wks	del 3p26.2-p26.3 (1.4 Mb)
Robberecht et al. (2009)	-	del Xp22.3 (787.5 kb)
Warren et al. (2009)	10-20 wks	dup Xp22.31 (289 kb), del 13q33.3 (115 kb), dup 5p15.33 (93 kb)
Menten et al. (2009)	-	del 7q36qter, del Xq28qter

*The specimens that failed to grow in culture were analyzed.

Table 1. Submicroscopic abnormalities detected by aCGH in spontaneous miscarriage specimens (Schaeffer, et al., 2004; Benkhalifa, et al., 2005; Shimokawa, et al., 2006; Robberecht, et al., 2009; Warren, et al., 2009; Menten, et al., 2009).

A potential drawback of this technique is inability to detect balanced structural abnormalities such as reciprocal/Robertsonian translocations and inversions. The change in ploidy is also not detectable, since the amount of sample DNA is adjusted to the same extent as the reference in the assay process (Lomax, et al., 2000). Another great concern of this technique is the detection of copy number variations (CNV) of unknown or uncertain clinical significance (de Ravel, et al., 2007; Bui, et al., 2011). CNVs extend across the whole chromosomes more frequently than previously expected and clinical interpretation of CNVs is difficult in case of lack of available information. Therefore, targeted arrays for aneuploidies and known microdeletion/duplication syndromes may be a current option in miscarriage analysis as a clinical use until the pathogenicity of CNVs assayed becomes elucidated.

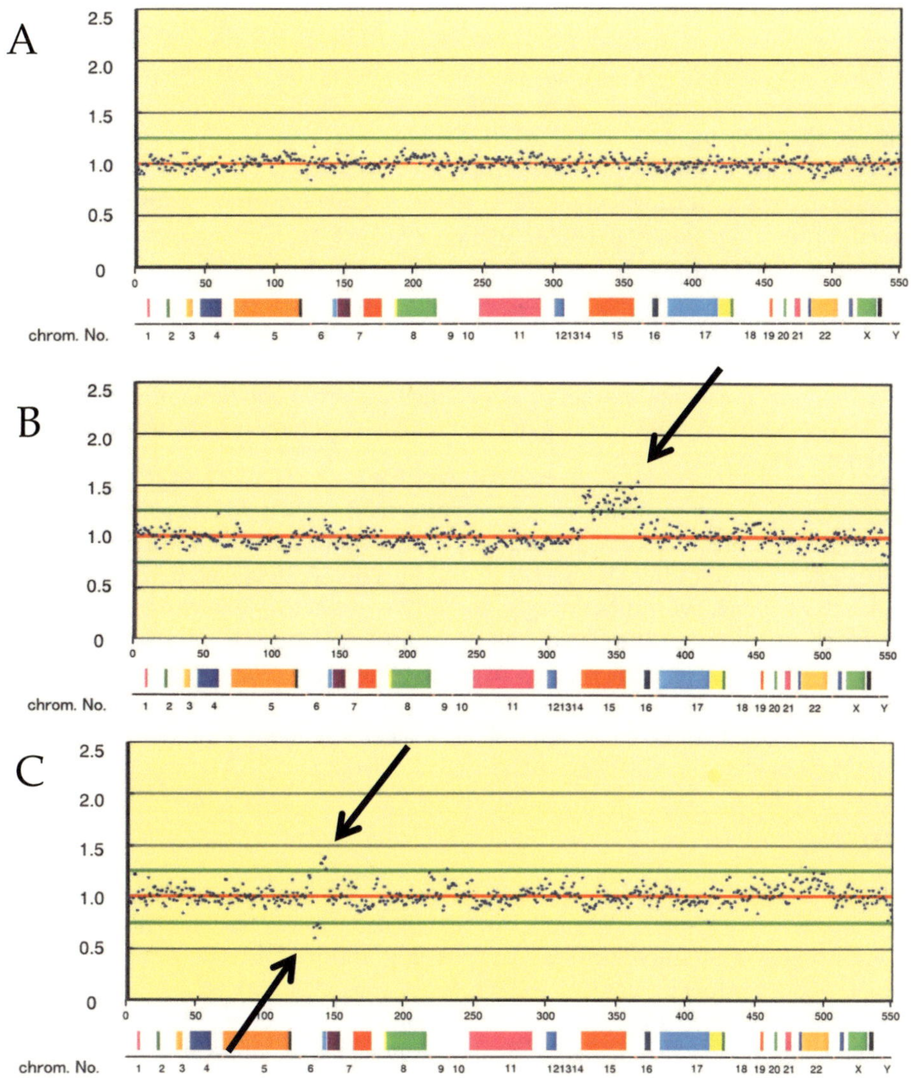

Fig. 6. The representative results of aCGH using Genome Disorder array.
Genome Disorder (GD) array analysis was performed by Aizu Y, Ph.D. at Division of Advanced Technology & Development, BML, Inc., Kawagoe, Japan. GD array was developed in Department of Molecular Cytogenetics, Medical Research Institute and School of Biomedical Science, Tokyo Medical and Dental University, Japan (Inazawa, et al., 2004; Udaka, et al., 2007; Hayashi, et al., 2011). This BAC array covers every subtelomeric region except p-arms of acrocentric chromosomes as well as responsible regions for microdeletion syndromes. Clones are horizontally ordered from chromosome 1 to 22. Thresholds of copy-number ratios are 1.25 for gain and 0.75 for loss, respectively.. A; Normal, B; gains at 15q11.2-13.1, 15q26.3 corresponding to trisomy 15, C; gain at 7p22.3-22.2 and loss at 6q27 corresponding to unbalanced reciprocal translocation between chromosome 6q and 7p.

4.4 Combined methods

Since every cytogenetic method has some drawbacks in miscarriage analysis, the combination assays have been encouraged in recent years. In MLPA and aCGH assays, ancillary FISH, microsatellite analysis, or flow-cytometry is performed to diagnose polyploidy in the event of normal assay results (Lomox, et al., 2000; Bruno, et al., 2006; Robberecht, et al., 2009; Menten, et al., 2009). On the other hand, aCGH assay could be additionally attempted to detect microabnormalities in normal karyotype cases judged by conventional analysis (Shimokawa, et al., 2006). Besides, FISH or polymorphism marker has been applied to exclude maternal contamination (Bell, et al., 1999; Jarrett, et al., 2001; Robberecht, et al., 2009), which is a troublesome issue in both classical karyotyping and DNA-based analysis of miscarriage. In FISH analysis, the demonstration of Y chromosome in cases with normal female karyotypes suggests maternal contamination, whereas it is impossible to distinguish maternal contamination in normal female fetus. Molecular approaches using microsatellite markers can evaluate maternal contamination irrespective of fetal sex by comparing maternal and putative fetal DNA polymorphism if both DNA are available (Jarrett, et al., 2001).

Recently, non-surgical managements have been performed for selected miscarriage cases to reduce patients' discomfort and avoid surgical complications such as uterine perforation, uterine adhesion, cervical trauma, hemorrhage and infection (Griebel, et al., 2005). It is also reported that the patients with miscarriages should be given the opportunity to choose a treatment option for their health-related quality of life (Wieringa-De Waard, et al., 2002). Since the specimens obtained by non-surgical managements are inappropriate for classical cytogenetics because of extensive degeneration and possible maternal contamination (Stephenson, et al., 2002). DNA-based analysis is a feasible strategy in patients who desire expectant management and cytogenetic analysis of miscarriage.

5. Conclusions

Cytogenetic study of miscarriage is of great significance for the management of RM patients as well as reproductive genetic research. As mentioned above, the currently-performed classical karyotyping has some drawbacks, possibly leading to failure of analysis or misdiagnosis. The introduction of new genetic techniques into miscarriage analysis could offer valuable information to RM patients and clinicians through more refined and complete diagnosis, and elucidate the genetic mechanism of early fetal development or demise as well as the precise incidence of genetic abnormalities associated with miscarriage.

6. References

Ahn, J. W., Ogilvie, C. M., Welch, A., Thomas, H., Madula, R., Hills, A., Donaghue, C. & Mann, K. (2007). Detection of subtelomere imbalance using MLPA: validation, development of an analysis protocol, and application in a diagnostic centre. *BMC Med Genet,* Vol.8, pp. 9, ISSN1471-2350 (Electronic)1471-2350 (Linking)

Bell, K. A., Van Deerlin, P. G., Haddad, B. R. & Feinberg, R. F. (1999). Cytogenetic diagnosis of "normal 46,XX" karyotypes in spontaneous abortions frequently may be misleading. *Fertil Steril,* Vol.71, No.2, pp. 334-41, ISSN 0015-0282 (Print)0015-0282 (Linking)

Benkhalifa, M., Kasakyan, S., Clement, P., Baldi, M., Tachdjian, G., Demirol, A., Gurgan, T., Fiorentino, F., Mohammed, M. & Qumsiyeh, M. B. (2005). Array comparative genomic hybridization profiling of first-trimester spontaneous abortions that fail to grow in vitro. *Prenat Diagn,* Vol.25, No.10, pp. 894-900, ISSN 0197-3851 (Print)0197-3851 (Linking)

Bielanska, M., Tan, S. L. & Ao, A. (2002). Chromosomal mosaicism throughout human preimplantation development in vitro: incidence, type, and relevance to embryo outcome. *Hum Reprod,* Vol.17, No.2, pp. 413-9, ISSN 0268-1161 (Print)0268-1161 (Linking)

Bruno, D. L., Burgess, T., Ren, H., Nouri, S., Pertile, M. D., Francis, D. I., Norris, F., Kenney, B. K., Schouten, J., Andy Choo, K. H. & Slater, H. R. (2006). High-throughput analysis of chromosome abnormality in spontaneous miscarriage using an MLPA subtelomere assay with an ancillary FISH test for polyploidy. *Am J Med Genet A,* Vol.140, No.24, pp. 2786-93, ISSN 1552-4825 (Print)1552-4825 (Linking)

Bui, T. H., Vetro, A., Zuffardi, O. & Shaffer, L. G. (2011). Current controversies in prenatal diagnosis 3: is conventional chromosome analysis necessary in the post-array CGH era? *Prenat Diagn,* Vol.31, No.3, pp. 235-43, ISSN 1097-0223 (Electronic)0197-3851 (Linking)

Carvalho, B., Doria, S., Ramalho, C., Brandao, O., Sousa, M., Matias, A., Barros, A. & Carvalho, F. (2010). Aneuploidies detection in miscarriages and fetal deaths using multiplex ligation-dependent probe amplification: an alternative for speeding up results? *Eur J Obstet Gynecol Reprod Biol,* Vol.153, No.2, pp. 151-5, ISSN 1872-7654 (Electronic)0301-2115 (Linking)

de Ravel, T. J., Devriendt, K., Fryns, J. P. & Vermeesch, J. R. (2007). What's new in karyotyping? The move towards array comparative genomic hybridisation (CGH). *Eur J Pediatr,* Vol.166, No.7, pp. 637-43, ISSN0340-6199 (Print)0340-6199 (Linking)

Diego-Alvarez, D., Garcia-Hoyos, M., Trujillo, M. J., Gonzalez-Gonzalez, C., Rodriguez de Alba, M., Ayuso, C., Ramos-Corrales, C. & Lorda-Sanchez, I. (2005). Application of quantitative fluorescent PCR with short tandem repeat markers to the study of aneuploidies in spontaneous miscarriages. *Hum Reprod,* Vol.20, No.5, pp. 1235-43, ISSN 0268-1161 (Print)0268-1161 (Linking)

Diego-Alvarez, D., Ramos-Corrales, C., Garcia-Hoyos, M., Bustamante-Aragones, A., Cantalapiedra, D., Diaz-Recasens, J., Vallespin-Garcia, E., Ayuso, C. & Lorda-Sanchez, I. (2006). Double trisomy in spontaneous miscarriages: cytogenetic and molecular approach. *Hum Reprod,* Vol.21, No.4, pp. 958-66, ISSN 0268-1161 (Print)0268-1161 (Linking)

Diego-Alvarez, D., Rodriguez de Alba, M., Cardero-Merlo, R., Diaz-Recasens, J., Ayuso, C., Ramos, C. & Lorda-Sanchez, I. (2007). MLPA as a screening method of aneuploidy and unbalanced chromosomal rearrangements in spontaneous miscarriages. *Prenat Diagn,* Vol.27, No.8, pp. 765-71, ISSN 0197-3851 (Print)0197-3851 (Linking)

Donaghue, C., Mann, K., Docherty, Z., Mazzaschi, R., Fear, C. & Ogilvie, C. (2010). Combined QF-PCR and MLPA molecular analysis of miscarriage products: an efficient and robust alternative to karyotype analysis. *Prenat Diagn,* Vol.30, No.2, pp. 133-7, ISSN 1097-0223 (Electronic)0197-3851 (Linking)

Doria, S., Lima, V., Carvalho, B., Moreira, M. L., Sousa, M., Barros, A. & Carvalho, F. (2010). Application of touch FISH in the study of mosaic tetraploidy and maternal cell contamination in pregnancy losses. *J Assist Reprod Genet,* Vol.27, No.11, pp. 657-62, ISSN 1573-7330 (Electronic)1058-0468 (Linking)

Griebel, C. P., Halvorsen, J., Golemon, T. B. & Day, A. A. (2005). Management of spontaneous abortion. *Am Fam Physician,* Vol.72, No.7, pp. 1243-50, ISSN 0002-838X (Print)0002-838X (Linking)

Hayashi, S., Imoto, I., Aizu, Y., Okamoto, N., Mizuno, S., Kurosawa, K., Okamoto, N., Honda, S., Araki, S., Mizutani, S., Numabe, H., Saitoh, S., Kosho, T., Fukushima, Y., Mitsubuchi, H., Endo, F., Chinen, Y., Kosaki, R., Okuyama, T., Ohki, H., Yoshihashi, H., Ono, M., Takada, F., Ono, H., Yagi, M., Matsumoto, H., Makita, Y., Hata, A. & Inazawa, J. (2011). Clinical application of array-based comparative genomic hybridization by two-stage screening for 536 patients with mental retardation and multiple congenital anomalies. *J Hum Genet,* Vol.56, No.2, pp. 110-24, ISSN 1435-232X (Electronic)1434-5161 (Linking)

Inazawa, J., Inoue, J. & Imoto, I. (2004). Comparative genomic hybridization (CGH)-arrays pave the way for identification of novel cancer-related genes. *Cancer Sci,* Vol.95, No.7, pp. 559-63, ISSN 1347-9032 (Print)1347-9032 (Linking)

Jarrett, K. L., Michaelis, R. C., Phelan, M. C., Vincent, V. A. & Best, R. G. (2001). Microsatellite analysis reveals a high incidence of maternal cell contamination in 46,XX products of conception consisting of villi or a combination of villi and membranous material. *Am J Obstet Gynecol,* Vol.185, No.1, pp. 198-203, ISSN 0002-9378 (Print)0002-9378 (Linking)

Jobanputra, V., Sobrino, A., Kinney, A., Kline, J. & Warburton, D. (2002). Multiplex interphase FISH as a screen for common aneuploidies in spontaneous abortions. *Hum Reprod,* Vol.17, No.5, pp. 1166-70, ISSN 0268-1161 (Print)0268-1161 (Linking)

Jobanputra, V., Esteves, C., Sobrino, A., Brown, S., Kline, J. & Warburton, D. (2011). Using FISH to increase the yield and accuracy of karyotypes from spontaneous abortion specimens. *Prenat Diagn,* Vol.31, No.8, pp. 755-9, ISSN 1097-0223 (Electronic)0197-3851 (Linking)

Kajii, T., Ferrier, A., Niikawa, N., Takahara, H., Ohama, K. & Avirachan, S. (1980). Anatomic and chromosomal anomalies in 639 spontaneous abortuses. *Hum Genet,* Vol.55, No.1, pp. 87-98, ISSN 0340-6717 (Print)0340-6717 (Linking)

Lomax, B., Tang, S., Separovic, E., Phillips, D., Hillard, E., Thomson, T. & Kalousek, D. K. (2000). Comparative genomic hybridization in combination with flow cytometry improves results of cytogenetic analysis of spontaneous abortions. *Am J Hum Genet,* Vol.66, No.5, pp. 1516-21, ISSN 0002-9297 (Print)0002-9297 (Linking)

Menten, B., Swerts, K., Delle Chiaie, B., Janssens, S., Buysse, K., Philippe, J. & Speleman, F. (2009). Array comparative genomic hybridization and flow cytometry analysis of spontaneous abortions and mors in utero samples. *BMC Med Genet,* Vol.10, pp. 89, ISSN 1471-2350 (Electronic)1471-2350 (Linking)

Morales, C., Sanchez, A., Bruguera, J., Margarit, E., Borrell, A., Borobio, V. & Soler, A. (2008). Cytogenetic study of spontaneous abortions using semi-direct analysis of chorionic villi samples detects the broadest spectrum of chromosome abnormalities. *Am J*

Med Genet A, Vol.146A, No.1, pp. 66-70, ISSN 1552-4833 (Electronic)1552-4825 (Linking)

Nikcevic, A. V., Tunkel, S. A., Kuczmierczyk, A. R. & Nicolaides, K. H. (1999). Investigation of the cause of miscarriage and its influence on women's psychological distress. *Br J Obstet Gynaecol,* Vol.106, No.8, pp. 808-13, ISSN 0306-5456 (Print)0306-5456 (Linking)

Ogasawara, M., Aoki, K., Okada, S. & Suzumori, K. (2000). Embryonic karyotype of abortuses in relation to the number of previous miscarriages. *Fertil Steril,* Vol.73, No.2, pp. 300-4, ISSN 0015-0282 (Print)0015-0282 (Linking)

Rai, R. & Regan, L. (2006). Recurrent miscarriage. *Lancet,* Vol.368, No.9535, pp. 601-11, ISSN 1474-547X (Electronic)0140-6736 (Linking)

Robberecht, C., Schuddinck, V., Fryns, J. P. & Vermeesch, J. R. (2009). Diagnosis of miscarriages by molecular karyotyping: benefits and pitfalls. *Genet Med,* Vol.11, No.9, pp. 646-54, ISSN 1530-0366 (Electronic)1098-3600 (Linking)

Schaeffer, A. J., Chung, J., Heretis, K., Wong, A., Ledbetter, D. H. & Lese Martin, C. (2004). Comparative genomic hybridization-array analysis enhances the detection of aneuploidies and submicroscopic imbalances in spontaneous miscarriages. *Am J Hum Genet,* Vol.74, No.6, pp. 1168-74, ISSN 0002-9297 (Print)0002-9297 (Linking)

Shaffer, L. G. & Bui, T. H. (2007). Molecular cytogenetic and rapid aneuploidy detection methods in prenatal diagnosis. *Am J Med Genet C Semin Med Genet,* Vol.145C, No.1, pp. 87-98, ISSN 1552-4868 (Print)1552-4868 (Linking)

Schouten, J. P., McElgunn, C. J., Waaijer, R., Zwijnenburg, D., Diepvens, F. & Pals, G. (2002). Relative quantification of 40 nucleic acid sequences by multiplex ligation-dependent probe amplification. *Nucleic Acids Res,* Vol.30, No.12, pp. e57, ISSN 1362-4962 (Electronic)0305-1048 (Linking)

Shimokawa, O., Harada, N., Miyake, N., Satoh, K., Mizuguchi, T., Niikawa, N. & Matsumoto, N. (2006). Array comparative genomic hybridization analysis in first-trimester spontaneous abortions with 'normal' karyotypes. *Am J Med Genet A,* Vol.140, No.18, pp. 1931-5, ISSN 1552-4825 (Print)1552-4825 (Linking)

Simpson, J. L. (2007). Causes of fetal wastage. *Clin Obstet Gynecol,* Vol.50, No.1, pp. 10-30, ISSN 0009-9201 (Print)0009-9201 (Linking)

Slater, H. R., Bruno, D. L., Ren, H., Pertile, M., Schouten, J. P. & Choo, K. H. (2003). Rapid, high throughput prenatal detection of aneuploidy using a novel quantitative method (MLPA). *J Med Genet,* Vol.40, No.12, pp. 907-12, ISSN 1468-6244 (Electronic)0022-2593 (Linking)

Snijders, A. M., Pinkel, D. & Albertson, D. G. (2003). Current status and future prospects of array-based comparative genomic hybridisation. *Brief Funct Genomic Proteomic,* Vol.2, No.1, pp. 37-45, ISSN 1473-9550 (Print)1473-9550 (Linking)

Stephenson, M. D., Awartani, K. A. & Robinson, W. P. (2002). Cytogenetic analysis of miscarriages from couples with recurrent miscarriage: a case-control study. *Hum Reprod,* Vol.17, No.2, pp. 446-51, ISSN 0268-1161 (Print)0268-1161 (Linking)

Stephenson, M. & Kutteh, W. (2007). Evaluation and management of recurrent early pregnancy loss. *Clin Obstet Gynecol,* Vol.50, No.1, pp. 132-45, ISSN 0009-9201 (Print)0009-9201 (Linking)

The ESHRE Capri Workshop Group (2008). Genetic aspects of female reproduction. *Hum Reprod Update,* Vol.14, No.4, pp. 293-307, ISSN 1460-2369 (Electronic)1355-4786 (Linking)

Udaka, T., Imoto, I., Aizu, Y., Torii, C., Izumi, K., Kosaki, R., Takahashi, T., Hayashi, S., Inazawa, J. & Kosaki, K. (2007). Multiplex PCR/liquid chromatography assay for screening of subtelomeric rearrangements. *Genet Test,* Vol.11, No.3, pp. 241-8, ISSN 1090-6576 (Print)1090-6576 (Linking)

Vorsanova, S. G., Kolotii, A. D., Iourov, I. Y., Monakhov, V. V., Kirillova, E. A., Soloviev, I. V. & Yurov, Y. B. (2005). Evidence for high frequency of chromosomal mosaicism in spontaneous abortions revealed by interphase FISH analysis. *J Histochem Cytochem,* Vol.53, No.3, pp. 375-80, ISSN 0022-1554 (Print)0022-1554 (Linking)

Warren, J. E., Turok, D. K., Maxwell, T. M., Brothman, A. R. & Silver, R. M. (2009). Array comparative genomic hybridization for genetic evaluation of fetal loss between 10 and 20 weeks of gestation. *Obstet Gynecol,* Vol.114, No.5, pp. 1093-102, ISSN 1873-233X (Electronic)0029-7844 (Linking)

Wieringa-De Waard, M., Hartman, E. E., Ankum, W. M., Reitsma, J. B., Bindels, P. J. & Bonsel, G. J. (2002). Expectant management versus surgical evacuation in first trimester miscarriage: health-related quality of life in randomized and non-randomized patients. *Hum Reprod,* Vol.17, No.6, pp. 1638-42, ISSN 0268-1161 (Print)0268-1161 (Linking)

Zou, G., Zhang, J., Li, X. W., He, L., He, G. & Duan, T. (2008). Quantitative fluorescent polymerase chain reaction to detect chromosomal anomalies in spontaneous abortion. *Int J Gynaecol Obstet,* Vol.103, No.3, pp. 237-40, ISSN 0020-7292 (Print)0020-7292 (Linking)